ECG Workout

Exercises in
Arrhythmia Interpretation

ECG Workout

Exercises in Arrhythmia Interpretation

3rd Edition

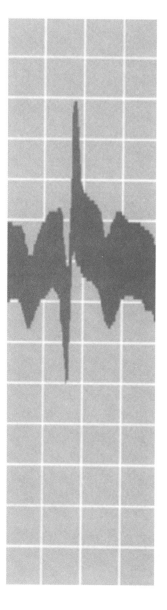

Jane Huff, RN, CCRN

Nurse Manager, Critical Care Unit
Arrhythmia Instructor
Advanced Cardiac Life Support (ACLS) Instructor
Central Arkansas Hospital
Searcy, Arkansas

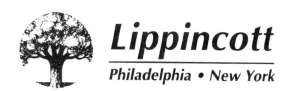

Lippincott
Philadelphia • New York

Acquisitions Editor: Lisa Stead
Editorial Assistant: Brian MacDonald
Project Editor: Barbara Ryalls
Production Manager: Helen Ewan
Production Coordinator: Pat McCloskey
Design Coordinator: Kathy Luedtke

Edition 3

9   8

Library of Congress Cataloging in Publications Data
RC685.A65 H84 1997
    ECG workout: exercises in arrhythmia interpretation / Jane Huff.
  —3rd ed.
      p.   cm.
    0-397-55371-4 (alk. paper)
    Includes bibliographical references and index.
    I. Title.
    [DNLM: 1. Arrhythmia—diagnosis—problems.
  2. Electrocardiography—problems. 3. Arrhythmia—diagnosis—
  problems. 4. Electrocardiography—problems. WG 18.2 H889e 1997]
  616.1′2807547—dc20
  DNLM/DLC
  for Library of Congress   96-29037
                                                         CIP

Care has been taken to confirm the accuracy of the information presented
and to describe generally accepted practices. However, the authors, editors, and
publisher are not responsible for errors or omissions or for any consequences
from application of the information in this book and make no warranty, express
or implied, with respect to the contents of the publication.

The authors, editors and publisher have exerted every effort to ensure that
drug selection and dosage set forth in this text are in accordance with current
recommendations and practice at the time of publication. However, in view of
ongoing research, changes in government regulations, and the constant flow of
information relating to drug therapy and drug reactions, the reader is urged to
check the package insert for each drug for any change in indications and dosage
and for added warnings and precautions. This is particularly important when
the recommended agent is a new or infrequently employed drug.

Some drugs and medical devices presented in this publication have Food
and Drug Administration (FDA) clearance for limited use in restricted research
settings. It is the responsibility of the health care provider to ascertain the FDA
status of each drug or device planned for use in their clinical practice.

To my mother, Willie, and my brother, Gene,
for their encouragement, devotion, and love.

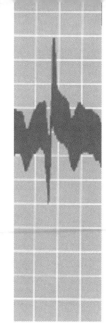

Reviewers

Marsha Coberly, RN, C, MSN
Lecturer, Medical-Surgical Section
College of Nursing
University of New Mexico
Albuquerque, New Mexico

Judith Ann Driscoll, RN, MSN
Assistant Professor
Deaconess College of Nursing
St. Louis, Missouri

Mary Ann O'Brien, RN
Instructor, Practical Nursing
James Lorenzo Walker Vocational–Technical Center
Naples, Florida

Cindy Roach, RN, DSN
Associate Professor
Chair, Department of Adult Health Nursing
Beth-el College of Nursing and Health Science
Colorado Springs, Colorado

Mary C. Shoemaker, PhD, RN
Level Coordinator, Associate Professor
Saint Francis Medical Center College of Nursing
Peoria, Illinois

Linda J. Ulak, RN, EdD, MS, CCRN
Assistant Professor, College of Nursing
Seton Hall University
South Orange, New Jersey

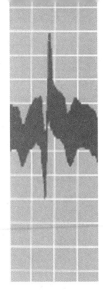

Preface

ECG Workout: Exercises in Arrhythmia Interpretation was written to assist medical, nursing, and paramedical personnel (physicians, nurses, medical and nursing students, paramedics, emergency medical technicians, telemetry technicians, and other allied health personnel) acquire the knowledge and skills essential for identification of basic arrhythmias. The text can also be used as a reference for ECG review for those already knowledgeable in ECG interpretation.

The text is written simply and illustrated with drawings, figures, tables, and ECG tracings. Each chapter is designed to build on the knowledge base from the previous chapters so the beginning student can quickly understand and grasp the basic concepts of electrocardiography. A great effort has been made not only to provide ECG tracings of good quality, but also to provide a sufficient number and variety of ECG practice strips so the reader feels confident in arrhythmia interpretation. There are 544 practice strips—more than any book currently on the market.

Chapter 1 presents a simplified discussion of anatomy and physiology of the heart, cardiopulmonary circulation, and coronary blood supply. The electrical basis of electrocardiology is discussed in Chapter 2. The components of the ECG tracing (waveforms, intervals, segments, complexes) are described in Chapter 3, in addition to practice tracings on waveform identification. Cardiac monitors, lead placements, and ECG artifacts are discussed in Chapter 4. A step-by-step guide to rhythm strip analysis is explained in Chapter 5, in addition to practice tracings on rhythm strip analysis. The individual arrhythmia chapters (Chapters 6 through 9) include a condensed description of each arrhythmia, arrhythmia examples, causes, and management protocols. Each arrhythmia chapter also includes 90 to 100 practice strips for self evaluation. Chapter 10 presents a general discussion of cardiac pacemakers (types, indications, function, pacemaker terminology, malfunctions, and pacemaker analysis), along with practice tracings on pacemaker rhythm strips. Chapter 11 includes two post-tests that can be used as a self-evaluation tool or for testing purposes.

The text has been reviewed and revised, replacing more than 50% of the ECG tracings. The ECG tracings are actual strips from patients, not computer-generated strips. Above each rhythm strip are 3-second indicators for rapid rate calculation. For more precise rate calculation, an ECG conversion table is provided on the inside back cover. For convenience, a removable ECG conversion table is also included with the text. The rates listed in the answer keys were determined by as precise a measurement as possible and will not always coincide with the rapid method of rate calculation.

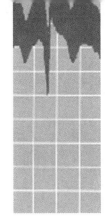

Contents

ECG Workout

**Exercises in
Arrhythmia Interpretation**

Anatomy and Physiology of the Heart

DESCRIPTION AND LOCATION OF THE HEART

The heart is a hollow, four-chambered muscular organ which lies in the mediastinal cavity between the right and left lungs, just behind the body of the sternum between the points of attachment of the 2nd through the 6th ribs (Figure 1-1). The lower border of the heart, which forms a blunt point known as the apex, lies on the diaphragm and points to the left. Approximately two thirds of its mass is to the left of the midline of the body, and one third is to the right. The average adult heart is 5 inches long and 3½ inches wide. This corresponds to an average man's clenched fist.

The primary function of the heart is to supply the body with enough blood to meet its metabolic demands. A normal adult heart contracts at a rate of 60–100 times per minute, pumping an average of 5.5 liters per minute. As metabolic demands increase, the heart responds by accelerating its rate to increase cardiac output. As a pump the heart has several unique properties: it expands and contracts without placing stress on the heart muscle; it can withstand continual activity without developing muscle fatigue; and it is capable of generating electrical impulses which maintain a proper heart rhythm.

HEART SURFACES

There are four main heart surfaces to consider when discussing the heart: anterior, posterior, inferior, and lateral (Figure 1-2). A simplified concept of the heart surfaces is listed on the next page.

Anterior: the front
Posterior: the back
Inferior: the bottom
Lateral: the side

STRUCTURE OF THE HEART WALL

The heart wall is arranged in three layers (Figure 1-3):

the pericardium—the outermost layer
the myocardium—the middle muscular layer
the endocardium—the inner layer

The pericardium consists of two parts: the fibrous pericardium and the serous pericardium. The fibrous pericardium is the tough, loosely fitting sac that surrounds the heart. It comes in direct contact

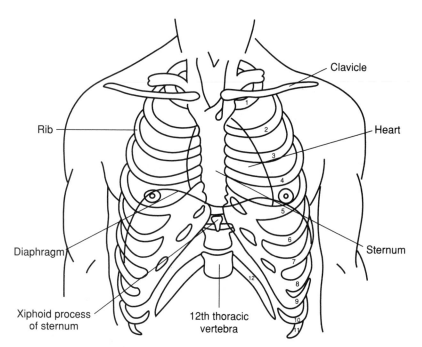

Figure 1-1. Thoracic projection of the boundaries of the heart on the chest wall.

cardium, and the visceral layer, which lines the outer surface of the myocardium. Between the two layers is a small space, the pericardial space or cavity, which normally contains 10–30ml of clear fluid secreted by the serous layers. This fluid lubricates the surface of the heart, allowing easy movement during contraction and expansion of the heart.

The middle muscular layer is responsible for the major pumping action of the ventricles and makes up the bulk of the heart wall. The myocardium contains the contractile fibers as well as the conduction system and blood supply.

The endocardium is a thin layer of tissue which lines the valves and inner chambers of the heart.

HEART CHAMBERS

The interior of the heart consists of four hollow chambers (Figure 1-4). The two upper chambers, the right atrium and the left atrium, are divided by a wall called the interatrial septum. The two lower chambers, the right ventricle and the left ventricle, are divided by a thicker wall called the interventricular septum. The two septa divide the heart into two pumping systems, a right heart and a left heart. The right heart pumps venous (deoxygenated) blood into the lungs. The left heart pumps arterial (oxygenated) blood into the systemic circulation. The heart cham-

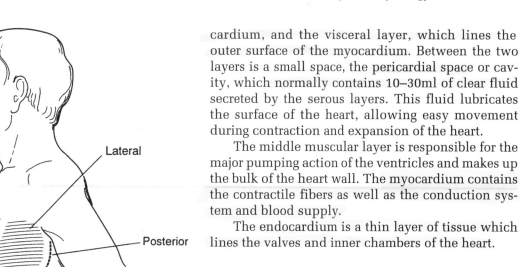

Figure 1-2. Heart surfaces.

with the covering of the lungs, the pleura. It is attached to the center of the diaphragm inferiorly, to the sternum anteriorly, and to the great vessels (the esophagus, trachea, and main bronchi) posteriorly. This position anchors the heart to the chest and prevents it from shifting about. The serous pericardium consists of two fluid-secreting layers: the parietal layer, which lines the inside of the fibrous peri-

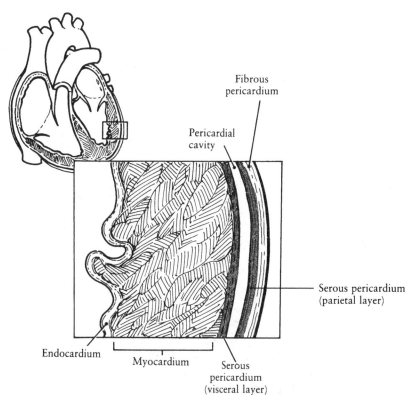

Figure 1-3. Heart wall. (From Bullock BL, Rosendahl PP: Pathophysiology, 3rd ed. Philadelphia: JB Lippincott, 1992).

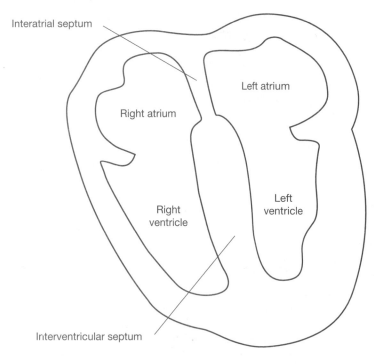

Figure 1-4. Chambers of the heart.

bers under highest pressure have the thickest musculature. Thus ventricular tissue is thicker than atrial tissue because the ventricles must achieve a higher pressure to eject blood. The left ventricle has the thickest musculature because it must eject blood against the pressure in the aorta, the vessel with the highest pressure.

HEART VALVES

There are four valves in the heart: the tricuspid valve, separating the right atrium from the right ventricle; the pulmonic valve, separating the right ventricle from the pulmonary artery; the mitral valve, separating the left atrium from the left ventricle; and the aortic valve, separating the left ventricle from the aorta (Figure 1-5). The primary function of the valves is to permit blood flow in one direction only, thereby preventing a backflow of blood. The opening and closing of the valves depends on pressure gradients within the cardiopulmonary system.

The tricuspid and mitral valves separate the atria from the ventricles and are referred to together as the atrioventricular valves (AV valves). As the atria fill with blood, pressure increases in the chambers, forcing the valves open and allowing blood to flow from the atria into the ventricles. The AV valves are forced shut during ventricular contraction (systole), preventing a backflow of blood into the atria. The AV

valves have cusps or leaflets which are connected to fingerlike projections (papillary muscles) in the ventricles by thin cords called chordae tendineae (Figure 1-6). The chordae tendineae and the papillary muscles stabilize the valves and prevent valve leaflet eversion. A dysfunction of the chordae tendineae or papillary muscles can cause an incomplete closure of an AV valve, resulting in a murmur. Closure of the AV valves constitutes the first heart sound (S_1).

The aortic and pulmonic valves, or semilunar valves, consist of half-moon-like flaps. The pulmonic valve is located just inside the orifice of the pulmonary artery and the aortic valve lies just inside the orifice of the aorta. Pressure inside the ventricles during ventricular systole forces the valves open so blood can be ejected into the pulmonary and systemic circulation. As the ventricular chambers empty, the loss of pressure causes the valves to close, preventing a backflow of blood into the ventricles. Closure of the semilunar valves constitutes the second heart sound (S_2).

BLOOD FLOW THROUGH THE HEART AND LUNGS

Blood flow through the heart and lungs can be traced from the right side to the left side (Figure 1-5). The right atrium receives unoxygenated blood from the superior vena cava, the inferior vena cava, and

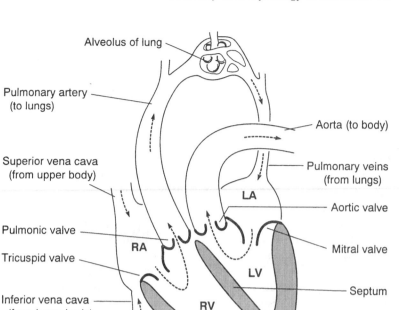

Figure 1-5. Chambers, valves, blood flow. *RA,* right atrium; *RV,* right ventricle; *LA,* left atrium; *LV,* left ventricle.

the coronary sinus. As the right atrium fills with blood the pressure in the chamber increases. When the pressure in the right atrium exceeds that of the right ventricle the tricuspid valve opens, allowing blood to flow into the right ventricle. Once filled, the right ventricle contracts, ejecting blood through the pulmonic valve into the lungs via the pulmonary

artery. In the lungs the blood picks up oxygen and releases excess carbon dioxide.

The left atrium receives the oxygenated blood from the lungs via the pulmonary veins. As the left atrium fills with blood the pressure in the chamber increases. When the pressure in the left atrium exceeds that of the left ventricle the mitral valve opens,

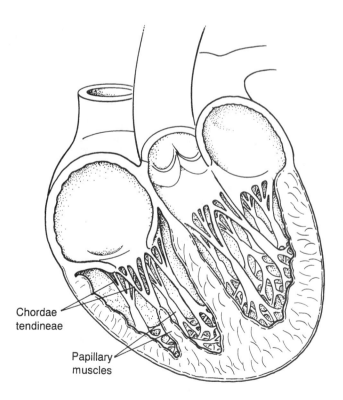

Figure 1-6. Papillary muscles and chordae tendineae.

allowing blood to flow into the left ventricle. Once filled, the left ventricle contracts, ejecting blood through the aortic valve into the aorta. The blood is then distributed throughout the body, where the blood releases oxygen to the cells and picks up carbon dioxide.

Even though blood flow can be traced, for simplicity's sake, from the right heart to the left heart, it must be remembered that right heart events and left heart events occur simultaneously: as the right atrium receives unoxygenated blood from the body, the left atrium receives oxygenated blood from the lungs. Increased pressures in the filled atria force the tricuspid and mitral valves open, allowing blood to enter both ventricles. Once filling is complete the ventricles contract simultaneously, ejecting blood through the pulmonic and aortic valves into the pulmonary and systemic circulation.

CORONARY CIRCULATION

The blood supply to the heart is provided by the right and left coronary arteries which arise from the aorta just above and behind the aortic valve (Figure 1-7; Table 1-1). The right coronary artery travels down the right side of the heart and curves around the bottom (inferior wall). It also supplies blood to the back (posterior wall) via the posterior descending

artery in 90% of the population. Occlusion of the right coronary artery results in an inferior or posterior wall myocardial infarction. The right coronary artery supplies blood to the following heart structures:

SA node in 50% of population
AV node in 90% of population
Right atrium and right ventricle
Inferior wall of the left ventricle
Posterior wall of the left ventricle in 90% of population

The left coronary artery has two branches: the left anterior descending (LAD) branch, which courses down the front (anterior wall) of the heart, and the circumflex, which travels down the side (lateral wall). Occlusion of the LAD results in an anterior wall myocardial infarction while occlusion of the circumflex results in a lateral wall myocardial infarction. The left anterior descending artery supplies blood to the following heart structures:

Anterior wall of the left ventricle
Interventricular septum
Bundle of His
Right bundle branch
Anterior fascicle of the left bundle branch

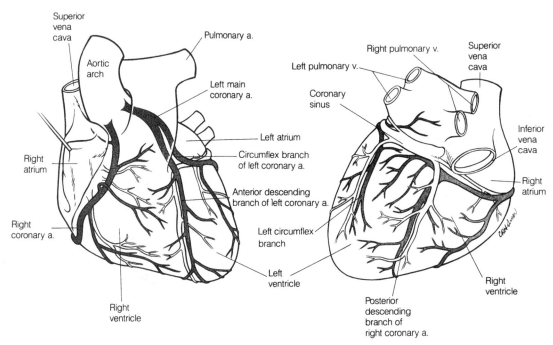

Figure 1-7. Coronary blood supply. (From Porth CM: Pathophysiology, 3rd ed. Philadelphia: JB Lippincott, 1990.)

Table 1-1. The Coronary Circulation and Heart Structures It Supplies

Artery	Structure Supplied
Right coronary artery	SA node in 50% of population
	AV node in 90% of population
	Right atrium
	Right ventricle
	Inferior wall of left ventricle
	Posterior wall of left ventricle in 90% of population
Left coronary artery	
Left anterior descending:	Anterior wall of left ventricle
	Intraventricular septum
	Bundle of His
	Right bundle branch
	Anterior fascicle of left bundle branch
Left circumflex:	SA node in 50% of population
	AV node in 10% of population
	Left atrium
	Lateral wall of left ventricle
	Posterior wall of left ventricle in 10% of population
	Posterior fascicle of left bundle branch

The circumflex artery supplies the following heart structures:

SA node in 50% of population

AV node in 10% of population

Left atrium

Lateral wall of the left ventricle

Posterior wall of the left ventricle in 10% of population

Posterior fascicle of the left bundle branch

Variations in blood distribution of the coronary arteries are common. Right or left coronary dominance denotes which artery system provides the posterior descending artery. When the right coronary artery (RCA) provides the posterior descending artery, the term *dominant RCA* is used. When it is the left coronary artery (LCA) that does this, the term *dominant LCA* is used. In most people the RCA is the dominant vessel. Although blood flow to the heart is continuous, blood flow is decreased during ventricular systole (when the coronary arteries are squeezed) and increased during ventricular filling (diastole). Whatever shortens filling time (e.g., increased heart rates) will diminish coronary blood flow.

AUTONOMIC INNERVATION OF THE HEART

The heart is controlled by the autonomic nervous system, which includes the sympathetic and parasympathetic nervous systems. Both systems are located in the medulla oblongata, a part of the brain stem, and work together to create a balance between heart rate, cardiac output, and blood pressure.

As body requirements change, multiple sensors in the body relay messages to the nerve centers in the brain. After analysis, the sympathetic and parasympathetic nerves transmit the appropriate impulses to the electrical conduction system of the heart, where they influence the automaticity, excitability, conductivity, and contractility of the heart's cardiac cells. Stimulation of the sympathetic nervous system causes a release of epinephrine, resulting in an increase in heart rate, cardiac output, and blood pressure. Stimulation of the parasympathetic nervous system causes a release of acetylcholine, resulting in a decrease in heart rate, cardiac output, and blood pressure.

2

Electrophysiology

CARDIAC CELLS

The heart consists of electrical cells and myocardial cells. The electrical cells are responsible for impulse formation and conduction, whereas the myocardial cells are responsible for muscular contraction.

The electrical cells are distributed in an orderly fashion along the conduction system of the heart. These cells possess three specific properties:

1. *Automaticity*—the ability of the cell to spontaneously generate and discharge an electrical impulse.

2. *Excitability*—the ability of the cell to respond to an electrical impulse.

3. *Conductivity*—the ability of the cell to transmit an electrical impulse from one cell to another.

The myocardial, or working cells, form the thin muscular layer of the atrial wall and the much thicker muscular layer of the ventricular wall. These cells possess two specific properties:

1. *Contractility*—the ability of the cell to shorten and lengthen its muscle fibers.

2. *Extensibility*—the ability of the cell to stretch.

DEPOLARIZATION AND REPOLARIZATION

The electrical cells generate and conduct electrical impulses that result in contraction and relaxation of the myocardial cells. These electrical impulses are generated by a flow of positively charged ions back and forth across the cardiac cell membrane, creating an electrical current which results in depolarization (electrical activation), contraction, and repolarization (recovery) of the cell (Figure 2-1).

Each cardiac cell is surrounded by and filled with a solution that contains positively charged ions (+) and negatively charged ions (−). Electrical charges are regulated primarily by two electrolytes: potassium (the primary intracellular ion) and sodium (the primary extracellular ion).

In the resting state of the cell, the inside of the cell membrane is considered negatively charged while the outside of the cell membrane is considered positively charged. Once an electrical impulse is generated, sodium moves rapidly into the cell and potassium begins to exit, converting the electrical forces inside the cell to a positive charge. The cell is then depolarized. As soon as the cardiac cell depolarizes, potassium reenters the cell and sodium exits,

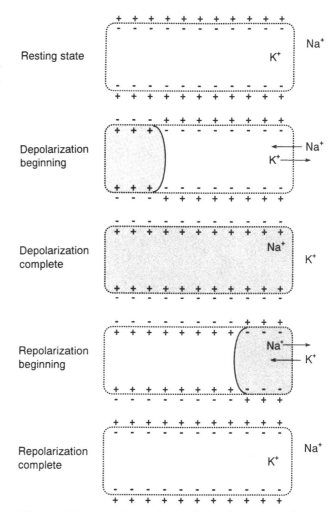

Figure 2-1. Depolarization and repolarization of a cardiac cell.

returning the inside of the cell to its resting negative charge. This process is called repolarization or the recovery phase.

Depolarization of one cardiac cell acts as a stimulus on adjacent cells and causes them to depolarize. Propagation of the electrical impulses from cell to cell produces an electric current which can be detected by skin electrodes and recorded as waves or deflections onto a graph paper called the electrocardiogram (ECG).

ELECTRICAL CONDUCTION SYSTEM OF THE HEART

The heart is endowed with an electrical conduction system that generates and conducts electrical impulses along specialized pathways to the atria and ventricles, causing them to contract (Figure 2-2). The system consists of the sinoatrial (SA) node, the inter-

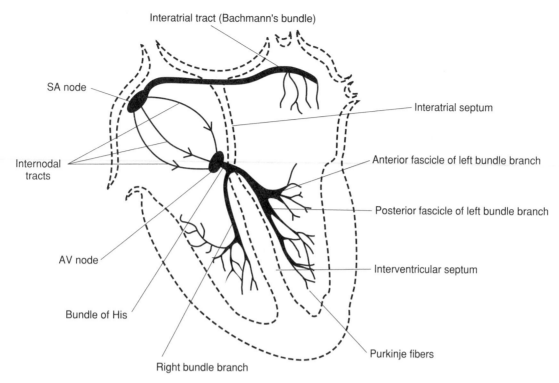

Figure 2-2. Electrical conduction system of the heart.

atrial tract (Bachmann's bundle), the internodal tracts, the atrio-ventricular (AV) node, the bundle of His, the right and left bundle branches, and the purkinje fibers.

The SA node is located in the wall of the right atrium near the inlet of the superior vena cava. Specialized electrical cells, called pacemaker cells, in the SA node discharge impulses at a rate of 60–100 times per minute in rhythmic fashion.

Pacemaker cells are located all along the conduction system, but the SA node is normally the primary pacemaker of the heart because it possesses the highest level of automaticity—that is, its inherent firing rate (60–100 times per minute) is usually greater than the other pacemaker sites (AV node pacemaker cells fire at 40–60 per minute and ventricular pacemaker cells at 30–40 per minute). If the SA node fails to generate electrical impulses at its normal rate or the conduction of these impulses is interrupted (blocked), pacemaker cells in other sites can assume control as pacemaker of the heart, but usually at a much slower rate. Such a pacemaker is called an escape pacemaker. A beat or series of beats arising from an escape pacemaker is called an escape beat or rhythm. In general, the farther away the impulse originates from the SA node, the slower the rate.

As the electrical impulse leaves the SA node it is conducted through the left atria by way of Bach-

mann's bundle, and through the right atria via the internodal tracts, causing electrical activation (depolarization) and contraction of the atria. The impulse is then conducted to the AV node, located in the lower right atrium near the interatrial septum, where it is delayed momentarily, awaiting the completion of atrial emptying and ventricular filling. Following the delay in the AV node the impulse moves rapidly through the bundle of His. The bundle of His splits into two important conducting pathways called the right bundle branch and the left bundle branch. The right bundle branch conducts the electrical impulse to the right ventricle while the left bundle branch divides into an anterior fascicle and a posterior fascicle, which conducts the impulse to the left ventricle. The impulse then enters the purkinje system where the purkinje fibers conduct the impulse to the ventricular muscle cells, causing ventricular depolarization and contraction. Repolarization then occurs.

The heart's electrical activity is represented on the monitor or ECG tracing by three basic waveforms: the P-wave, the QRS complex, and the T-wave (Figure 2-3). Between the waveforms are the following segments and intervals: the PR interval, the ST segment, and the QT interval. A U-wave is sometimes present. While the letters themselves have no special significance, each component represents a particular event in the depolarization-repolarization cycle. The

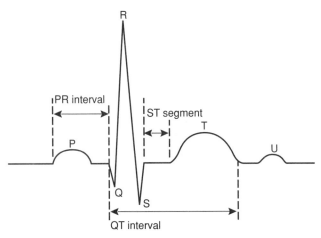

Figure 2-3. Relationship of the electrical conduction system to the ECG.

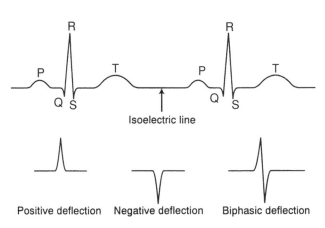

Figure 2-5. Relationship between waveforms and the isoelectric line.

P-wave depicts atrial depolarization, or the spread of the impulse from the SA node throughout the atria. The PR interval represents the time required for the impulse to travel through the atria, AV node, bundle of His, bundle branches, and purkinje fibers. The QRS complex depicts ventricular depolarization, or the spread of the impulse throughout the ventricles. The ST segment represents the end of ventricular depolarization and the beginning of ventricular repolarization. The T-wave represents the latter phase of ventricular repolarization. The U-wave, which is not always present, may represent further repolarization of the ventricles. The QT interval represents both ventricular depolarization and repolarization.

THE CARDIAC CYCLE

A cardiac cycle consists of one heart beat or one P–QRS–T sequence. It represents a sequence of atrial

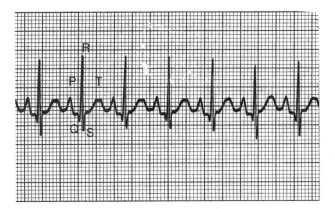

Figure 2-4. The cardiac cycle.

contraction (systole) and relaxation (diastole) followed by ventricular contraction and relaxation. The basic cycle repeats itself again and again (Figure 2-4). On the ECG, a cardiac cycle is measured from one heartbeat to the beginning of the next (from one R-wave to the next R-wave). Between cardiac cycles the monitor or ECG recorder returns to a baseline called the isoelectric line, a flat line between the T-wave and the P-wave (Figure 2-5). Any waveform above the isoelectric line is considered a positive (upright) deflection and any waveform below this line is considered a negative (downward) deflection. A deflection having both a positive and negative component is called a biphasic deflection. This basic concept can be applied to the P-wave, the QRS complex, and the T-wave deflections.

WAVEFORMS AND CURRENT FLOW

A monitor lead or ECG lead provides a particular view of the heart's electrical activity between two points (or poles). Each lead consists of a positive (+) pole and a negative (−) pole. The direction in which the electric current flows determines how the waveforms appear on the ECG tracing (Figure 2-6). An electric current flowing toward the positive pole will produce a positive deflection; an electric current flowing away from the positive pole will produce a negative deflection. When an electric current flows partly toward and partly away from the positive pole, a biphasic deflection is produced. The size of the wave deflection will depend on the magnitude of the electrical current flowing toward the individual pole.

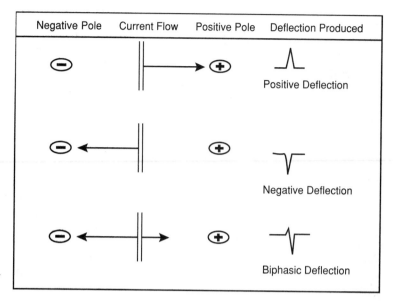

Figure 2-6. Relationship between current flow and waveform deflections.

REFRACTORY AND SUPERNORMAL PERIODS OF THE CARDIAC CYCLE

There is a period of time during the cardiac cycle when the cardiac cells may or may not be depolarized by an electrical stimulus, depending on the strength of the electrical impulse. This period is called the refractory period and is divided into the absolute refractory period (ARP) and the relative refractory period (RRP), as shown in Figure 2-7. The absolute refractory period extends from the onset of the QRS complex to the peak of the T-wave. During

this time the cardiac cells have depolarized and are in the process of repolarizing. Because the cardiac cells have not repolarized to their threshold potential (the level at which a cell must be repolarized before it can be depolarized again), they cannot be stimulated to depolarize—in other words, the electrical cells cannot conduct an impulse nor can the myocardial cells contract during the absolute refractory period. The relative refractory period begins at the peak of the T-wave and ends with the end of the T-wave. During this time the cardiac cells have repolarized sufficiently to respond to a strong electrical stimulus. This period is also called the vulnera-

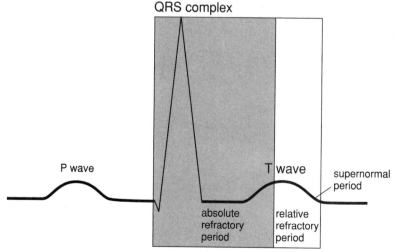

Figure 2-7. Refractory and supernormal periods.

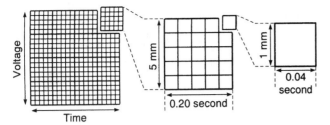

Figure 2-8. Electrocardiographic paper.

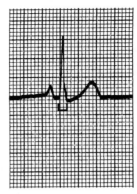

Figure 2-9. QRS width: 0.08 seconds; QRS height: 16 mm.

ble period of repolarization. A strong stimulus occurring during the vulnerable period may usurp the primary pacemaker of the heart (usually the SA node) and take over pacemaker control. The supernormal period occurs near the end of the T-wave just before the cells have completely repolarized. During this period the cardiac cells will respond to a weak stimulus.

ECG GRAPH PAPER

The P–QRS–T sequence is recorded on special graph paper made up of horizontal and vertical lines (Figure 2-8). The horizontal lines measure the duration of the waveforms in seconds of time. Each small square measured horizontally represents 0.04 seconds in time. The width of the QRS complex in Figure 2-9 extends across for 2 squares and represents 0.08 seconds (0.04 seconds × 2 squares). The vertical lines measure the voltage or amplitude of the waveform in millimeters (mm). Each small square measured vertically represents 1 mm in height. The height of the QRS complex in Figure 2-9 extends upward from baseline 16 small squares and represents 16 mm voltage (1 mm × 16 squares).

3

Wave Forms, Intervals, Segments, and Complexes

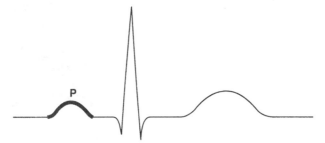

Figure 3-1. The P wave.

Much of the information provided by the ECG tracing is contained in the examination and/or measurement of the three principal waveforms (the P-wave, QRS complex, and T-wave) and their associated intervals and segments. Collection of this data provides the facts necessary for an accurate cardiac rhythm interpretation.

P-WAVE

The first deflection of the cardiac cycle, the P-wave, is caused by depolarization of the atria. The onset of the waveform begins as the deflection leaves baseline and ends when the deflection returns to baseline (Figure 3-1). Normal P-waves are small, rounded, and positive (upright) in Lead II, with an amplitude between 0.5 mm–2.5 mm and duration of 0.10 seconds or less. There should be one P-wave preceding each QRS complex. A P-wave of normal size, shape, and direction indicates that the electrical impulse originated in the SA node and that normal depolarization of the atria has occurred. Abnormal P-waves indicate that the sinus impulse traveled through altered or damaged atria, or that the electrical impulse responsible for the P-wave originated in a site outside the SA node (ectopic pacemaker site). Several P-wave examples are shown in Figure 3-2.

PR INTERVAL

The PR interval represents the time required for the electrical impulse to leave the SA node and travel through the atria, AV node, the bundle branches, and the purkinje network. The PR interval includes a P-wave and the short, flat (isoelectric) line that follows

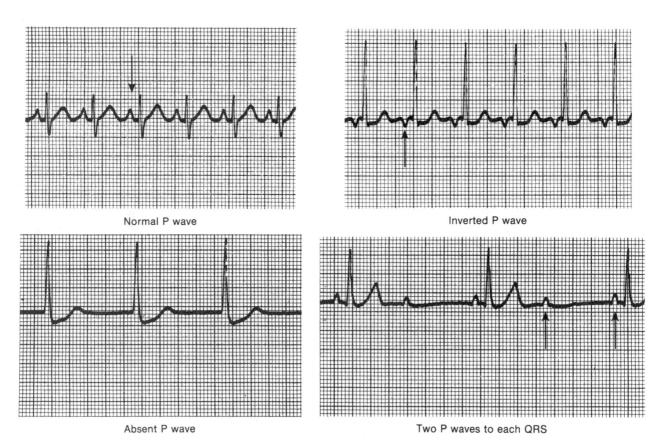

Normal P wave

Inverted P wave

Absent P wave

Two P waves to each QRS

Figure 3-2. P wave examples.

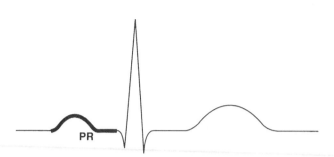

Figure 3-3. The PR interval.

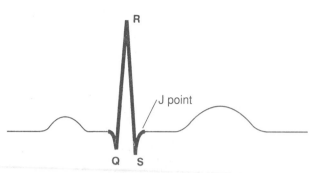

Figure 3-5. The QRS complex.

it (Figure 3-3). The PR interval is measured from the beginning of the P-wave as it leaves baseline to the beginning of the QRS complex. The duration of the normal PR interval is 0.12–0.20 seconds. A normal PR interval indicates that the electrical impulse leaving the SA node was conducted through the entire electrical conduction system within a normal amount of time. The PR interval may be shorter than normal if the electrical impulse was conducted through an abnormal conduction pathway that bypasses the AV node, or if the impulse originated in an ectopic site close to or in the AV junction. The PR interval may be longer than normal if the electrical impulse is delayed traveling through the AV node and bundle of His. Examples of PR intervals are shown in Figure 3-4.

QRS COMPLEX

The QRS complex represents the time required for the electrical impulse to depolarize the ventricles. The QRS is measured from the beginning of the QRS as the first wave leaves baseline to the point where the last wave of the complex begins to flatten out at, above, or below baseline (Figure 3-5). This point, the junction between the QRS and the ST segment, is called the "junction" or "J" point. Elevation or depression of the ST segment makes ending the QRS more difficult. The QRS ends as soon as the straight line of the ST segment begins, even though the straight line may be above or below baseline. The normal QRS complex is predominantly positive in Lead II, with a duration of 0.10 seconds or less. The abnormal QRS is wide with a duration of 0.12 seconds or more.

The QRS complex is composed of three wave deflections: the Q-, R-, and S-waves. The R-wave is a positive deflection; the Q-wave is a negative deflection that precedes an R-wave; the S-wave is a negative deflection following an R-wave. Many variations exist, however, in the configuration of the QRS, and you may not always see all three QRS waveforms (Figure 3-6). Whatever the variation, the complex is still called the QRS complex. It is possible to have more than one R-wave or S-wave in a QRS complex.

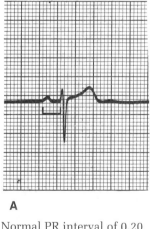

A

Normal PR interval of 0.20 seconds (0.04 seconds × 5 squares).

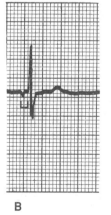

B

Short PR interval of 0.08 seconds (0.04 seconds × 2 squares).

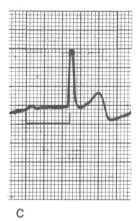

C

Long PR interval of 0.48 seconds (0.04 seconds × 12 squares).

Figure 3-4. PR interval examples.

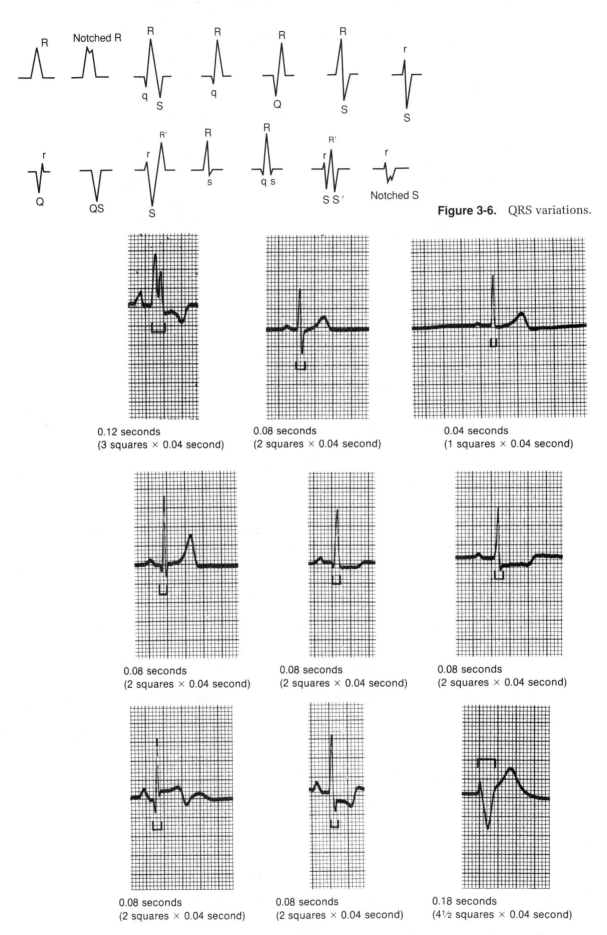

Figure 3-6. QRS variations.

0.12 seconds
(3 squares × 0.04 second)

0.08 seconds
(2 squares × 0.04 second)

0.04 seconds
(1 squares × 0.04 second)

0.08 seconds
(2 squares × 0.04 second)

0.08 seconds
(2 squares × 0.04 second)

0.08 seconds
(2 squares × 0.04 second)

0.08 seconds
(2 squares × 0.04 second)

0.08 seconds
(2 squares × 0.04 second)

0.18 seconds
(4½ squares × 0.04 second)

Figure 3-7. QRS examples.

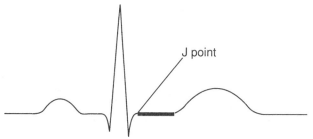

Figure 3-8. The ST segment.

The second R-wave is labeled R prime (R′) and the second S-wave is labeled S prime (S′). To be labeled separately, a wave must cross the baseline. A wave that changes direction but does not cross the baseline is called a notch. Upper-case letters are used to designate waves of large amplitude, while lower-case letters are used to label small waveforms.

A normal QRS complex indicates that depolarization of the ventricles occurred within a normal amount of time. An abnormal (wide) QRS indicates that abnormal depolarization of the ventricles has occurred, either due to a block in one of the bundle branches, or because the electrical impulse was conducted through an abnormal conduction pathway, or because the electrical impulse originated in an ectopic site in the ventricles. Examples of QRS complexes are shown in Figure 3-7.

ST SEGMENT

The ST segment represents the end of ventricular depolarization and the beginning of ventricular repolarization. The ST segment begins with the end of the QRS complex and ends with the onset of the T-wave (Figure 3-8). The point marking the end of the QRS is known as the J point. The normal ST segment is flat (isoelectric). Elevation or depression of the ST segment by 1 mm or more above or below baseline (measured 0.08 seconds or 2 squares past the J point) is considered abnormal. If elevated, the ST segment may be horizontal (straight across), convex (arched upward), or concave (arched inward). If depressed, the ST segment may be horizontal, downsloping, or upsloping. An elevated ST segment is an ECG sign of myocardial injury, as seen in acute myocardial infarction. Other causes of ST segment elevation include coronary vasospasm (Prinzmetal's angina) and pericarditis. A depressed ST segment is an ECG sign of myocardial ischemia. Although ST segment depression is most often associated with myocardial ischemia, other common causes include left and right ventricular hypertro-

phy, left and right bundle branch block, and the administration of digitalis (which causes a sagging ST depression known as "digitalis effect"). A normal ST segment indicates that the early phase of ventricular repolarization is normal. Abnormalities in the ST segment indicate abnormal ventricular repolarization has occurred. Examples of ST segments are shown in Figure 3-9.

T-WAVE

The T-wave represents the latter phase of ventricular repolarization. The onset of the normal T-wave begins as the deflection slopes upward from the ST segment and ends when the waveform returns to baseline (Figure 3-10). With fast heart rates, the onset and end of the T-wave is sometimes difficult to determine with certainty. Normal T-waves are rounded, slightly asymmetrical (with the first, upward part ascending more slowly than the second, downward part) and positive in lead II, with an amplitude less than 5 mm and a duration of 0.10–0.25 seconds or greater. Abnormal T-waves are symmetrical and may be tall and peaked, biphasic (both positive and negative), or deeply inverted. Abnormal T-waves are seen in myocardial ischemia, myocardial infarction, hyperkalemia, pericarditis, ventricular hypertrophy, and in the administration of certain drugs (quinidine, procainamide). A normal T-wave indicates that the latter phase of ventricular repolarization is normal. Abnormalities in the T-wave indicate abnormal ventricular repolarization has occurred. Examples of T-waves are shown in Figure 3-11.

QT INTERVAL

The QT interval represents the time between the onset of ventricular depolarization and the end of ventricular repolarization. The QT interval is measured from the beginning of the QRS complex to the end of the T-wave (Figure 3-12). The duration of the QT interval is dependent on the heart rate. In general, a QT interval less than half the distance between consecutive R-waves (called the R-R interval) is normal, one that is greater than half is abnormal, and one that is about half is "borderline." The QT interval is shorter with fast heart rates and longer when the heart rate is slow. The determination of the QT interval should be made in a lead where the T-wave is most prominent and should not include the U-wave. Also, if the QRS is widened beyond 0.08 sec-

(text continues on page 23)

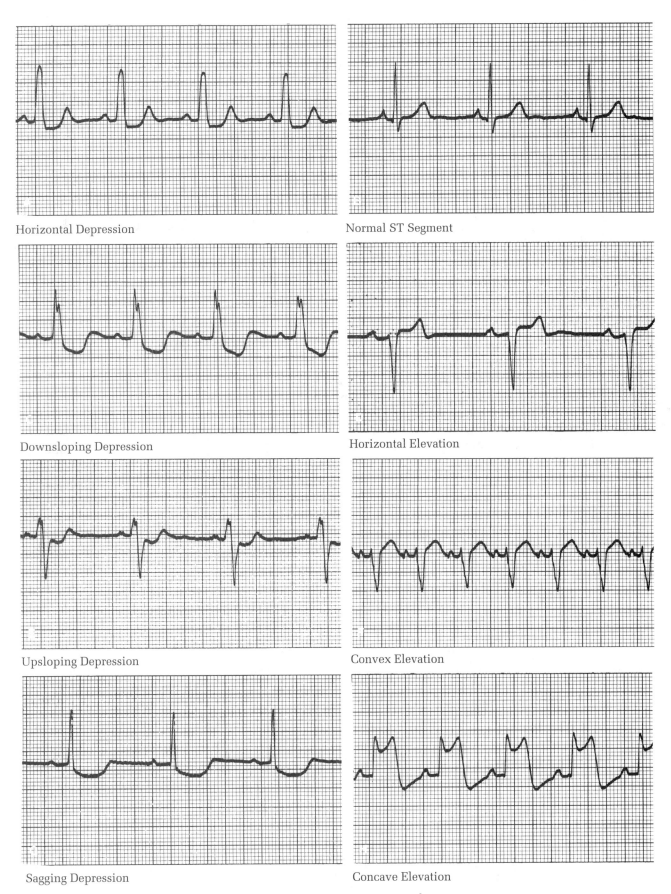

Horizontal Depression

Normal ST Segment

Downsloping Depression

Horizontal Elevation

Upsloping Depression

Convex Elevation

Sagging Depression

Concave Elevation

Figure 3-9. ST segment examples.

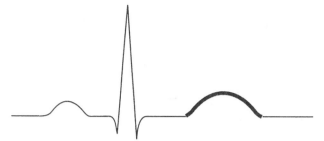

Figure 3-10. The T wave.

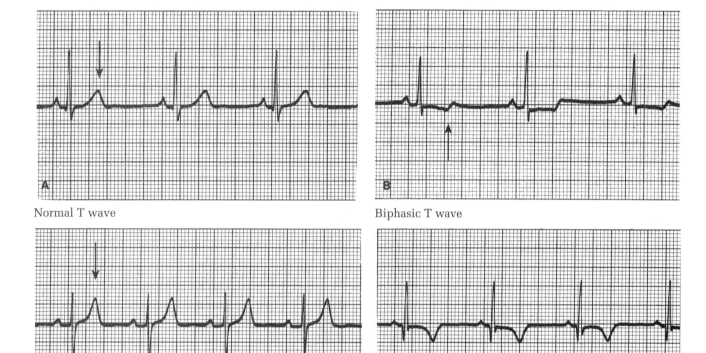

Normal T wave

Biphasic T wave

Tall, peaked T wave

Inverted T wave

Figure 3-11. T wave examples.

Table 3-1. QT Interval Normals

Heart Rate (per minute)	QT Normal Range (seconds)
40	0.41–0.51
50	0.38–0.46
60	0.35–0.43
70	0.33–0.41
80	0.32–0.39
90	0.30–0.36
100	0.28–0.34
120	0.26–0.32
150	0.23–0.28
180	0.21–0.25
200	0.20–0.24

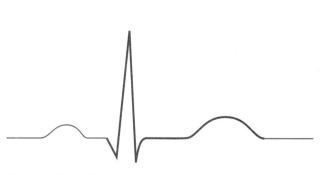

Figure 3-12. QT interval.

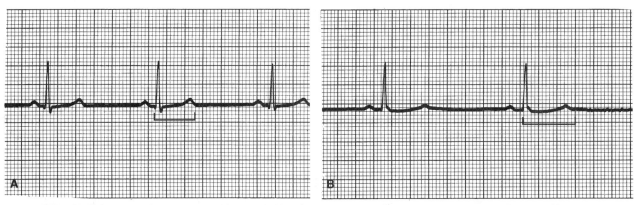

Normal QT interval of 0.44 sec (11 squares × .04 sec = 0.44 sec). Heart rate of 48 (31 small squares between consecutive R waves = 48

Prolonged QT interval of 0.56 sec (14 squares × .04 sec = 0.56 sec). Heart rate of 40 (38 small squares between consecutive R waves = 40)

Figure 3-13. QT interval examples.

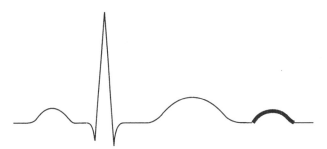

Figure 3-14. The U wave.

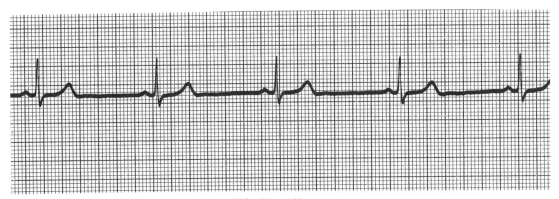

ECG without U wave

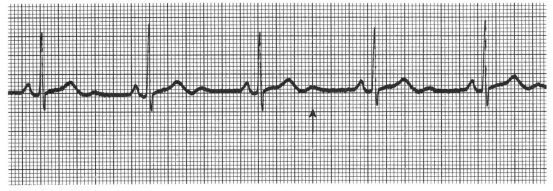

ECG with U wave

Figure 3-15. U wave example.

onds, the excess widening beyond 0.08 seconds must be subtracted from the actual measurement to obtain the correct QT interval.

The normal range of the QT interval expected at a given heart rate is shown in Table 3-1. A normal QT interval indicates that ventricular depolarization and repolarization has occurred within a normal amount of time. A prolonged QT interval indicates that ventricular repolarization time is slowed, which means that the relative refractory period or vulnerable period of the cardiac cycle is longer, predisposing patients to potentially lethal ventricular dysrhythmias (see discussion of *torsade de pointes,* Chapter 9). Electrolyte abnormalities (hypocalcemia, hypokalemia), slow heart rates, liquid protein diets, pericarditis, left ventricular hypertrophy, hypothermia, central nervous system disorders, and an excess of certain drugs (quinidine, procainamide, tricyclic antidepressants, disopyramide, amiodarone, phenothiazines) can prolong the QT interval. Examples of QT intervals are shown in Figure 3-13.

U-WAVE

A U-wave, if present, represents a part of the latter phase of ventricular repolarization. The U-wave is a small deflection seen after the T-wave and occurring before the next P-wave. A U-wave can best be seen when the heart rate is slow. The onset of the waveform begins as the deflection leaves baseline and ends when the deflection returns to baseline (Figure 3-14). Normal U-waves are small, round, symmetrical, and positive in Lead II, with an amplitude less than 2 mm. Abnormal U-waves may be abnormally tall (as seen in hypokalemia) or inverted. Normal U-waves indicate that the latter phase of ventricular repolarization is normal. Abnormalities in the size or direction of the U-wave indicate that an abnormality in the latter phase of ventricular repolarization has occurred. Examples of U-waves are shown in Figure 3-15.

Waveform Practice: Labeling Waves

Directions: For each of the following rhythm strips (strips 3-1 through 3-11) label the P, Q, R, S, T, and U waves. Some of the strips may not have all of these waveforms. Check your answers with the answer keys in the Appendix.

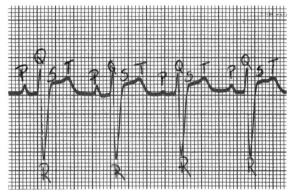

Strip 3-1.

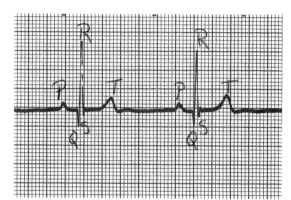

Strip 3-2.

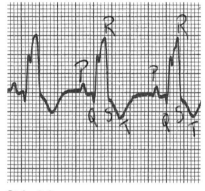

Strip 3-3.

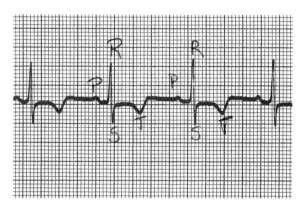

Strip 3-4.

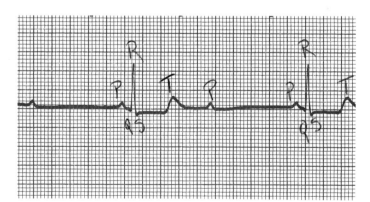

Strip 3-5.

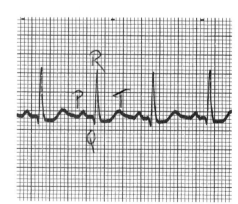

Strip 3-6.

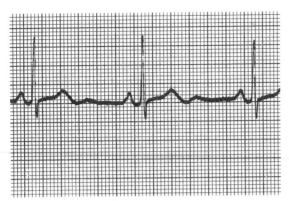

Strip 3-7.

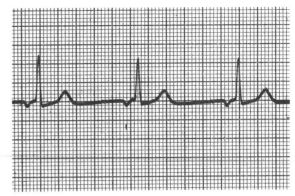

Strip 3-8.

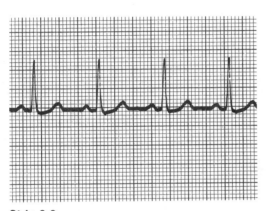

Strip 3-9.

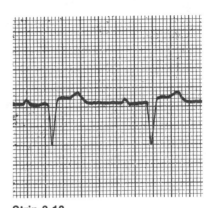

Strip 3-10.

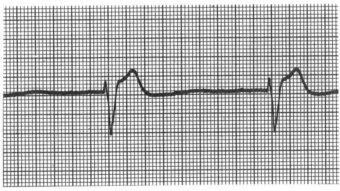

Strip 3-11.

4

Cardiac Monitors

PURPOSE OF ECG MONITORING

The electrocardiogram (ECG) is a recording of cardiac electrical activity (not mechanical function). The ECG records the following two basic electrical processes:

1. Depolarization (the spread of the electrical stimulus through the heart muscle) producing the P-wave from the atria and the QRS from the ventricles.

2. Repolarization (the return of the stimulated muscle to the resting state) producing the ST segment, the T-wave, and the U-wave.

The depolarization-repolarization process produces electrical currents which are transmitted to the surface of the body. This electrical activity is readily detected by electrodes attached to the skin. After the electric current is detected it is amplified, displayed on a monitor screen (oscilloscope), and recorded on ECG graph paper as waves and complexes. The waveforms can then be analyzed in a systematic manner and the "cardiac rhythm" identified.

The 12-lead ECG provides 12 different views of the heart's electrical activity and is used for cardiac rhythm interpretation as well as to help diagnose many cardiac conditions. Single-lead monitoring is used to monitor the patient's cardiac rhythm continuously from a single lead. Single-lead monitoring is used to monitor patients in critical care units, cardiac stepdown units, outpatient surgery departments, emergency rooms, post-anesthesia recovery units, and so forth. Single-lead monitoring allows continuous observation of the heart's electrical activity, which is essential for identification of abnormal heart rhythms (arrhythmias). Continuous monitoring is also useful in evaluating the effects of therapy.

TYPES OF SINGLE-LEAD MONITORING

There are two types of single-lead monitoring: hardwire and telemetry. With hardwire monitoring, conductive gel discs (electrodes) are placed on the patient's chest and attached to a lead-cable system which is then connected to a bedside monitor. With telemetry (wireless monitoring), electrodes are attached to the patient's chest and the leads connected to a portable monitor transmitter.

Hardwire Monitoring

You may perform hardwire monitoring using one of several systems available. The most common

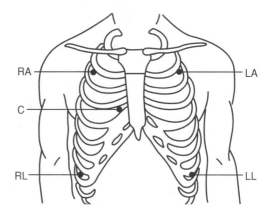

Figure 4-1. Five-leadwire system
This illustration shows you where to place the electrodes and attach lead wires using a five-leadwire system. The lead wires are color-coded as follows:
white—right arm (RA)
black—left arm (LA)
green—right leg (RL)
red—left leg (LL)
brown—chest (C)
The five-leadwire system allows you to monitor your patients in any of the standard 12 leads using a lead selector on the monitor. In this example the brown chest lead is in V_1 position. The chest lead can be placed in any of the six chest lead positions (Figure 4-2).

hardwire monitoring systems are the 5-leadwire system and the 3-leadwire system.

1. *Five-leadwire system* (Figure 4-1). With the 5-leadwire system, five electrodes and five leadwires are used. One electrode is placed below the right clavicle (2nd interspace, right midclavicular line), one below the left clavicle (2nd interspace, left midclavicular line), one on the right lower rib cage (8th interspace, right midclavicular line), one on the left lower rib cage (8th interspace, left midclavicular line), and one in a chest lead position (V_1–V_6). The six chest lead positions (Figure 4-2) include:

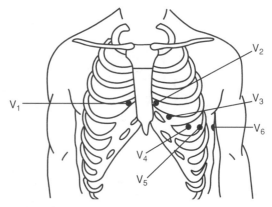

Figure 4-2. Chest lead positions.

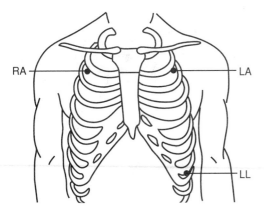

Figure 4-3. Three-leadwire system
This illustration shows you where to place the electrodes and attach leadwires using a three-leadwire system. The lead wires are color-coded as follows:
    white—right arm (RA)
    black—left arm (LA)
    red—left leg (LL)
Leads placed in this position will allow you to monitor leads I, II, or III using the lead selector on the monitor.

V_1—4th intercostal space, right sternal border

V_2—4th intercostal space, left sternal border

V_3—midway between V_2 and V_4

V_4—5th intercostal space, left midclavicular line

V_5—5th intercostal space, left anterior axillary line

V_6—5th intercostal space, left midaxillary line

The right arm (RA) lead is attached to the electrode below the right clavicle, the left arm (LA) lead is attached to the electrode below the left clavicle, the right leg (RL) lead is attached to the electrode on the right lower rib cage, the left leg (LL) lead is attached to the electrode on the left lower rib cage, and the chest lead is attached to the chest electrode. The 5-leadwire system allows you to monitor your patients in any of the standard 12 leads (Leads I, II, III, AVR, AVL, AVF, and V_1 through V_6) using a lead selector on the monitor.

    2. *Three-leadwire system* (Figure 4-3). With the 3-leadwire system, three electrodes and three leadwires are used. One electrode is placed below the right clavicle (2nd interspace, right midclavicular line), one below the left clavicle (2nd interspace, left midclavicular line), and one on the left lower rib cage (8th interspace, left midclavicular line). The right arm (RA) lead is attached to the electrode below the right clavicle, the left arm (LA) lead is attached to the electrode below the left clavicle, and the left leg (LL) lead is attached to the electrode on the left lower rib cage. You can monitor either limb leads I, II, or III by turning the lead selector on the monitor. Although you can't monitor chest leads (V_1–V_6) with a 3-leadwire system, you can monitor modified chest leads which provide similar information. To monitor any of these leads, reposition the left leg (LL) lead to the appropriate position for the chest lead you want to monitor, and turn the lead selector on the monitor to lead III. Examples of modified chest lead V_1 (MCL$_1$) and modified chest lead V_6 (MCL$_6$) are shown in Figure 4-4.

Telemetry Monitoring

    Wireless monitoring, or telemetry (Figure 4-5), gives your patient more freedom than the hardwire monitoring system. Instead of being connected to a bedside monitor, the patient is connected to a portable monitor transmitter which can be placed in a pajama pocket or in a telemetry pouch and secured with a strap around the neck, chest, or waist. With the telemetry monitoring system you will have three

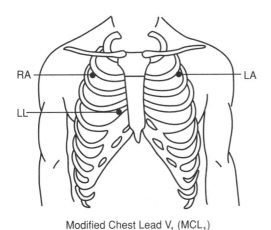

Modified Chest Lead V_1 (MCL$_1$)

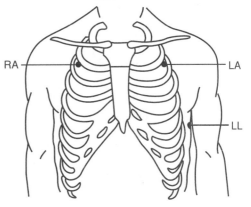

Modified Chest Lead V_6 (MCL$_6$)

Figure 4-4. Three-leadwire system: Leads MCL$_1$ and MCL$_6$
Modified chest leads can be monitored with the three-leadwire system by repositioning the left leg (LL) lead to chest position desired and turning the lead selector on the monitor to lead III.

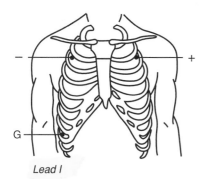

Lead I

Negative lead – 2nd interspace
right midclavicular line

Positive lead – 2nd interspace
left midclavicular line

Ground lead – 8th interspace
right midclavicular line

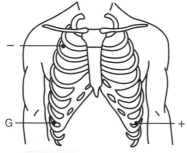

Lead II

Negative lead – 2nd interspace
right midclavicular line

Positive lead – 8th interspace
left midclavicular line

Ground lead – 8th interspace
right midclavicular line

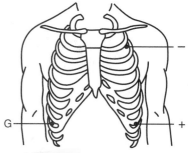

Lead III

Negative lead – 2nd interspace
left midclavicular line

Positive lead – 8th interspace
left midclavicular line

Ground lead – 8th interspace
right midclavicular line

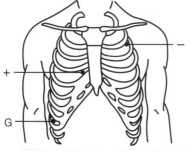

Modified Chest Lead V₁ (MCL₁)

Negative lead – 2nd interspace
left midclavicular line

Positive lead – 4th interspace
right sternal border

Ground lead – 8th interspace
right midclavicular line

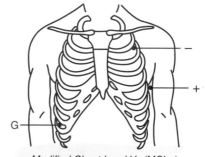

Modified Chest Lead V₆ (MCL₆)

Negative lead – 2nd interspace
left midclavicular line

Positive lead – 5th interspace
left midaxillary line

Ground lead – 8th interspace
right midclavicular line

Figure 4-5. Telemetry lead positions.

electrodes and three lead wires—one positive (+), one negative (−), and one ground (G). The electrodes and lead wires are placed on the chest in positions which approximate those used in the 12-lead ECG. Telemetry monitoring allows you to monitor your patients in limb leads I, II, III, and modified chest lead V_1 (MCL₁) and modified chest lead V_6 (MCL₆).

APPLYING THE ELECTRODE PADS

Proper attachment of the electrodes to the skin is the most important step in obtaining a good quality ECG tracing. Unless there is good contact between the skin and the electrode pad, distortions of the ECG tracing (artifacts) may appear. An artifact is any abnormal wave, spike, or movement on the ECG tracing that is not generated by the electrical activity of the heart. The procedure for attaching the electrodes is as follows:

1. *Choose monitor lead position.* It is helpful to assess the 12-lead ECG to ascertain which lead provides the best QRS voltage and P-wave identification.

2. *Prepare the skin:*

   a. Shave the sites, if necessary, with a razor. Hair interferes with good contact between the electrode pad and the skin.

   b. Wipe sites with alcohol or acetone pad to remove skin oil. Allow to dry.

   c. Gently abrade skin. A dry washcloth may be used. Some companies produce electrode pads with a small amount of abrasive material attached to the pad's peel-off section—these work extremely well.

  d. If the patient is perspiring, apply a thin coat of tincture of benzoin and allow it to dry.

3. *Attach electrode pads:*

  a. Avoid placing pads over bony areas, such as the clavicles or prominent rib markings.

  b. Remove pads from packaging. Check electrode disc for presence of moist conductive gel. Dried gel can cause loss of the ECG signal.

  c. Place electrode pad on prepared sites, pressing firmly around periphery of the pad.

4. *Connect lead wires.* Attach appropriate lead wires to the electrode pads according to established electrode-lead positions.

TROUBLESHOOTING MONITOR PROBLEMS

Many problems may be encountered during cardiac monitoring. The most common problems are related to patient movement, interference from equipment in or near the patient room, weak ECG signals, poor choice of monitor lead or electrode placement, and poor contact between the skin and electrode-lead attachments. Monitor problems can cause artifacts on the ECG tracing, making identification of the cardiac rhythm difficult or triggering false monitor alarms (high rate alarms and low rate alarms). Some problems are potentially serious and require intervention, whereas others are transient, non-life-threatening occurrences that will correct themselves. The nurse or monitor technician needs to develop sufficient troubleshooting skills to be able to recognize the monitoring problems, identify probable causes, and seek solutions to correct the problem. The most common monitoring problems are discussed below:

False High Rate Alarms

High voltage artifact potentials are often interpreted by the monitor as QRS complexes and activate the high rate alarm (Figure 4-6). Most high voltage artifacts are related to muscle movements from turning in bed or moving the extremities. Seizure activity can also produce high voltage artifact potentials.

False Low Rate Alarms

Any disturbance in the transmission of the electrical signal from the skin electrode to the monitoring system can activate a false low rate alarm (Figures 4-7 through 4-9). This problem is usually caused by ineffective contact between the skin and the electrode or lead wire due to dried conductive gel, a loose electrode, or a disconnected lead wire. The low rate alarm can also be activated by low voltage QRS complexes. If the ventricular waveforms are not tall enough, the monitor detects no electrical activity and will sound the low rate alarm.

Muscle Tremors

Muscle tremors (Figures 4-10 and 4-11) can occur in tense, nervous patients or those shivering from cold or having a chill. The ECG baseline has an uneven, coarsely jagged appearance obscuring the components of the ECG tracing. The problem may be continuous or intermittent.

Telemetry-Related Interference

This type of artifact occurs when the ECG signals are poorly received over a telemetry monitoring system (Figure 4-12). Weak ECG signals are caused by weak batteries or by the transmitter being used in the outer fringes of the reception area of the base station receiver, resulting in sharp spikes or straight lines on the ECG tracing.

Electrical Interference (AC Interference)

Electrical interference (Figure 4-13) can occur when multiple electrical equipment is in use in the patient room, when the patient is using an electrical appliance such as an electric razor or hair dryer, when improperly grounded equipment is in use, or when loose or exposed wiring is present. This type of artifact results in a wide baseline consisting of a continuous series of fine, even, rapid spikes which can obscure the components of the ECG tracing.

Wandering Baseline

A wandering baseline (Figure 4-14) (a monitor pattern that wanders up and down on the monitor screen or ECG tracing) is caused by exaggerated respiratory movements commonly seen in patients with respiratory distress. This type of artifact makes it difficult to identify the cardiac rhythm as well as changes in the ST segment and T-wave.

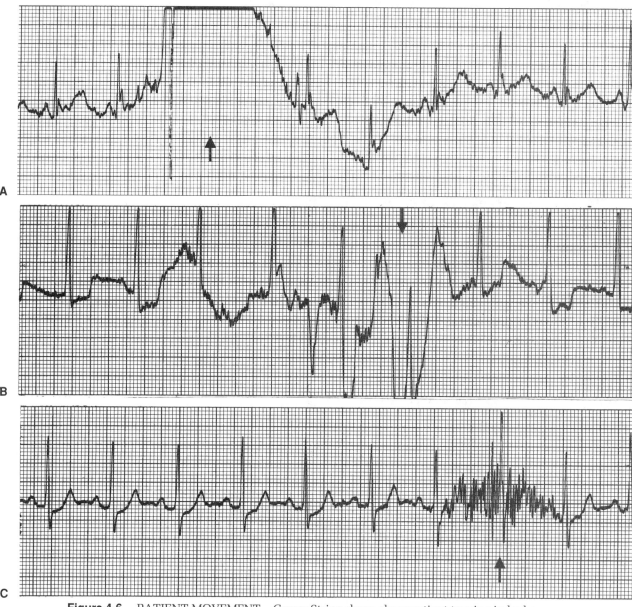

Figure 4-6. PATIENT MOVEMENT—*Cause:* Strips above show patient turning in bed or extremity movement. *Solution:* Problem is usually intermittent and no correction is necessary. Movement artifact can be reduced by avoiding placement of electrode pads in areas where extremity movement is greatest (bony areas such as the clavicles).

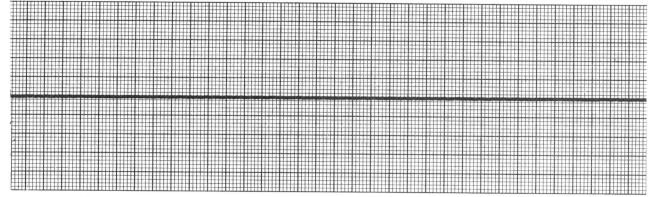

Figure 4-7. CONTINUOUS STRAIGHT LINE—*Cause:* dried conductive gel, disconnected lead wire, or disconnected electrode pad. *Solution:* Check electrode/lead system; re-prep and re-attach electrodes and leads as necessary. Note: A straight line may also indicate the absence of electrical activity in the heart—the patient must be evaluated immediately for the presence of a pulse.

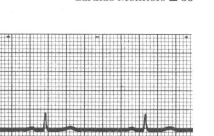

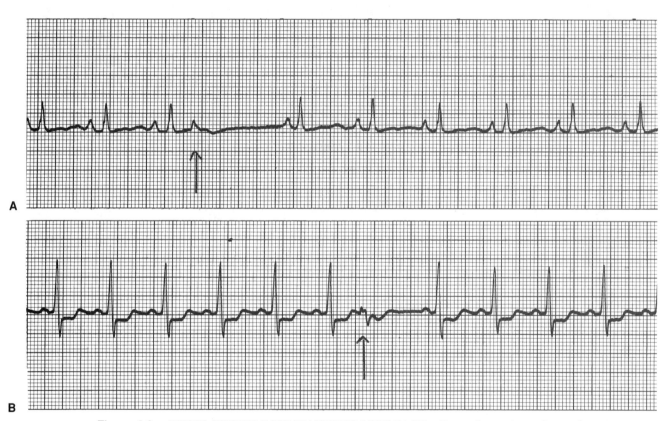

Figure 4-8. CONTINUOUS LOW WAVEFORM VOLTAGE—*Cause:* Low voltage QRS complexes. *Solution*: Turn up amplitude (gain) knob on monitor or change lead positions.

Figure 4-9. INTERMITTENT LOW WAVEFORM VOLTAGE—*Cause*: Intermittent low voltage QRS complexes are seen in both strips above. *Solution*: If problem is frequent and activates the low rate alarm, change lead positions.

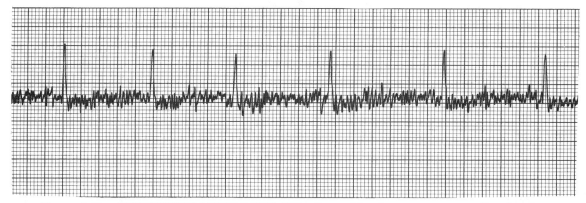

Figure 4-10. CONTINUOUS MUSCLE TREMOR—*Cause:* Muscle tremors are usually related to tense or nervous patients or those shivering from cold or a chill. *Solution:* Treat cause.

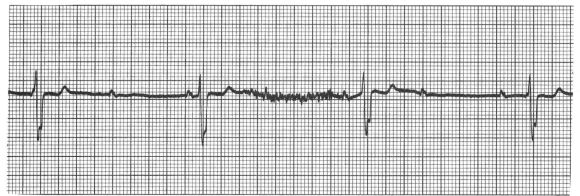

Figure 4-11. INTERMITTENT MUSCLE TREMOR—*Cause:* Muscle tremors that occur intermittently. *Solution:* Correction is usually not necessary.

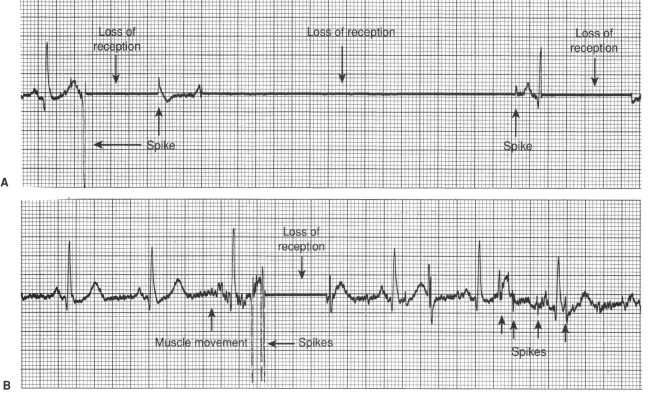

Figure 4-12. TELEMETRY-RELATED INTERFERENCE—*Cause:* ECG signals are poorly received over the telemetry system causing sharp spikes and sometimes loss of signal reception. This problem is usually related to weak batteries or the transmitter being used in the outer fringes of the reception area for the base station receiver. *Solution:* Change batteries; keep patient in reception area of base station receivers.

Figure 4-13. ELECTRICAL INTERFERENCE (AC Interference)—*Cause*: Patient using electrical equipment (electric razor, hair dryer); multiple electrical equipment in use in room; improperly grounded equipment; loose electrical connections or exposed wiring. *Solution:* If patient is using electrical equipment, problem is transient and will correct itself. If patient is not using electrical equipment a) unplug all equipment not in continuous use b) remove from service and report any equipment with breaks or wires showing c) ask the electrical engineer to check the wiring.

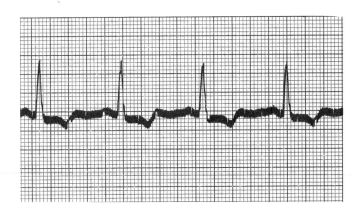

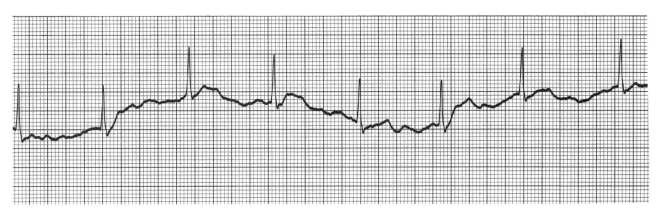

Figure 4-14. WANDERING BASELINE—*Cause:* Exaggerated respiratory movements usually seen in patients in respiratory distress (COPD patients). *Solution:* Avoid placing electrode pads in areas where movements of the accessory muscles are most exaggerated (which can be anywhere on the anterior chest wall). Place the pads on the upper back or top of the shoulders if necessary.

Analyzing a Rhythm Strip

Shortest R wave variation

Longest R wave variation

Measure between here

1st two R waves

R wave variations

Figure 5-1. Index card.

There are five basic steps to be followed in analyzing a rhythm strip. Each step should be followed in sequence. Eventually, this will become a habit and will enable you to identify a strip quickly and accurately.

STEP 1: DETERMINE THE REGULARITY (RHYTHM) OF THE R-WAVES

Starting at the left side of the rhythm strip, place an index card above the first two QRS complexes (Figure 5-1). Using a sharp pencil, mark on the index card the top of the two R-waves. Measure from R-wave to R-wave across the rhythm strip, marking on the index card any variation in R-wave regularity. If the rhythm varies by 0.12 seconds (3 squares) or more between the shortest and longest R-wave variation marked on the index card, the rhythm is irregular. If the rhythm does not vary, or varies by less than 0.12 seconds, the rhythm is considered regular.

Calipers may also be used, instead of an index card, to determine regularity of the rhythm strip. The R-wave regularity is assessed in the same manner as with the index card, by placing the two caliper points on top of two consecutive R-waves and proceeding left to right across the rhythm strip, noting any variation in the R-R regularity.

The author prefers the index card method, as each R-wave variation (however slight) can be marked and a specific measurement done to determine if a 0.12 second or greater variance exists between the shorter and longer R-wave variations. With calipers, a variation in the R-wave regularity may be noted, but without marking and measuring between the shortest and longest R-wave variations, there is no way to determine how irregular the rhythm is. Examples of rhythm measurements are shown in Figures 5-2 through 5-4.

STEP 2: CALCULATE THE HEART RATE

This measurement will always refer to the ventricular rate unless the atrial and ventricular rates differ, in which case both will be given. The ventricular rate is the number of QRS complexes in a 6-second rhythm strip. The top of the electrocardiogram paper is marked at 3-second intervals; two intervals equals 6 seconds (Figure 5-5). There are two ways to calculate heart rate. One is given to use with regular rhythms and one to use with irregular rhythms.

Regular Rhythms

Count the number of small squares between two R-waves (Figure 5-6) and refer to the conversion table (text continues on page 40)

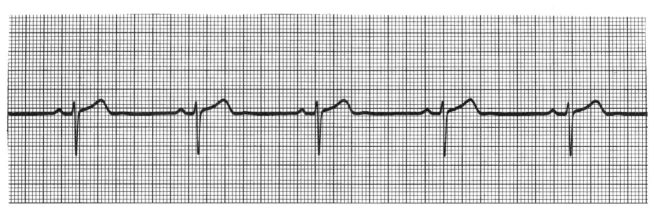

Figure 5-2. Regular rhythm; R-R intervals do not vary.

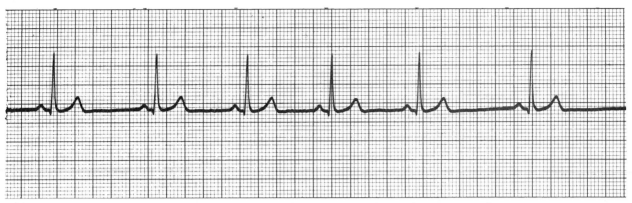

Figure 5-3. Irregular rhythm; R-R intervals vary by 0.32 seconds.

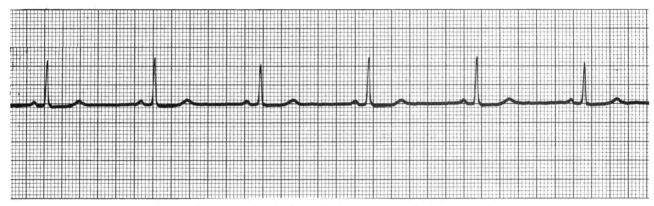

Figure 5-4. Regular rhythm; R-R intervals vary by 0.04 seconds.

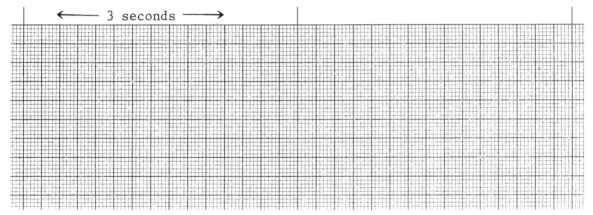

Figure 5-5. ECG graph paper.

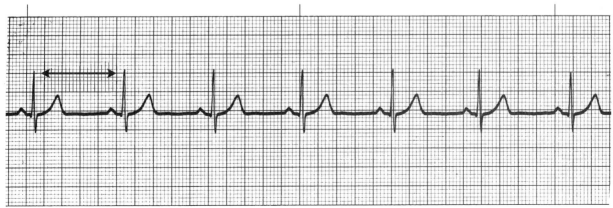

Figure 5-6. Regular rhythm; 25 small squares between R waves = 60 heart rate.

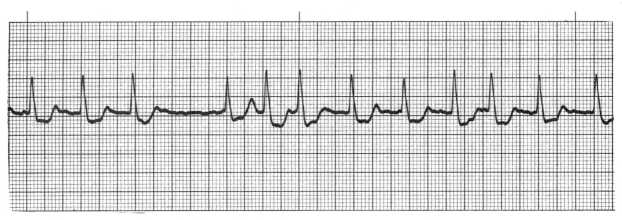

Figure 5-7. Irregular rhythm—11 R waves × 10 = 110 heart rate.

printed on the back inside cover. If a conversion table is not at hand, divide the number of small squares between two R-waves into 1500.

Irregular Rhythms

Count the number of R-waves in a 6-second strip and multiply by 10 (6 seconds × 10 = 60 seconds, or the heart rate per minute) (Figure 5-7), or count the number of R-waves in a 3-second strip and multiply by 20 (3 seconds × 20 = 60 seconds, or the heart rate per minute).

The following are other hints:

When rhythm strips have premature beats (Figure 5-8), the premature beats are not included in the calculation of the rate. Count the rate in the uninterrupted section—this is the underlying rhythm. In this example, the uninterrupted section is regular and the heart rate is 68 (22 squares between R-waves = 68).

When rhythm strips have more than one rhythm on a 6-second strip (Figure 5-9), rates must be calculated for each rhythm. This will aid in the identification of each rhythm. In the example, the first rhythm is irregular and the heart rate is 180 (9 R-waves in 3 seconds × 20 = 180). The second rhythm is regular and the heart rate is 214 (7 squares between R-waves = 214).

When a rhythm covers less than 3 seconds on a rhythm strip (Figure 5-10), rate calculation is diffcult but not impossible. In the example, the first rhythm takes up half of a 3-second interval. There are only two R-waves—therefore you can't determine if the rhythm is regular or irregular. In this situation, multiply the two R-waves by 40 (1.5 seconds × 40 = 60 seconds, or the heart rate per minute) to obtain an approximate heart rate of 80. The second rhythm is regular, with a heart rate of 167 (9 small squares between R-waves = 167).

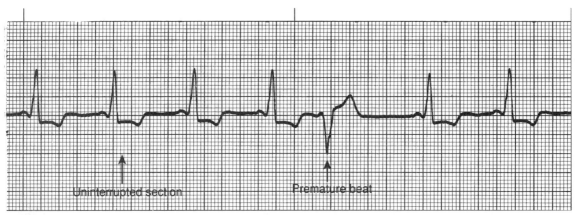

Figure 5-8. Rhythm with premature beat.

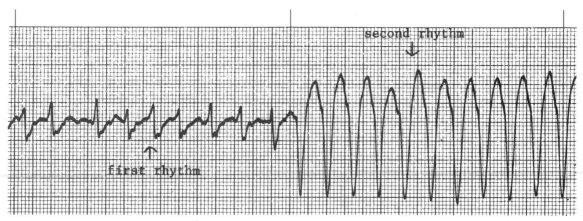

Figure 5-9. Rhythm strip with two different rhythms.

STEP 3: IDENTIFY AND EXAMINE P-WAVES

Analyze the P-waves—one P-wave should precede each QRS complex. All P-waves should be identical (or nearly identical) in size, shape, and position. In Figure 5-11 there is one P-wave to each QRS complex, and all P-waves are identical in size, shape, and position. In Figure 5-12 there is one P-wave to each QRS, but the P-waves vary in size, shape, and position.

STEP 4: MEASURE THE PR INTERVAL

Measure from the beginning of the P-wave as it leaves baseline to the beginning of the QRS complex. Count the number of squares contained in this interval and multiply by 0.04 seconds. In Figure 5-13 the PR interval is 0.16 seconds (4 squares × 0.04 seconds = 0.16 seconds).

STEP 5: MEASURE THE QRS COMPLEX

Measure from the beginning of the QRS as it leaves baseline until the end of the QRS when the ST segment begins. Count the number of squares in this measurement and multiply by 0.04 seconds. In Figure 5-14 the QRS takes up 3 squares and represents 0.12 seconds (3 squares × 0.04 seconds = 0.12 seconds). In Figure 5-15 the QRS takes up 2½ squares and represents 0.10 seconds (2½ squares × 0.04 seconds = 0.10 seconds).

If rhythm strips are analyzed using a systematic step-by-step approach, accurate interpretation will be achieved most of the time (Box 5-1).

Box 5-1. Summary: Rhythm Strip Analysis
1. Determine regularity (rhythm)
2. Calculate rate
3. Examine P-waves
4. Measure PR interval
5. Measure QRS complex

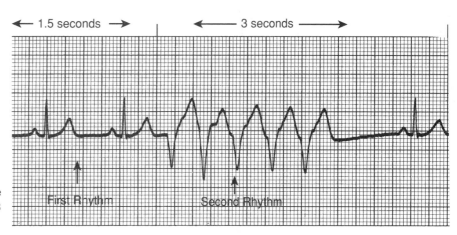

Figure 5-10. Calculating rate when a rhythm covers less than 3 seconds.

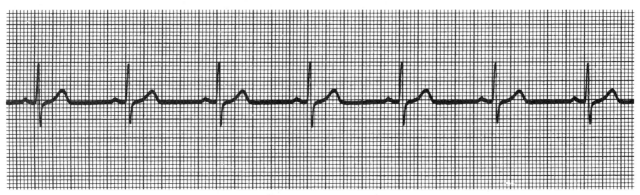

Figure 5-11. Normal P waves.

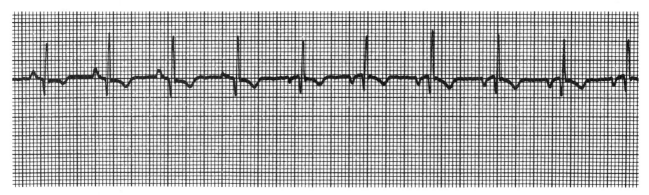

Figure 5-12. Abnormal P waves.

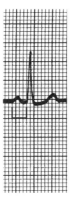

Figure 5-13. PR 0.16 seconds.

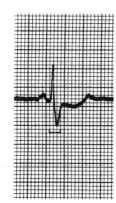

Figure 5-14. QRS 0.12 seconds.

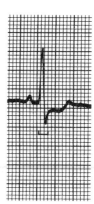

Figure 5-15. QRS 0.10 seconds.

Waveform Practice—
Analyzing Rhythm Strips

Directions: Analyze the following rhythm strips using the 5-step process discussed in this chapter. Check your answers with the answer keys in the appendix.

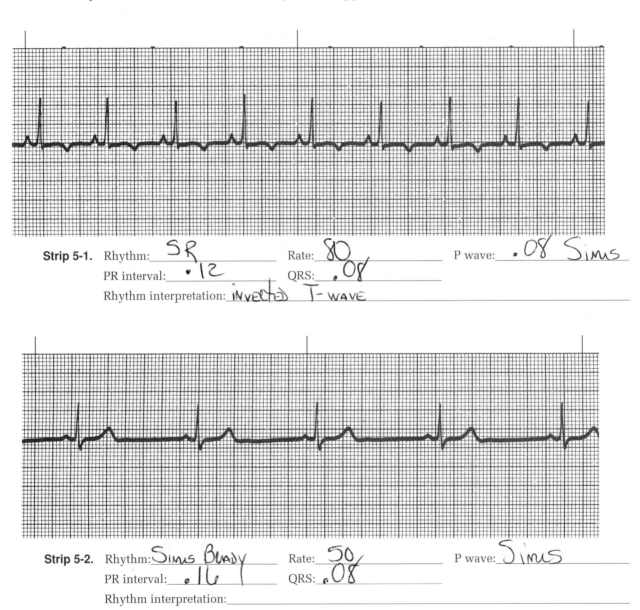

Strip 5-1. Rhythm: _SR_ Rate: _80_ P wave: _.08 Sinus_

PR interval: _.12_ QRS: _.08_

Rhythm interpretation: _INVECTED T-WAVE_

Strip 5-2. Rhythm: _Sinus Brady_ Rate: _50_ P wave: _Sinus_

PR interval: _.16_ QRS: _.08_

Rhythm interpretation: _____

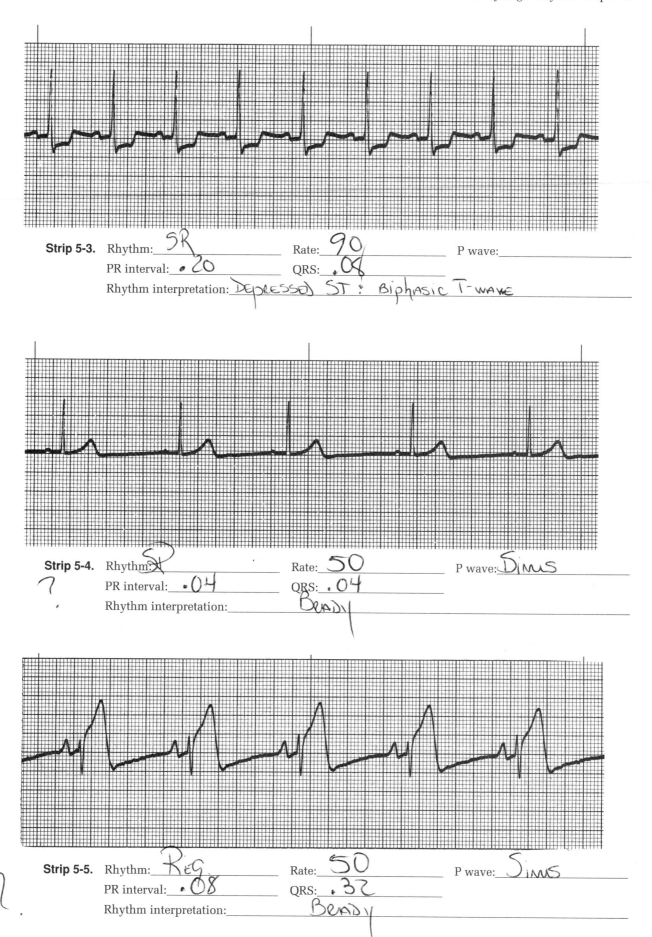

Strip 5-3. Rhythm: SR   Rate: 90   P wave: _____

PR interval: .20   QRS: .08

Rhythm interpretation: Depressed ST : Biphasic T-wave

Strip 5-4. Rhythm: SR   Rate: 50   P wave: Sinus

PR interval: .04   QRS: .04

Rhythm interpretation: Brady

Strip 5-5. Rhythm: Reg   Rate: 50   P wave: Sinus

PR interval: .08   QRS: .32

Rhythm interpretation: Brady

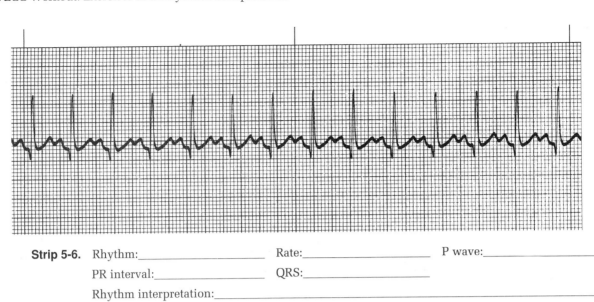

Strip 5-6. Rhythm:_____ Rate:_____ P wave:_____

PR interval:_____ QRS:_____

Rhythm interpretation:_____

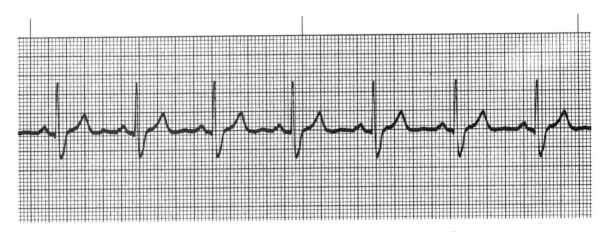
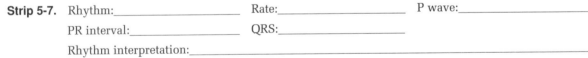

Strip 5-7. Rhythm:_____ Rate:_____ P wave:_____

PR interval:_____ QRS:_____

Rhythm interpretation:_____

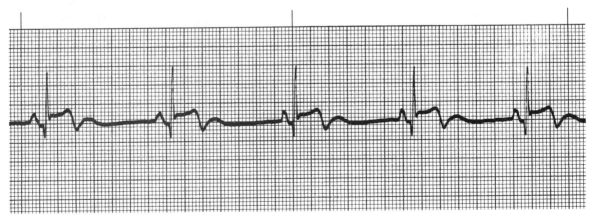

Strip 5-8. Rhythm:_____ Rate:_____ P wave:_____

PR interval:_____ QRS:_____

Rhythm interpretation:_____

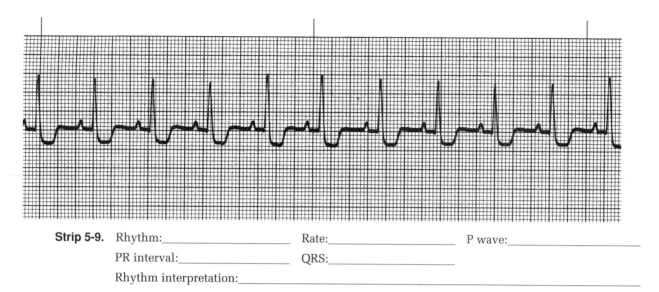

Strip 5-9. Rhythm:_____ Rate:_____ P wave:_____

PR interval:_____ QRS:_____

Rhythm interpretation:_____

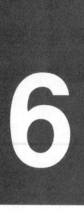

Sinus Arrhythmias

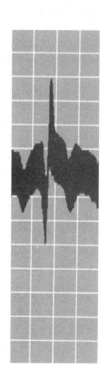

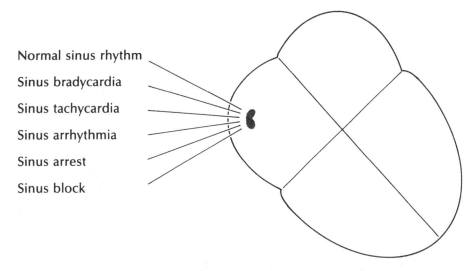

Normal sinus rhythm
Sinus bradycardia
Sinus tachycardia
Sinus arrhythmia
Sinus arrest
Sinus block

Figure 6-1. Sinus arrhythmias.

The term arrhythmia (also known as dysrhythmia) refers to any heart rhythm other than the normal rhythm of the heart (normal sinus rhythm). Sinus arrhythmias (Figure 6-1) result from disturbances in impulse discharge or impulse conduction from the sinus node. The sinus node retains its role as pacemaker of the heart but discharges impulses too fast (sinus tachycardia) or too slow (sinus bradycardia); discharges impulses irregularly (sinus arrhythmia); fails to discharge an impulse (sinus arrest); or the impulses discharged are blocked as they exit the SA node (sinus exit block), thus preventing conduction to the atria. Impulse formation is under the control of the sympathetic and parasympathetic nervous systems. The sympathetic nervous system is responsible for speeding up the heart rate, whereas the parasympathetic nervous system (chiefly the vagus nerve) produces a slowing of the heart rate. Normally these

systems are balanced, maintaining a heart rate between 60–100 times a minute.

Sinus bradycardia, sinus tachycardia, sinus arrhythmia, sinus arrest, and sinus block are all considered arrhythmias. However, sinus bradycardia at rest, sinus tachycardia with exercise, and respiratory sinus arrhythmia are all normal findings.

NORMAL SINUS RHYTHM

In a normal sinus rhythm (Figure 6-2) (Box 6-1), the electrical impulses are formed in the sinoatrial (SA) node and discharged regularly at a rate of 60–100 times per minute. The P-waves are normal in configuration and direction, and precede each QRS complex. The PR interval and QRS duration are within normal limits. Normal sinus rhythm (NSR) is

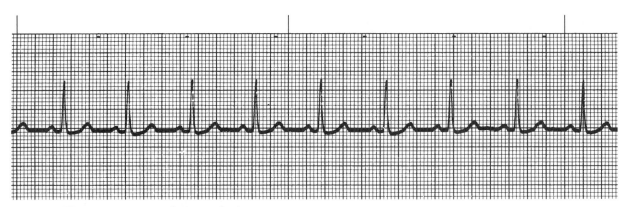

Figure 6-2. **Normal Sinus Rhythm**

Rhythm:	Regular
Rate:	84
P waves:	Normal and precede each QRS
PR:	0.14 to 0.16 seconds
QRS:	0.06 to 0.08 seconds

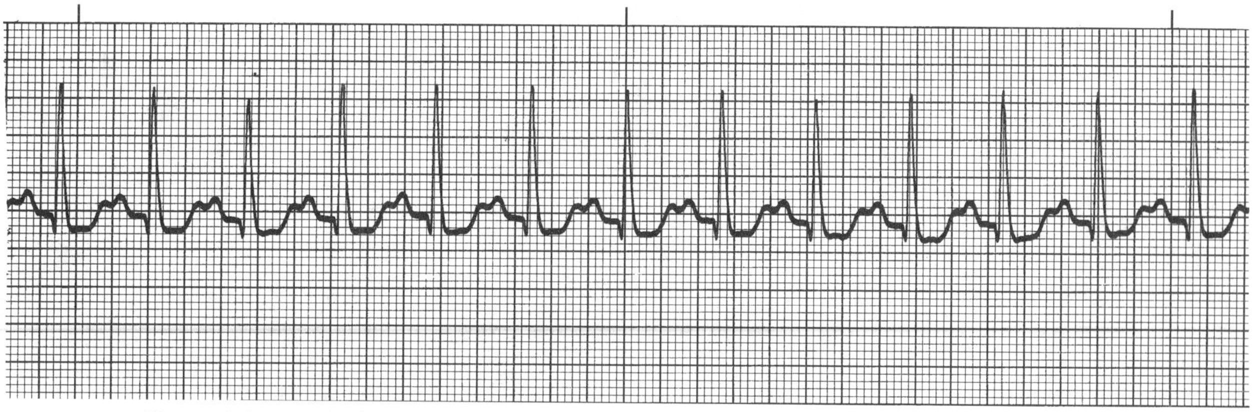

Figure 6-3. Sinus Tachycardia

Rhythm:	Regular
Rate:	115
P waves:	Sinus
PR:	0.16 to 0.18 seconds
QRS:	0.08 to 0.10 seconds

Box 6-1. Normal Sinus Rhythm: Identifying ECG Features

Rhythm:	Regular
Rate:	60–100
P-waves:	Normal in configuration and direction; one P-wave precedes each QRS complex
PR:	Normal (0.12–0.20 seconds)
QRS:	Normal (0.10 seconds or less)

the normal rhythm of the heart and is of no clinical significance. No treatment is indicated.

SINUS TACHYCARDIA

Sinus tachycardia (Figure 6-3) (Box 6-2) originates in the SA node and discharges impulses regularly at a rate between 100–160 times per minute. The P-waves are normal in configuration and direction, and precede each QRS complex. The PR and QRS duration is within normal limits. The distinguishing feature of this rhythm is the sinus origin and the rate between 100–160.

Sinus tachycardia is a normal response of the heart to the body's demand for an increase in blood flow (e.g., exercise). The sinus node increases its rate in response to the needs of the body. When these needs no longer exist, the heart rate slows down. Sinus tachycardia begins and ends gradually in contrast to other tachycardias, which begin and end abruptly.

Sinus tachycardia can be caused by any condition that produces an increase in sympathetic tone or a decrease in parasympathetic (vagal) tone. Conditions commonly associated with sinus tachycardia include: exercise, fever, anxiety, pain, anemia, hypoxia, hypovolemia, hypotension, heart failure, shock, pulmonary embolism, myocardial ischemia, alcohol intoxication or withdrawal, ingestion of caffeine, smoking, drugs that increase sympathetic tone (epinephrine, dopamine, tricyclic antidepressants, cocaine), and drugs that cause a decrease in vagal tone (atropine).

A rapid heart rate increases myocardial oxygen demands, thus increasing the heart's workload. In the setting of acute myocardial infarction this could lead to an increase in myocardial ischemia, angina, or an extension in infarct size. In addition, shortened diastolic filling time can result in reduced stroke volume and may lead to heart failure.

Sinus tachycardia in healthy individuals is more likely to be caused by exercise, fever, anxiety, pain, and so forth, and does not require treatment. How-

Box 6-2. Sinus Tachycardia: Identifying ECG Features

Rhythm:	Regular
Rate:	100–160
P-waves:	Normal in configuration and direction; one P-wave precedes each QRS complex
PR:	Normal (0.12–0.20 seconds)
QRS:	Normal (0.10 seconds or less)

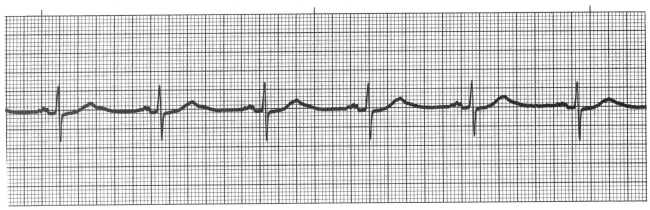

Figure 6-4. Sinus Bradycardia

Rhythm:	Regular
Rate:	54
P waves:	Sinus
PR:	0.20 seconds
QRS:	0.06 to 0.08 seconds
Note:	A notched P wave is usually indicative of left atrial hypertrophy

ever, in unhealthy individuals the development of sinus tachycardia signifies that a need exists for increased oxygen requirements and serves as a significant warning sign. Sinus tachycardia is often the earliest sign of left ventricular failure, shock, or infarct extension. Treatment of sinus tachycardia must be directed, not at the rapid heart rate itself, but at the underlying cause.

SINUS BRADYCARDIA

Sinus bradycardia (Figure 6-4) (Box 6-3) originates in the SA node and discharges impulses regularly at a rate between 40–60 times per minute. The P-waves are normal in configuration and direction, and precede each QRS complex. The PR and QRS duration is within normal limits. The distinguishing feature of this rhythm is the sinus origin and a rate between 40–60.

Sinus bradycardia occurs normally in trained athletes and during sleep. During sleep, enhanced vagal activity can result in sinus rates of less than 40 beats per minute, and this is considered normal. Sinus bradycardia is commonly seen in acute inferior myocardial infarction involving the right coronary artery, which supplies blood to the SA node. It has also been noted as a "reperfusion rhythm" during and/or following treatment with thrombolytic agents (TPA and streptokinase). In general, sinus bradycardia can be caused by any condition that produces an increase in parasympathetic (vagal) tone and a decrease in sympathetic tone.

Conditions commonly associated with sinus bradycardia include: fright, carotid sinus massage, carotid sinus hypersensitivity syndrome, sleep apnea syndrome, hypothermia, hypothyroidism, vomiting, straining (Valsalva maneuver), ocular pressure, increased intracranial pressure, and sudden movement from a recumbent to an upright position. Drugs that may cause sinus bradycardia include beta blockers, calcium-channel blockers, digitalis, and morphine. Vasovagal reactions (a sudden increase in vagal tone accompanied by vascular dilation) are commonly seen with vomiting or pain and are often precipitated by sudden stressful situations. These reactions may result in marked bradycardia (heart rates <40/min) and hypotension, leading to a decrease in cardiac output which may cause dizziness, lightheadedness, or fainting (vasovagal syncope). Vasovagal reactions are usually transient and require no treatment once the cause (e.g. pain, vomiting) has been removed.

Treatment of sinus bradycardia is usually not necessary unless the patient becomes symptomatic

Box 6-3.	**Sinus Bradycardia: Identifying ECG Features**
Rhythm:	Regular
Rate:	40–60
P-waves:	Normal in configuration and direction; one P-wave precedes each QRS complex
PR:	Normal (0.12–0.20 seconds)
QRS:	Normal (0.10 seconds or less)

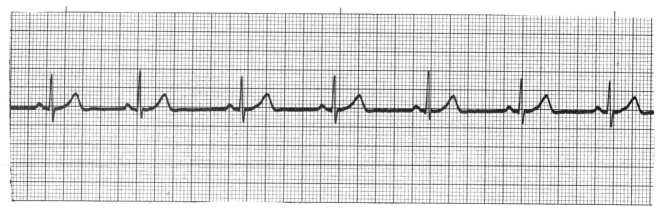

Figure 6-5. **Sinus Arrhythmia**

Rhythm:	Irregular
Rate:	60
P waves:	Normal in configuration; precede each QRS
PR:	0.12 to 0.14 seconds
QRS:	0.06 to 0.08 seconds

(e.g., develops hypotension, heart failure, anginal pain, syncope, or mental status changes). A simple maneuver such as asking the patient to cough, which decreases vagal tone, might be tried initially in an attempt to increase the heart rate. If sinus bradycardia is persistent and produces symptoms the treatment of choice is atropine, a parasympatholytic drug which prevents the vagus nerve from slowing the heart rate. The usual dose is 0.5mg IV push every 5 minutes until the bradycardia is resolved or a maximum dose of 0.04 mg/kg (usually between 2–3 mg) is given. Atropine must be administered correctly—atropine administered too slowly or in doses less than 0.5 mg exert a sympatholytic effect and can further decrease the heart rate. Atropine should be given cautiously, particularly in acute myocardial infarction, because oxygen demands caused by the increase in heart rate could extend the infarction. If the arrhythmia still does not resolve following the administration of atropine, a transcutaneous (external) or transvenous pacemaker may be needed. All medications that cause a decrease in heart rate should be reviewed and discontinued if indicated. For chronic bradycardia, permanent pacing may be indicated.

SINUS ARRHYTHMIA

Sinus arrhythmia (Figure 6-5) (Box 6-4) originates in the sinus node and discharges impulses irregularly. The heart rate may be normal (60–100), but is often associated with sinus bradycardia. The P-waves are normal in configuration and direction, and precede each QRS. The PR and QRS duration are

Box 6-4. **Sinus Arrhythmia: Identifying ECG Features**

Rhythm:	Irregular
Rate:	Normal (60–100) or slow (less than 60)
P-waves:	Normal in configuration and direction; one P-wave precedes each QRS complex
PR:	Normal (0.12–0.20 seconds)
QRS:	Normal (0.10 seconds or less)

within normal limits. The distinguishing feature of this rhythm is the sinus origin and the rhythm irregularity.

Sinus arrhythmia is a normal variation in sinus rhythm, most commonly caused by the respiratory cycle. With inspiration the heart rate increases slightly, and with expiration it decreases slightly due to changes in vagal tone occurring during the different phases of respiration. Respiratory sinus arrhythmia is most pronounced in children and young adults. Nonrespiratory sinus arrhythmia (sinus arrhythmia not associated with respiration) occurs rarely and has been observed in patients with heart disease.

Sinus arrhythmia is of no clinical significance and does not require treatment.

SINUS ARREST AND SINUS EXIT BLOCK

Sinus arrest and sinus exit block (two separate arrhythmias with different pathophysiologies) (Fig-

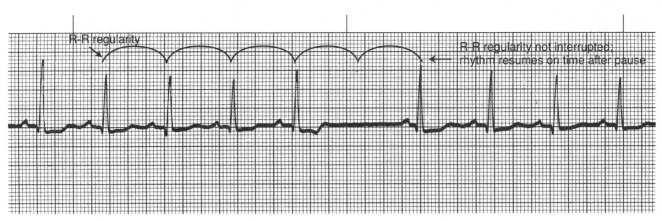

Figure 6-6. **Normal Sinus Rhythm with Sinus Block**

Rhythm: Basic rhythm regular, irregular during pause

Rate: Basic rhythm 84

P waves: Normal in basic rhythm, absent during pause

PR: 0.16 to 0.18 seconds in basic rhythm, absent during pause

QRS: 0.08 to 0.10 seconds in basic rhythm, absent during pause

Comment: ST segment depression is present

ures 6-6 and 6-7) (Box 6-5) are discussed together here because distinguishing between them is at times difficult, and because their treatment and clinical significance are the same. Both sinus arrest and SA exit block originate in the sinus node and are characterized by a pause in the sinus rhythm in which one or more beats (cardiac cycles) is missing. The P-waves in the underlying rhythm will be normal in configuration and direction, with one P-wave preceding each QRS complex. The PR and QRS duration in the underlying rhythm is within normal limits. The distinguishing feature of both rhythms is the abrupt pause in the underlying sinus rhythm in which one or more P-QRS-T sequences is missing, followed by a resumption of the basic rhythm following the pause.

Sinus arrest is caused by a failure of the SA node to discharge an impulse. This failure in the automaticity of the SA node upsets the timing of the sinus node discharge, and the underlying rhythm will not resume on time following the pause. Therefore, the length of the pause will not be a multiple of the underlying P-P (or R-R) interval. With sinus exit block, an electrical impulse is generated by the SA node but is blocked as it exits the sinus node, preventing conduction of the impulse to the atria. Because the regularity of the sinus node discharge is not interrupted (just blocked), the underlying rhythm will resume on time following the pause and the length of the pause will be a multiple of the underlying P-P (or R-R) interval.

Differentiating between the two rhythms involves comparing the length of the pause with the underlying P-P (or R-R) interval to determine if the underlying rhythm resumes on time following the pause. This is only useful if the underlying rhythm is regular. If the underlying rhythm is irregular, as in sinus arrhythmia (Figure 6-8), it is impossible to distinguish SA arrest from SA block on the surface electrocardiogram. In this case the rhythm would best be

---

Box 6-5. **Sinus Arrest and Sinus Exit Block: Identifying ECG Features**

Rhythm: Underlying rhythm usually regular; irregular during pause

Rate: Underlying rhythm may be normal (60–100) or slow (less than 60)

P-waves: Sinus P-waves present with underlying rhythm; P-waves absent during pause

PR: Normal duration (0.12–0.20 seconds) with underlying rhythm; PR absent during pause

QRS: Normal (0.10 seconds or less) with underlying rhythm; QRS absent during pause

Differentiating Features

Sinus block: Underlying rhythm resumes on time following the pause, with the length of the pause being a multiple of the underlying P-P (or R-R) interval

Sinus arrest: Underlying rhythm does not resume on time following the pause; the length of the pause is not a multiple of the underlying P-P (or R-R) interval

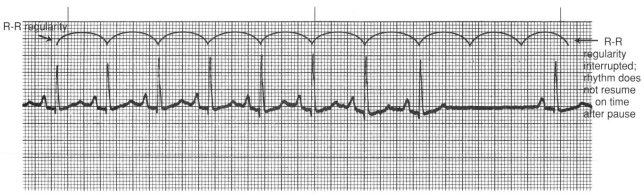

Figure 6-7. **Normal Sinus Rhythm with Sinus Arrest**

Rhythm: Basic rhythm regular, irregular during pause

Rate: Basic rhythm 94

P waves: Normal in basic rhythm, absent during pause

PR: 0.16 to 0.18 seconds in basic rhythm, absent during pause

QRS: 0.06 to 0.08 seconds in basic rhythm, absent during pause

interpreted as sinus arrest/block, indicating that either rhythm could be present.

Sinus arrest or sinus exit block may be caused by an increase in vagal tone, damage to the SA node, hypoxia, hyperkalemia, or by drugs such as digitalis, the beta-blockers, or the calcium-channel blockers. The pauses may be short and produce no symptoms, or long and produce symptoms of hypotension, dizziness, or syncope. If the pause is long enough, es-

cape beats or rhythms from the AV node and ventricles may appear. As in sinus bradycardia, asking the patient to cough might cause a decrease in vagal tone and result in sinus node recovery. If sinus arrest or sinus exit block produce symptoms, the arrhythmias are treated the same as in symptomatic sinus bradycardia. In addition, all medications that depress sinus node discharge or conduction should be stopped.

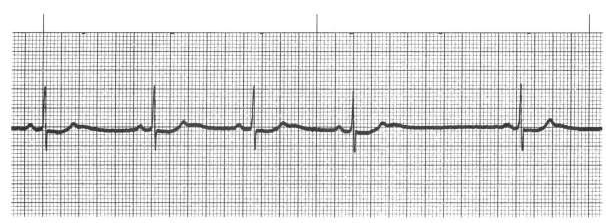

Figure 6-8. **Sinus Arrhythmia with Sinus Arrest/Block**

Rhythm: Basic rhythm irregular

Rate: Basic rhythm 60

P waves: Normal in basic rhythm, absent during pause

PR: 0.16 to 0.18 seconds in basic rhythm, absent during pause

QRS: 0.06 seconds in basic rhythm, absent during pause

Comment: Due to the irregularity of the basic rhythm, sinus arrest cannot be differentiated from sinus block, and the rhythm is interpreted as sinus arrest/block

Comment: ST segment depression and a U wave are present.

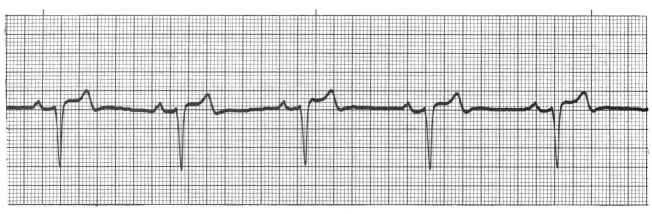

Strip 6-1. Rhythm:_____ Rate:_____ P wave:_____

PR interval:_____ QRS:_____

Rhythm interpretation:_____

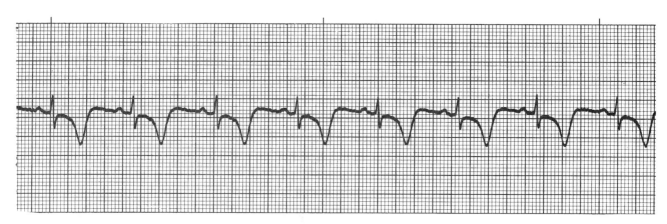

Strip 6-2. Rhythm:_____ Rate:_____ P wave:_____

PR interval:_____ QRS:_____

Rhythm interpretation:_____

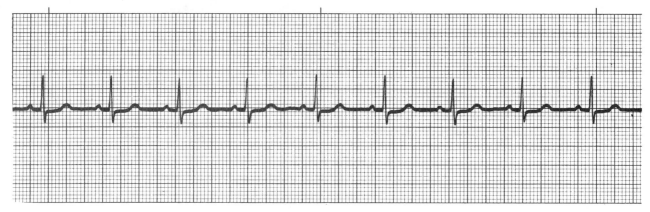

Strip 6-3. Rhythm:_____ Rate:_____ P wave:_____

PR interval:_____ QRS:_____

Rhythm interpretation:_____

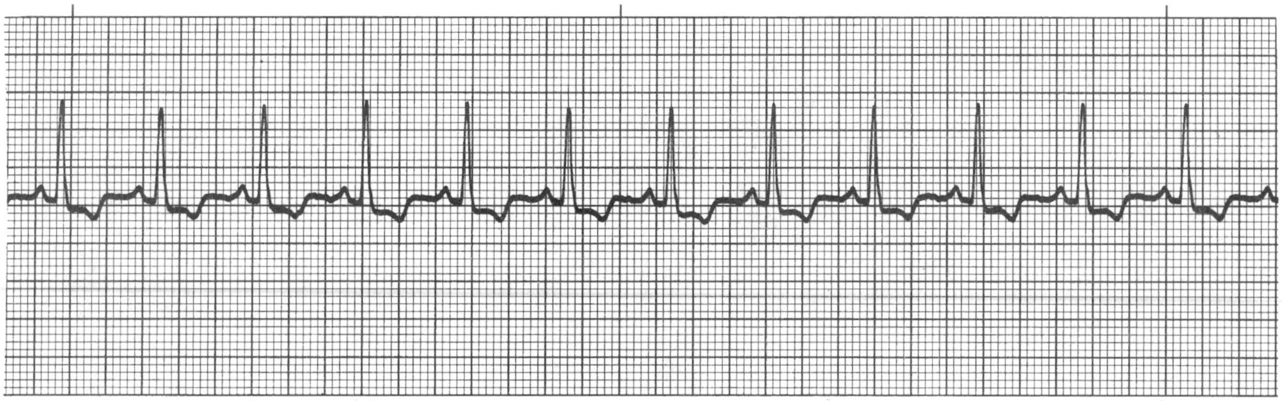

Strip 6-4. Rhythm:_____ Rate:_____ P wave:_____

PR interval:_____ QRS:_____

Rhythm interpretation:_____

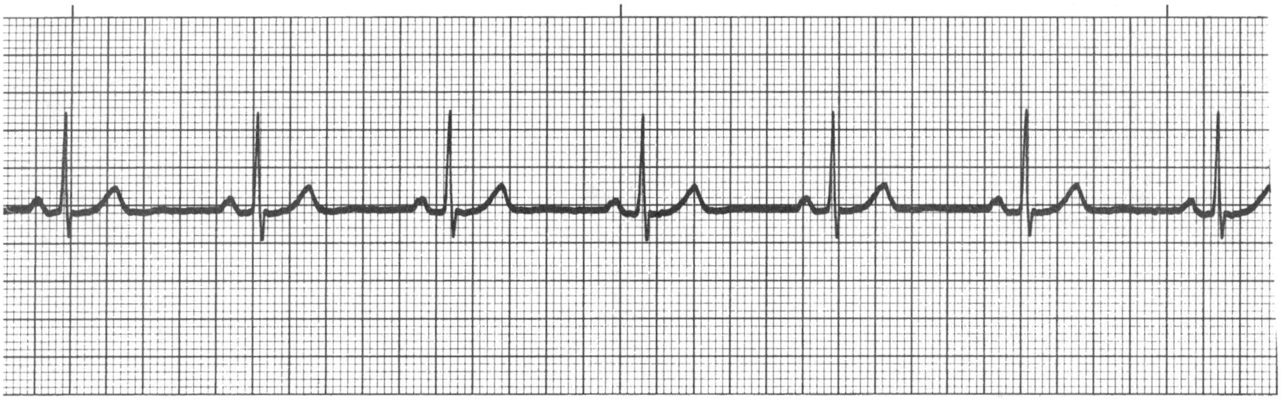

Strip 6-5. Rhythm:_____ Rate:_____ P wave:_____

PR interval:_____ QRS:_____

Rhythm interpretation:_____

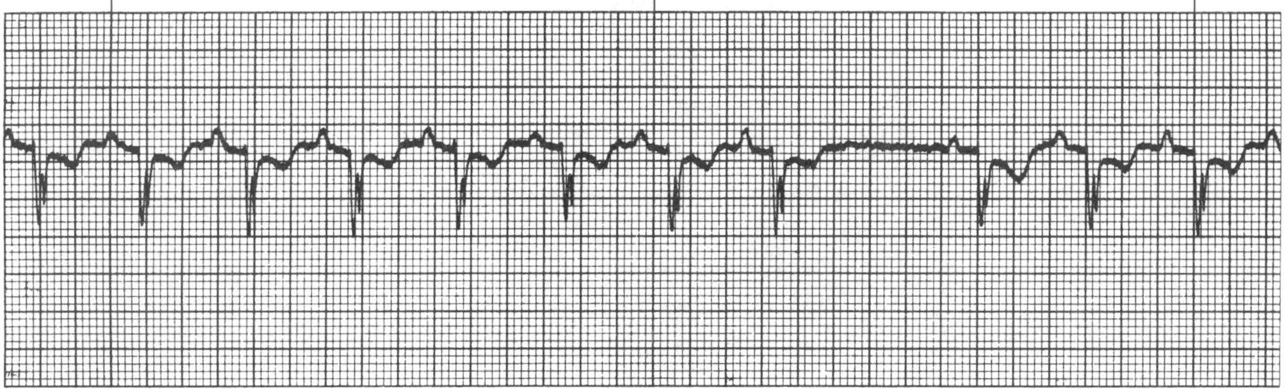

Strip 6-6. Rhythm:_____ Rate:_____ P wave:_____

PR interval:_____ QRS:_____

Rhythm interpretation:_____

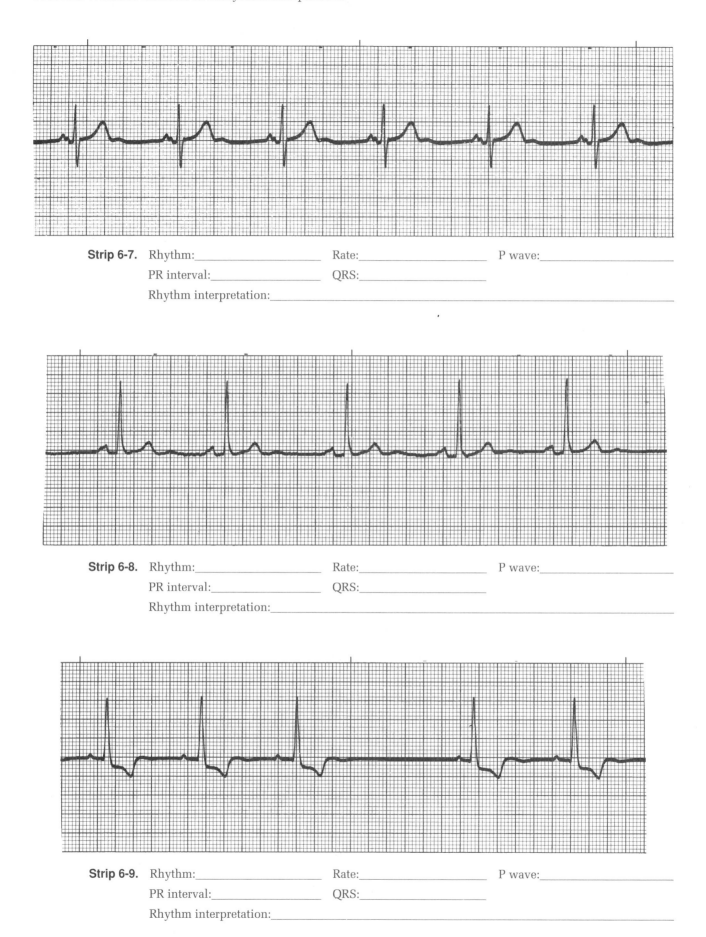

Strip 6-7. Rhythm:_____ Rate:_____ P wave:_____

PR interval:_____ QRS:_____

Rhythm interpretation:_____

Strip 6-8. Rhythm:_____ Rate:_____ P wave:_____

PR interval:_____ QRS:_____

Rhythm interpretation:_____

Strip 6-9. Rhythm:_____ Rate:_____ P wave:_____

PR interval:_____ QRS:_____

Rhythm interpretation:_____

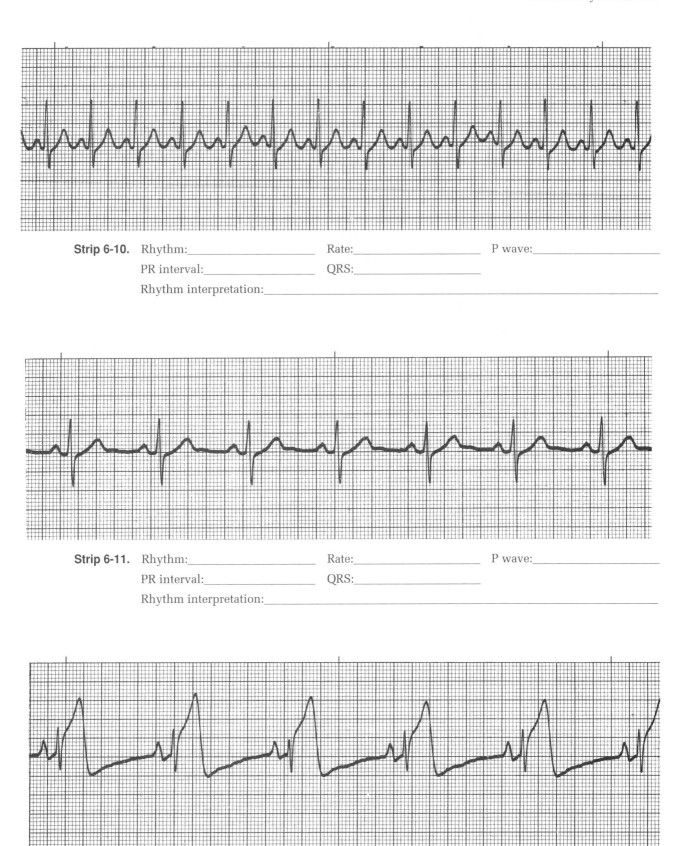

Strip 6-10. Rhythm:_____ Rate:_____ P wave:_____

PR interval:_____ QRS:_____

Rhythm interpretation:_____

Strip 6-11. Rhythm:_____ Rate:_____ P wave:_____

PR interval:_____ QRS:_____

Rhythm interpretation:_____

Strip 6-12. Rhythm:_____ Rate:_____ P wave:_____

PR interval:_____ QRS:_____

Rhythm interpretation:_____

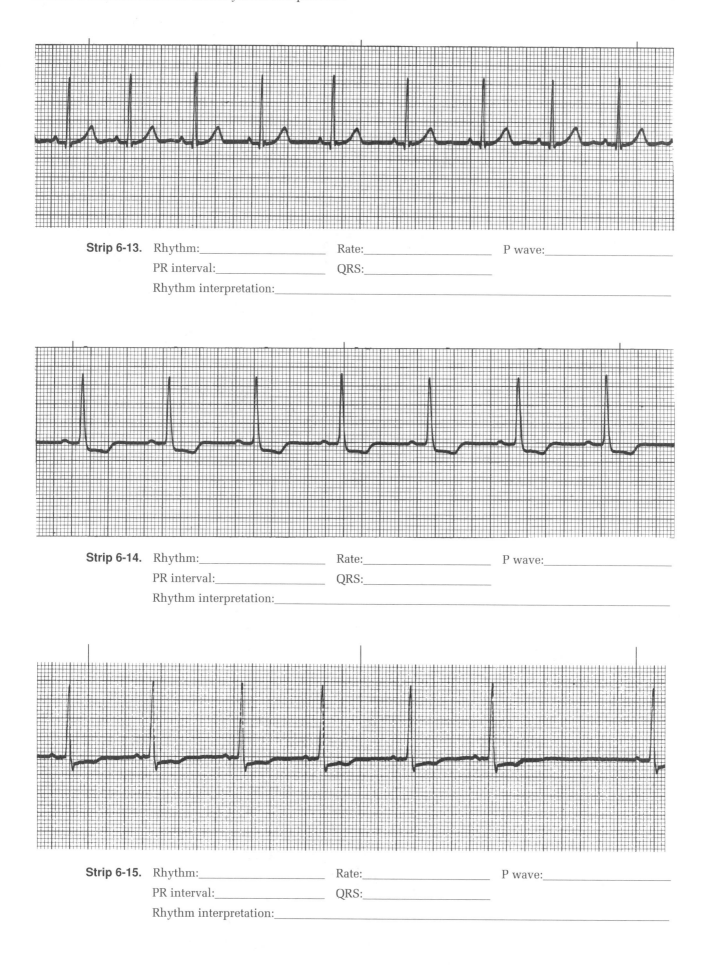

Strip 6-13. Rhythm:_____ Rate:_____ P wave:_____

PR interval:_____ QRS:_____

Rhythm interpretation:_____

Strip 6-14. Rhythm:_____ Rate:_____ P wave:_____

PR interval:_____ QRS:_____

Rhythm interpretation:_____

Strip 6-15. Rhythm:_____ Rate:_____ P wave:_____

PR interval:_____ QRS:_____

Rhythm interpretation:_____

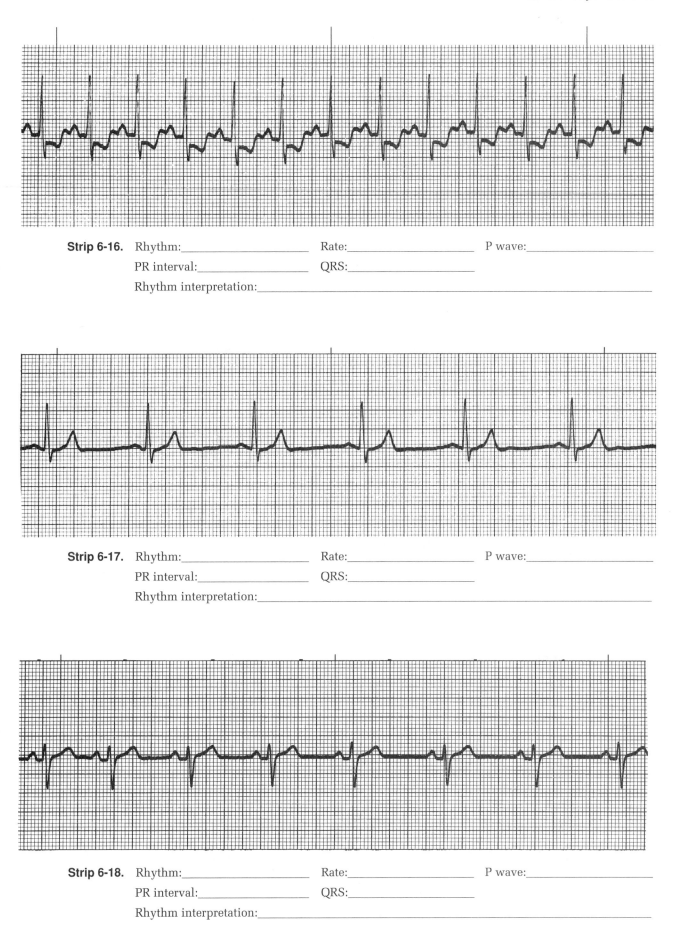

Strip 6-16. Rhythm:_____ Rate:_____ P wave:_____

PR interval:_____ QRS:_____

Rhythm interpretation:_____

Strip 6-17. Rhythm:_____ Rate:_____ P wave:_____

PR interval:_____ QRS:_____

Rhythm interpretation:_____

Strip 6-18. Rhythm:_____ Rate:_____ P wave:_____

PR interval:_____ QRS:_____

Rhythm interpretation:_____

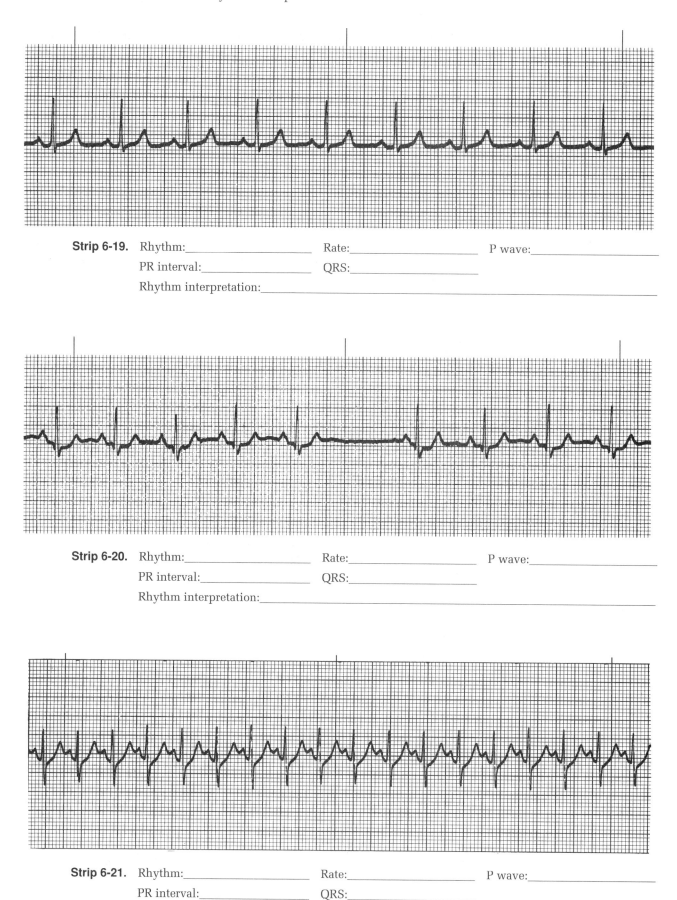

Strip 6-19. Rhythm:_____ Rate:_____ P wave:_____

PR interval:_____ QRS:_____

Rhythm interpretation:_____

Strip 6-20. Rhythm:_____ Rate:_____ P wave:_____

PR interval:_____ QRS:_____

Rhythm interpretation:_____

Strip 6-21. Rhythm:_____ Rate:_____ P wave:_____

PR interval:_____ QRS:_____

Rhythm interpretation:_____

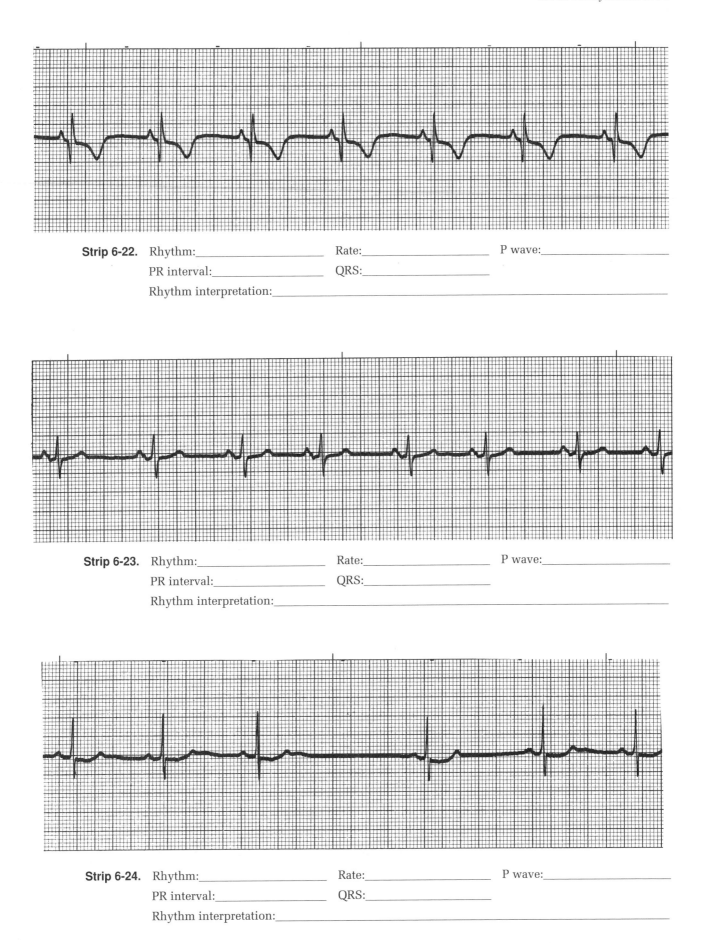

Strip 6-22. Rhythm:_____ Rate:_____ P wave:_____

PR interval:_____ QRS:_____

Rhythm interpretation:_____

Strip 6-23. Rhythm:_____ Rate:_____ P wave:_____

PR interval:_____ QRS:_____

Rhythm interpretation:_____

Strip 6-24. Rhythm:_____ Rate:_____ P wave:_____

PR interval:_____ QRS:_____

Rhythm interpretation:_____

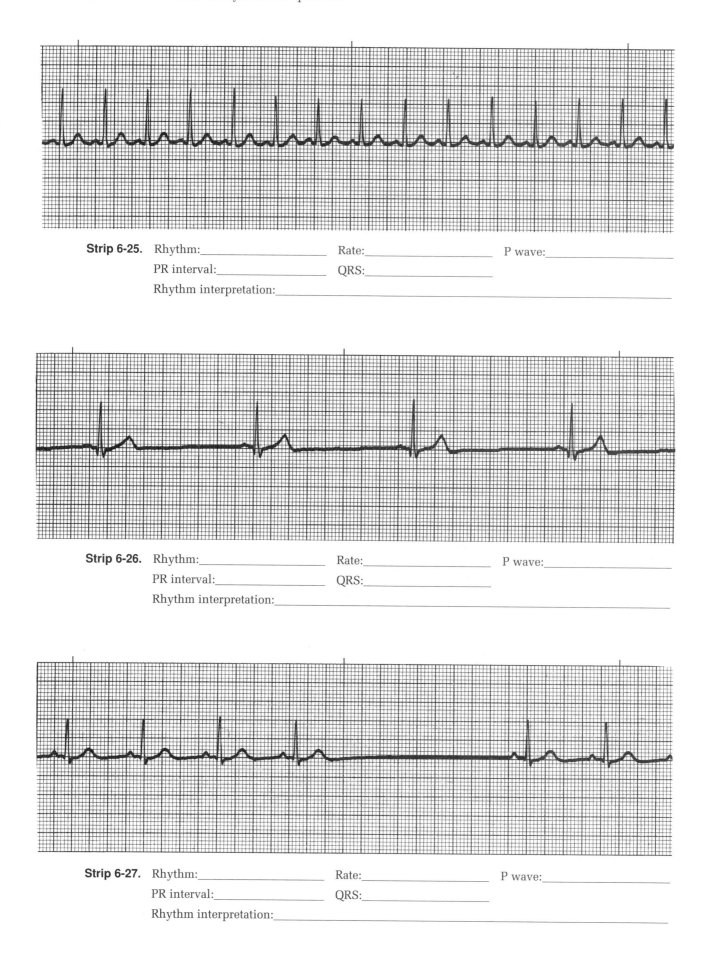

Strip 6-25. Rhythm:_____ Rate:_____ P wave:_____

PR interval:_____ QRS:_____

Rhythm interpretation:_____

Strip 6-26. Rhythm:_____ Rate:_____ P wave:_____

PR interval:_____ QRS:_____

Rhythm interpretation:_____

Strip 6-27. Rhythm:_____ Rate:_____ P wave:_____

PR interval:_____ QRS:_____

Rhythm interpretation:_____

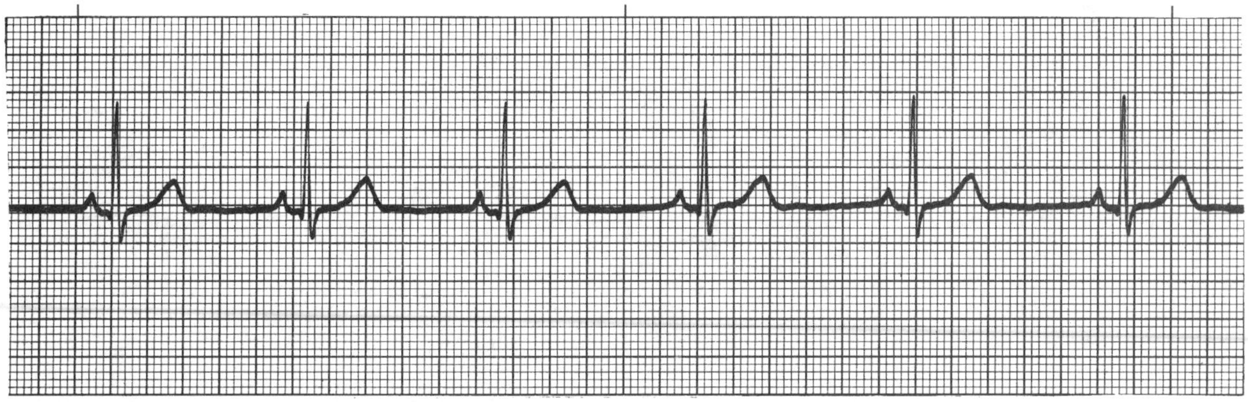

Strip 6-28. Rhythm:_____ Rate:_____ P wave:_____

PR interval:_____ QRS:_____

Rhythm interpretation:_____

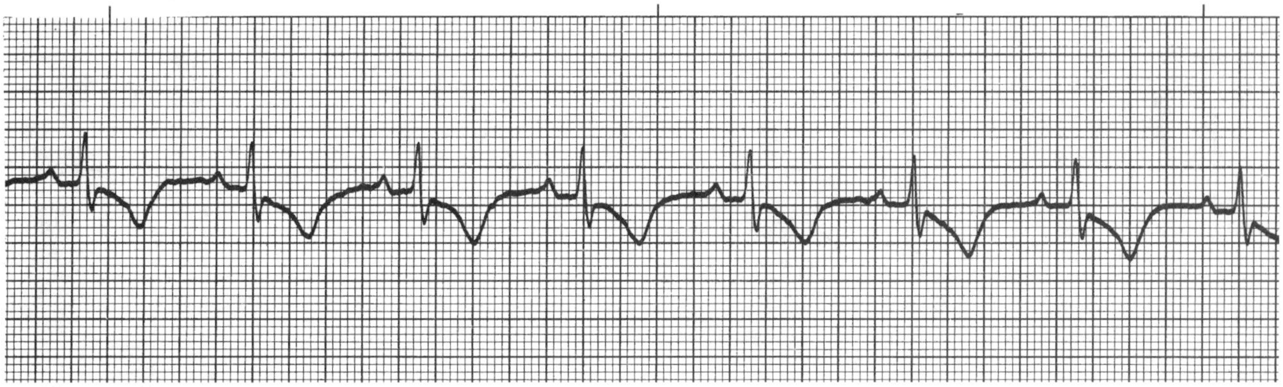

Strip 6-29. Rhythm:_____ Rate:_____ P wave:_____

PR interval:_____ QRS:_____

Rhythm interpretation:_____

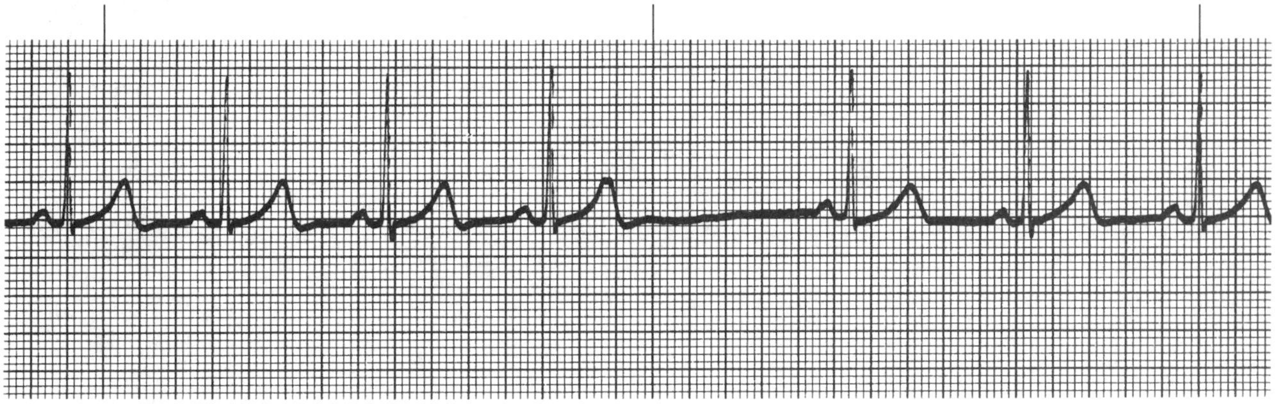

Strip 6-30. Rhythm:_____ Rate:_____ P wave:_____

PR interval:_____ QRS:_____

Rhythm interpretation:_____

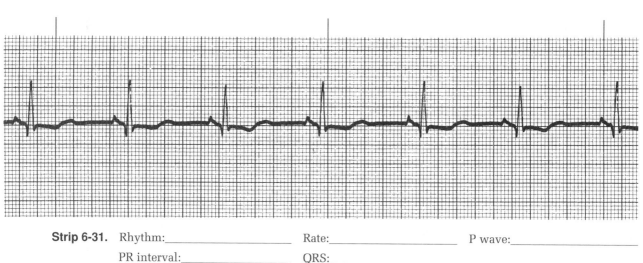

Strip 6-31. Rhythm:_____ Rate:_____ P wave:_____

PR interval:_____ QRS:_____

Rhythm interpretation:_____

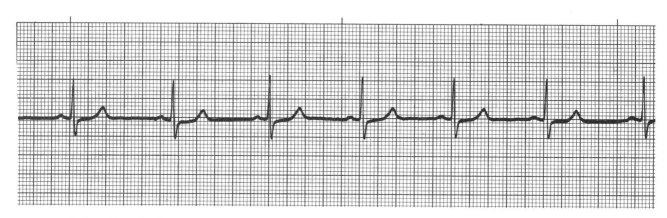

Strip 6-32. Rhythm:_____ Rate:_____ P wave:_____

PR interval:_____ QRS:_____

Rhythm interpretation:_____

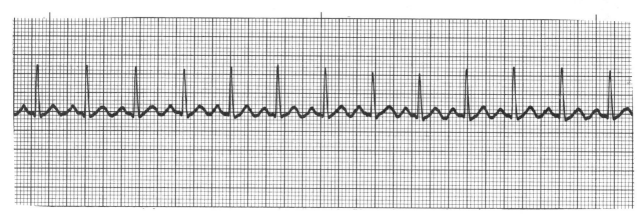

Strip 6-33. Rhythm:_____ Rate:_____ P wave:_____

PR interval:_____ QRS:_____

Rhythm arterpretation:_____

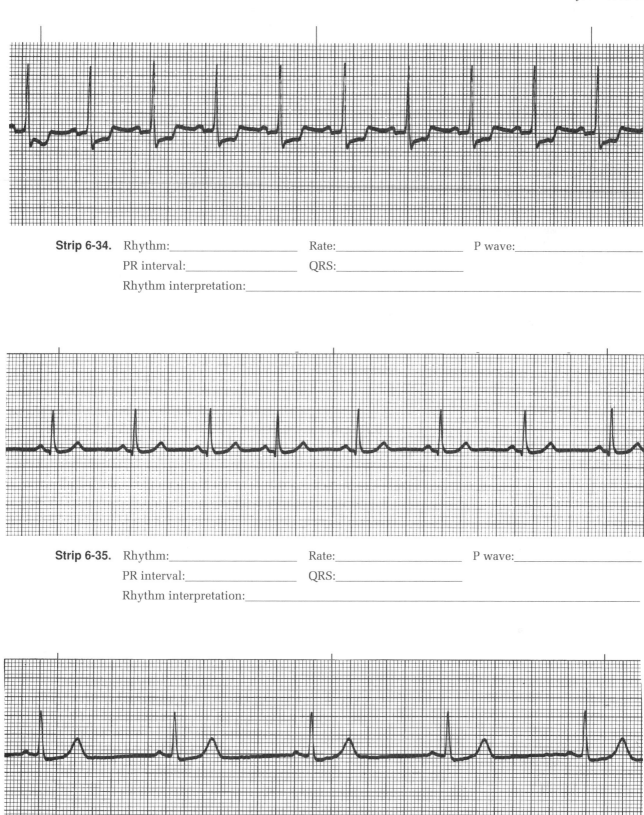

Strip 6-34. Rhythm:_____ Rate:_____ P wave:_____

PR interval:_____ QRS:_____

Rhythm interpretation:_____

Strip 6-35. Rhythm:_____ Rate:_____ P wave:_____

PR interval:_____ QRS:_____

Rhythm interpretation:_____

Strip 6-36. Rhythm:_____ Rate:_____ P wave:_____

PR interval:_____ QRS:_____

Rhythm interpretation:_____

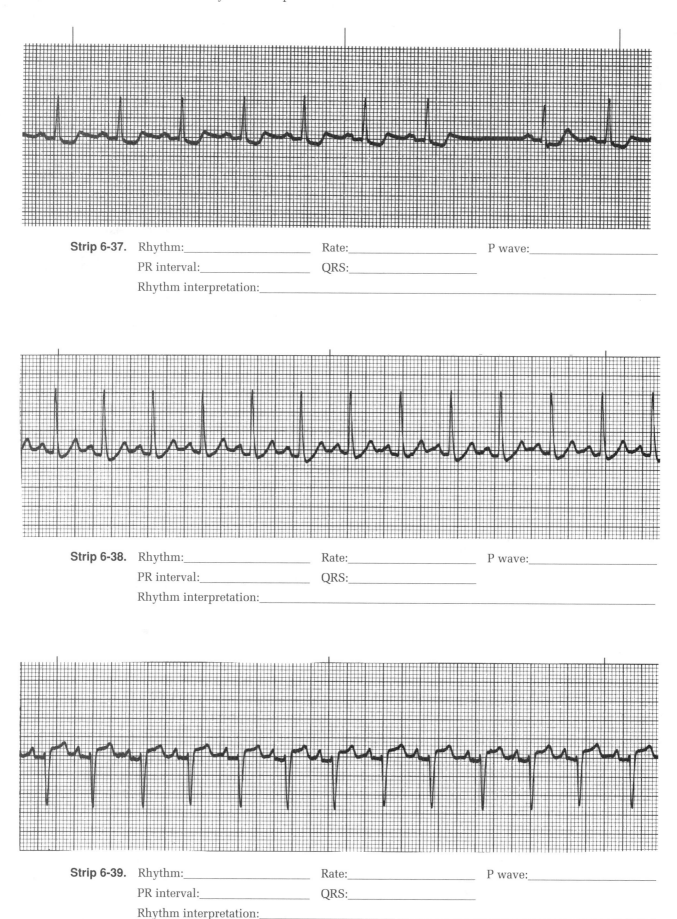

Strip 6-37. Rhythm:_____ Rate:_____ P wave:_____

PR interval:_____ QRS:_____

Rhythm interpretation:_____

Strip 6-38. Rhythm:_____ Rate:_____ P wave:_____

PR interval:_____ QRS:_____

Rhythm interpretation:_____

Strip 6-39. Rhythm:_____ Rate:_____ P wave:_____

PR interval:_____ QRS:_____

Rhythm interpretation:_____

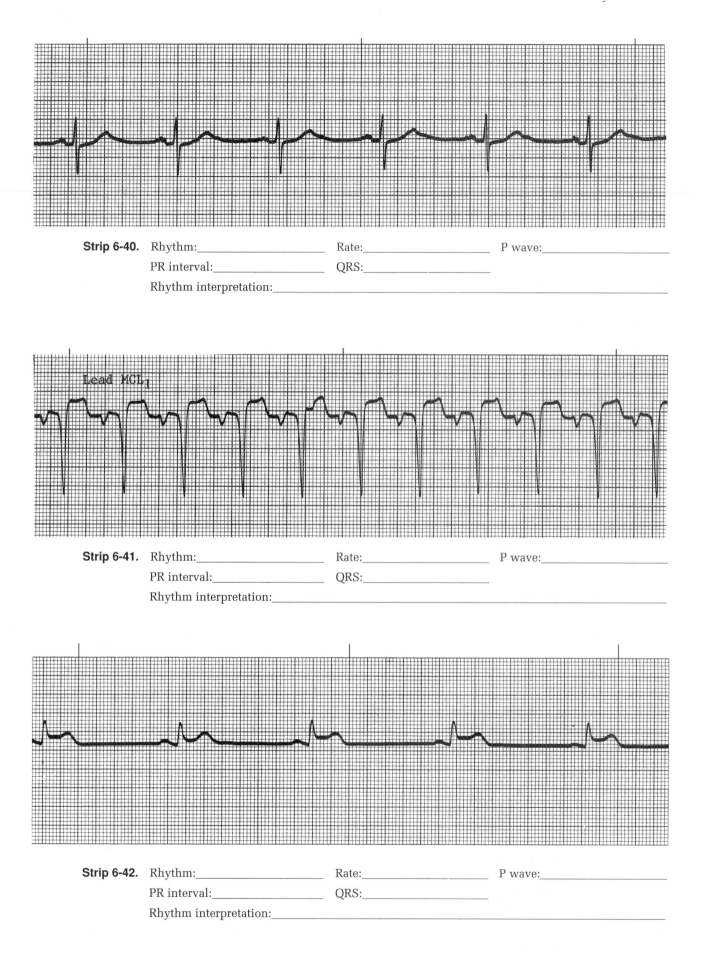

Strip 6-40. Rhythm:_____ Rate:_____ P wave:_____

PR interval:_____ QRS:_____

Rhythm interpretation:_____

Strip 6-41. Rhythm:_____ Rate:_____ P wave:_____

PR interval:_____ QRS:_____

Rhythm interpretation:_____

Strip 6-42. Rhythm:_____ Rate:_____ P wave:_____

PR interval:_____ QRS:_____

Rhythm interpretation:_____

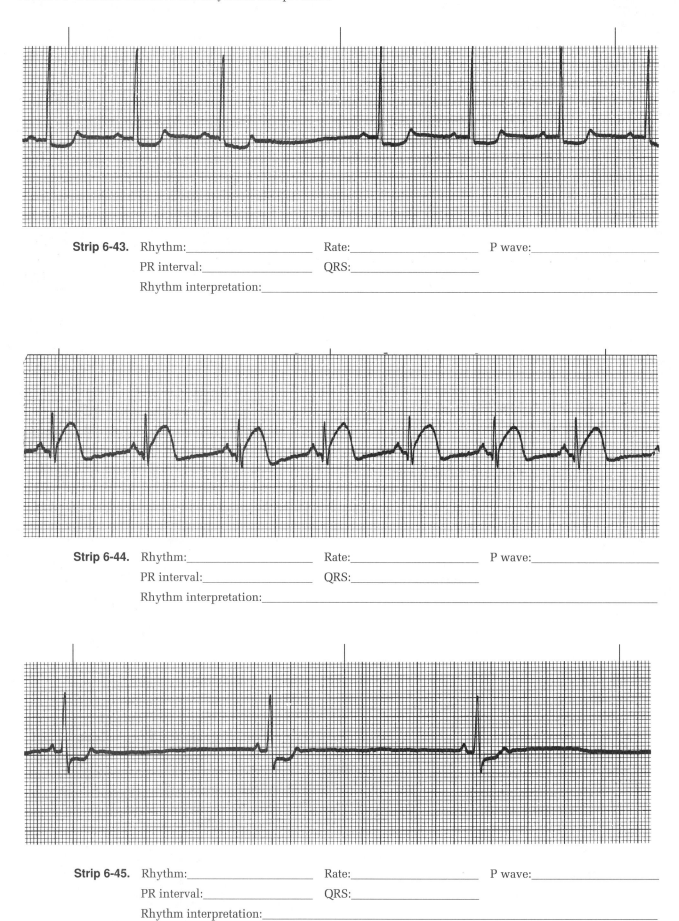

Strip 6-43. Rhythm:_____ Rate:_____ P wave:_____

PR interval:_____ QRS:_____

Rhythm interpretation:_____

Strip 6-44. Rhythm:_____ Rate:_____ P wave:_____

PR interval:_____ QRS:_____

Rhythm interpretation:_____

Strip 6-45. Rhythm:_____ Rate:_____ P wave:_____

PR interval:_____ QRS:_____

Rhythm arrterpretation:_____

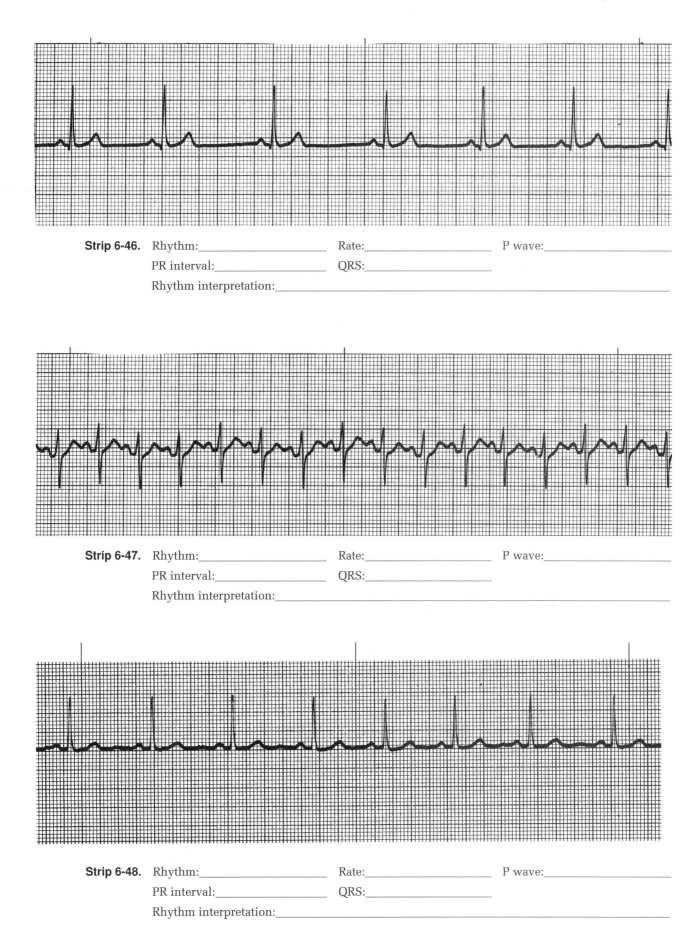

Strip 6-46. Rhythm:_____ Rate:_____ P wave:_____

PR interval:_____ QRS:_____

Rhythm interpretation:_____

Strip 6-47. Rhythm:_____ Rate:_____ P wave:_____

PR interval:_____ QRS:_____

Rhythm interpretation:_____

Strip 6-48. Rhythm:_____ Rate:_____ P wave:_____

PR interval:_____ QRS:_____

Rhythm interpretation:_____

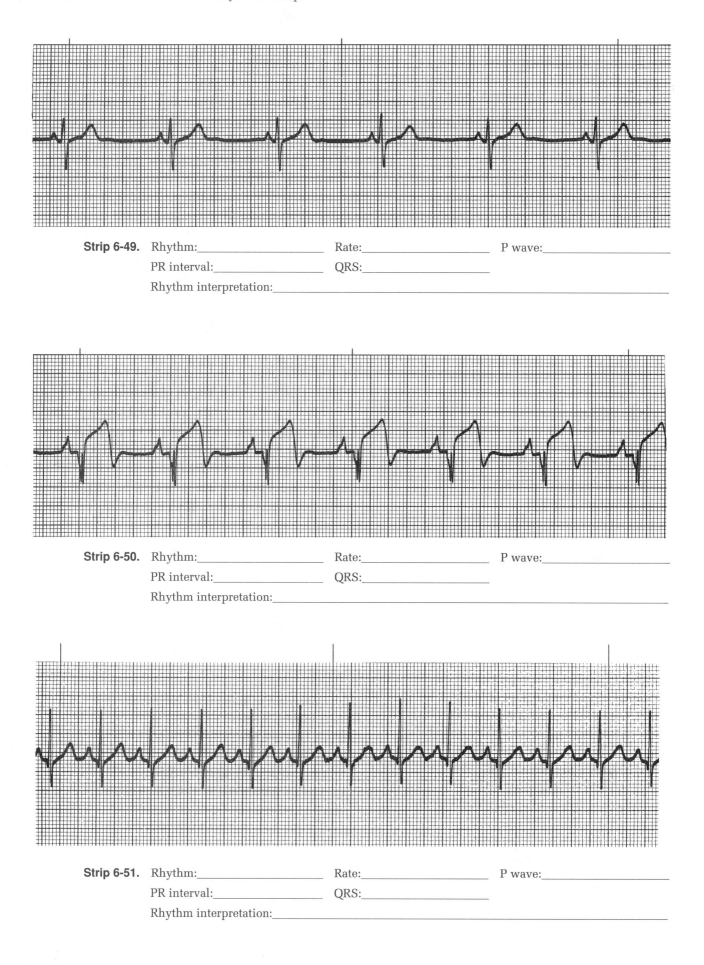

Strip 6-49. Rhythm:_____ Rate:_____ P wave:_____

PR interval:_____ QRS:_____

Rhythm interpretation:_____

Strip 6-50. Rhythm:_____ Rate:_____ P wave:_____

PR interval:_____ QRS:_____

Rhythm interpretation:_____

Strip 6-51. Rhythm:_____ Rate:_____ P wave:_____

PR interval:_____ QRS:_____

Rhythm interpretation:_____

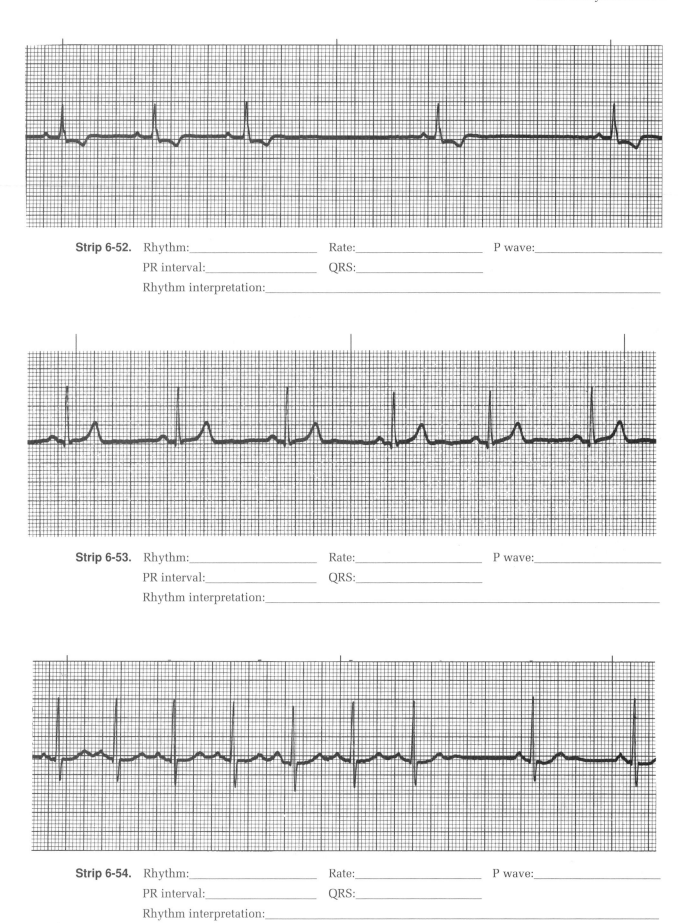

Strip 6-52. Rhythm:_____ Rate:_____ P wave:_____

PR interval:_____ QRS:_____

Rhythm interpretation:_____

Strip 6-53. Rhythm:_____ Rate:_____ P wave:_____

PR interval:_____ QRS:_____

Rhythm interpretation:_____

Strip 6-54. Rhythm:_____ Rate:_____ P wave:_____

PR interval:_____ QRS:_____

Rhythm interpretation:_____

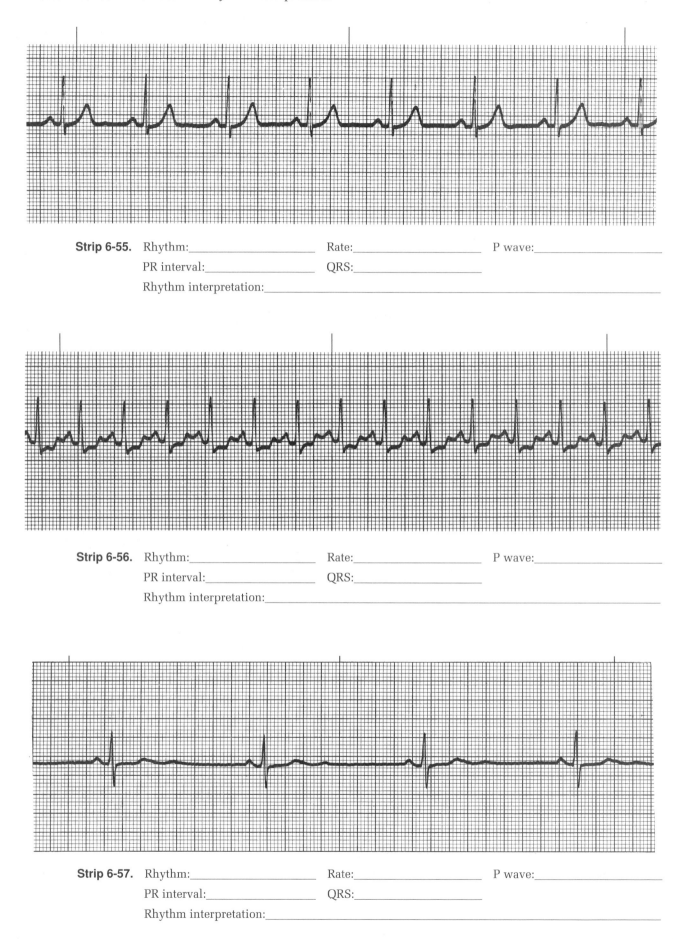

Strip 6-55. Rhythm:_____ Rate:_____ P wave:_____

PR interval:_____ QRS:_____

Rhythm interpretation:_____

Strip 6-56. Rhythm:_____ Rate:_____ P wave:_____

PR interval:_____ QRS:_____

Rhythm interpretation:_____

Strip 6-57. Rhythm:_____ Rate:_____ P wave:_____

PR interval:_____ QRS:_____

Rhythm arrpretation:_____

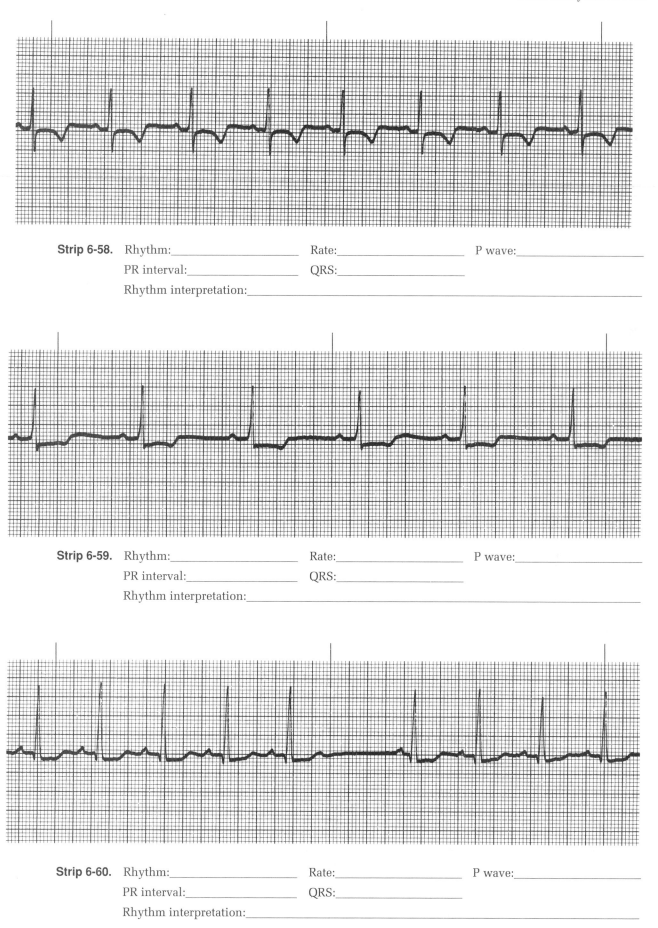

Strip 6-58. Rhythm:_____ Rate:_____ P wave:_____

PR interval:_____ QRS:_____

Rhythm interpretation:_____

Strip 6-59. Rhythm:_____ Rate:_____ P wave:_____

PR interval:_____ QRS:_____

Rhythm interpretation:_____

Strip 6-60. Rhythm:_____ Rate:_____ P wave:_____

PR interval:_____ QRS:_____

Rhythm interpretation:_____

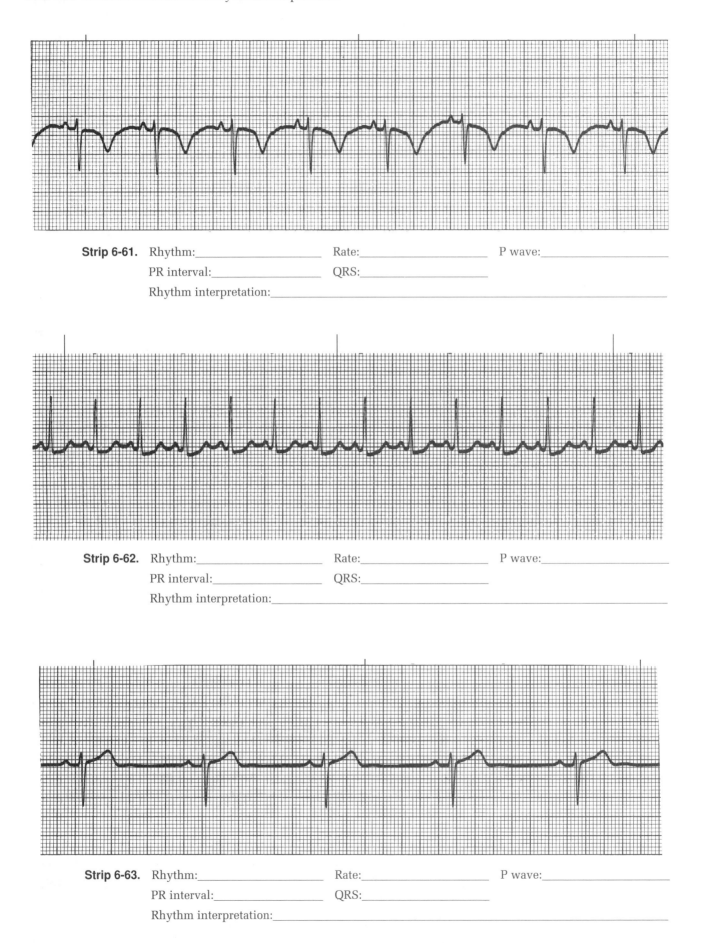

Strip 6-61. Rhythm:_____ Rate:_____ P wave:_____

PR interval:_____ QRS:_____

Rhythm interpretation:_____

Strip 6-62. Rhythm:_____ Rate:_____ P wave:_____

PR interval:_____ QRS:_____

Rhythm interpretation:_____

Strip 6-63. Rhythm:_____ Rate:_____ P wave:_____

PR interval:_____ QRS:_____

Rhythm arterpretation:_____

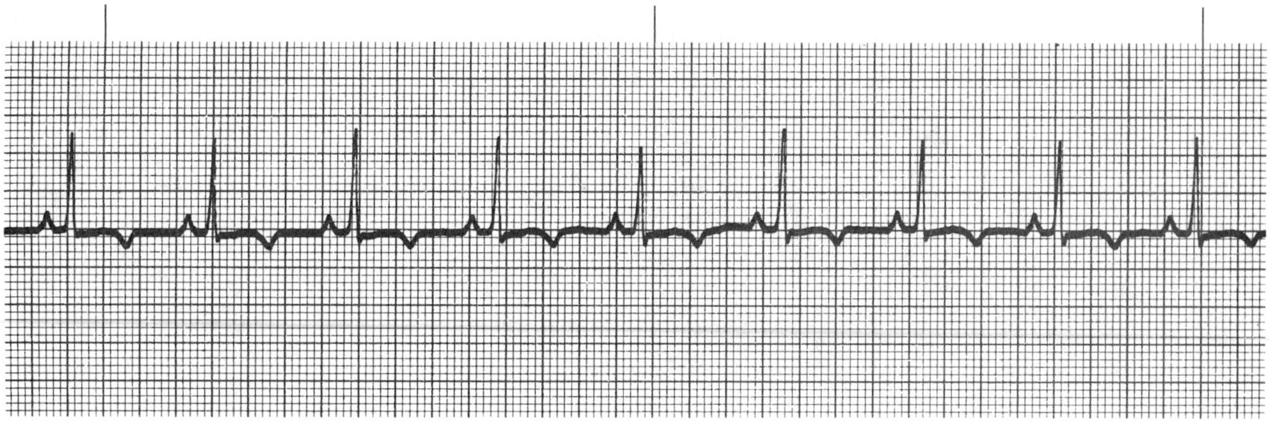

Strip 6-64. Rhythm:_____ Rate:_____ P wave:_____

PR interval:_____ QRS:_____

Rhythm interpretation:_____

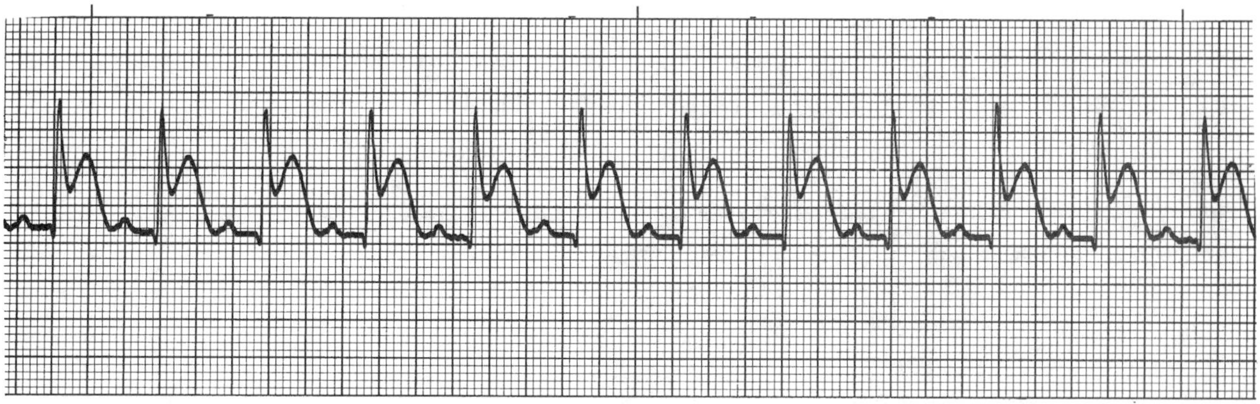

Strip 6-65. Rhythm:_____ Rate:_____ P wave:_____

PR interval:_____ QRS:_____

Rhythm interpretation:_____

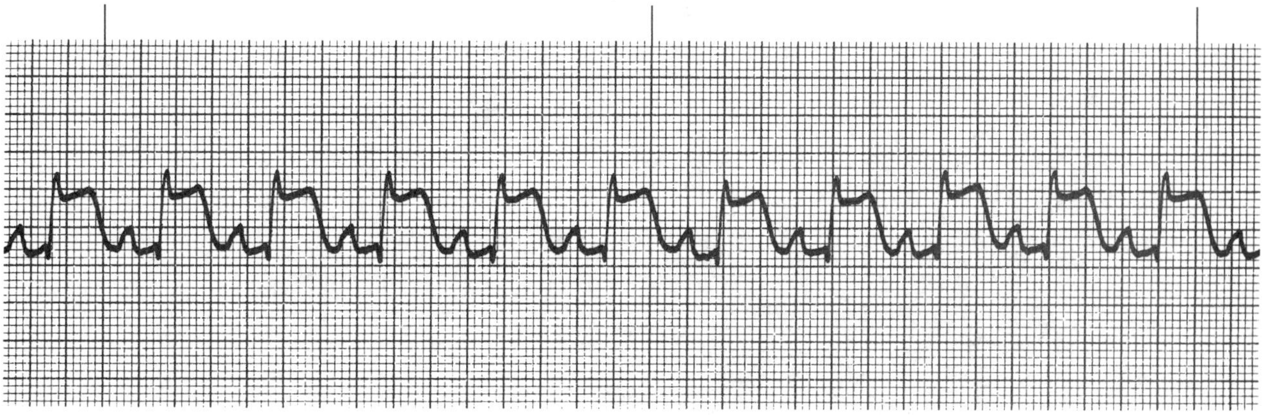

Strip 6-66. Rhythm:_____ Rate:_____ P wave:_____

PR interval:_____ QRS:_____

Rhythm interpretation:_____

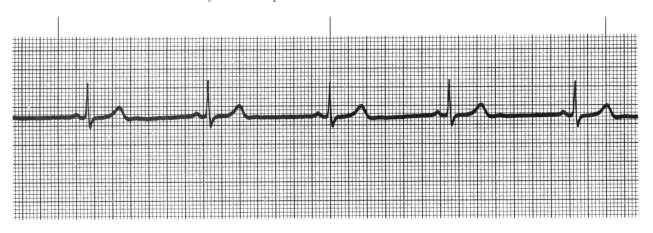

Strip 6-67. Rhythm:_____ Rate:_____ P wave:_____

PR interval:_____ QRS:_____

Rhythm interpretation:_____

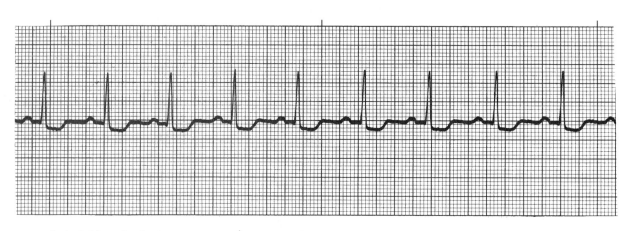

Strip 6-68. Rhythm:_____ Rate:_____ P wave:_____

PR interval:_____ QRS:_____

Rhythm interpretation:_____

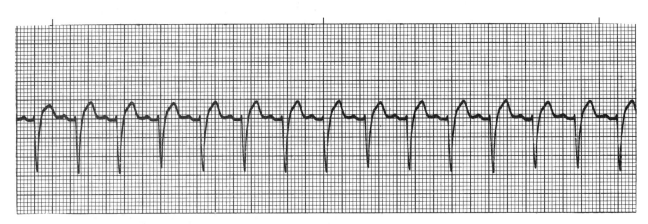

Strip 6-69. Rhythm:_____ Rate:_____ P wave:_____

PR interval:_____ QRS:_____

Rhythm interpretation:_____

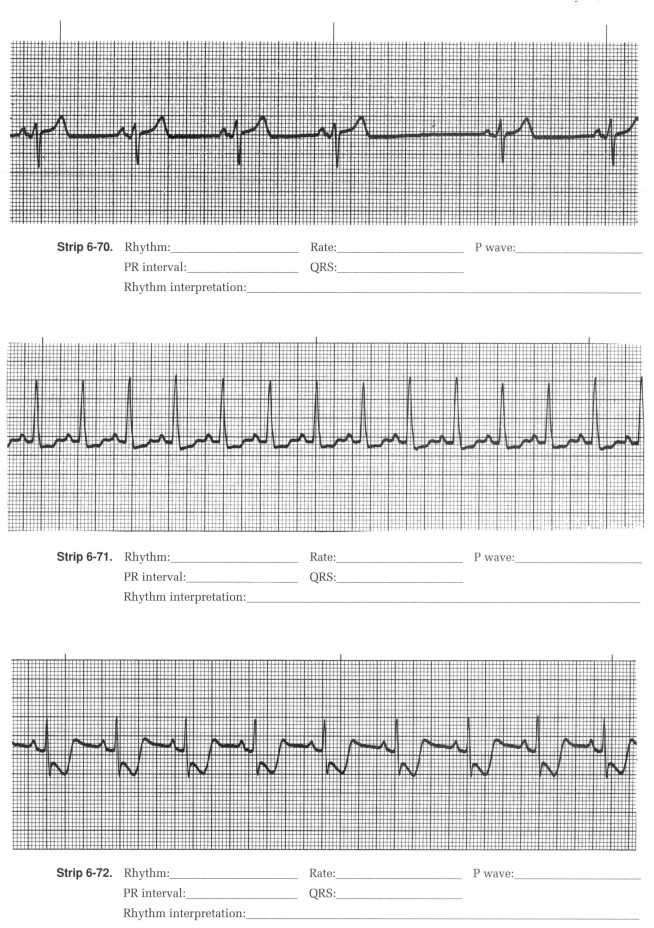

Strip 6-70. Rhythm:_____ Rate:_____ P wave:_____

PR interval:_____ QRS:_____

Rhythm interpretation:_____

Strip 6-71. Rhythm:_____ Rate:_____ P wave:_____

PR interval:_____ QRS:_____

Rhythm interpretation:_____

Strip 6-72. Rhythm:_____ Rate:_____ P wave:_____

PR interval:_____ QRS:_____

Rhythm interpretation:_____

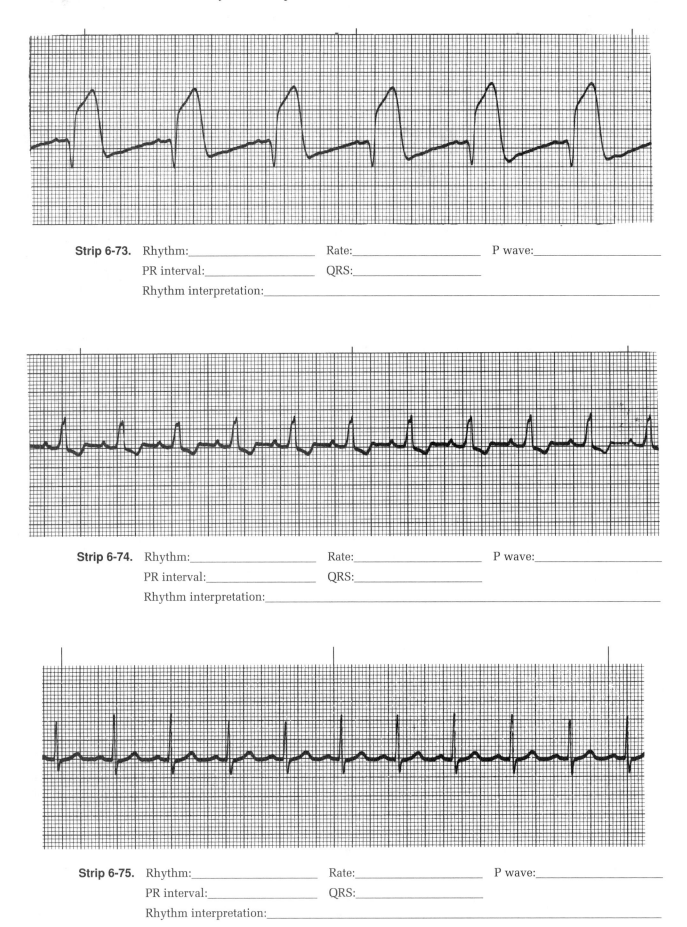

Strip 6-73. Rhythm:_____ Rate:_____ P wave:_____

PR interval:_____ QRS:_____

Rhythm interpretation:_____

Strip 6-74. Rhythm:_____ Rate:_____ P wave:_____

PR interval:_____ QRS:_____

Rhythm interpretation:_____

Strip 6-75. Rhythm:_____ Rate:_____ P wave:_____

PR interval:_____ QRS:_____

Rhythm arterpretation:_____

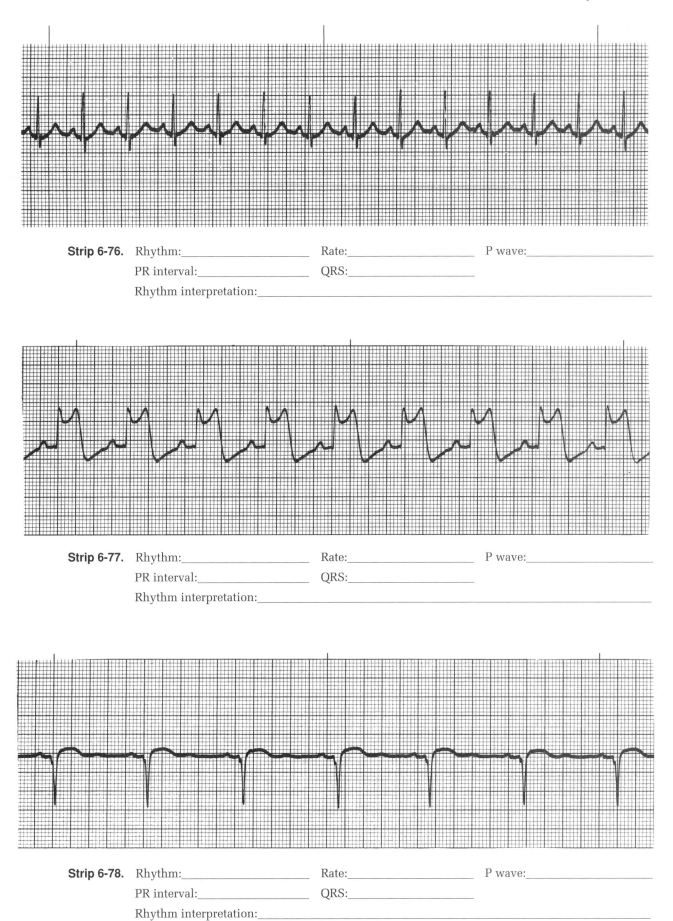

Strip 6-76. Rhythm:_____ Rate:_____ P wave:_____

PR interval:_____ QRS:_____

Rhythm interpretation:_____

Strip 6-77. Rhythm:_____ Rate:_____ P wave:_____

PR interval:_____ QRS:_____

Rhythm interpretation:_____

Strip 6-78. Rhythm:_____ Rate:_____ P wave:_____

PR interval:_____ QRS:_____

Rhythm interpretation:_____

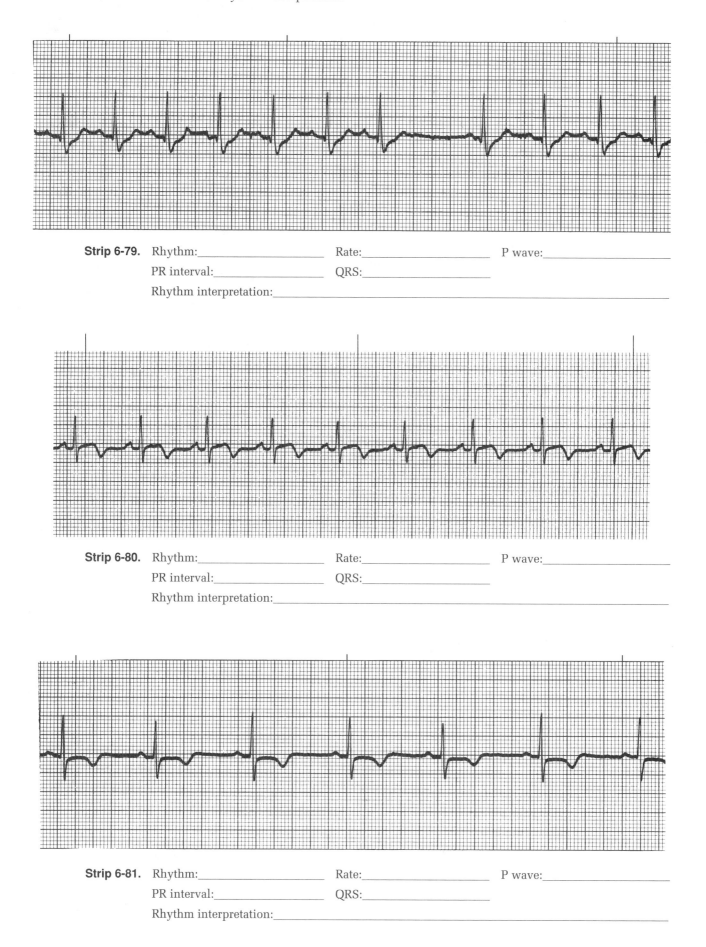

Strip 6-79. Rhythm:_____ Rate:_____ P wave:_____

PR interval:_____ QRS:_____

Rhythm interpretation:_____

Strip 6-80. Rhythm:_____ Rate:_____ P wave:_____

PR interval:_____ QRS:_____

Rhythm interpretation:_____

Strip 6-81. Rhythm:_____ Rate:_____ P wave:_____

PR interval:_____ QRS:_____

Rhythm interrpretation:_____

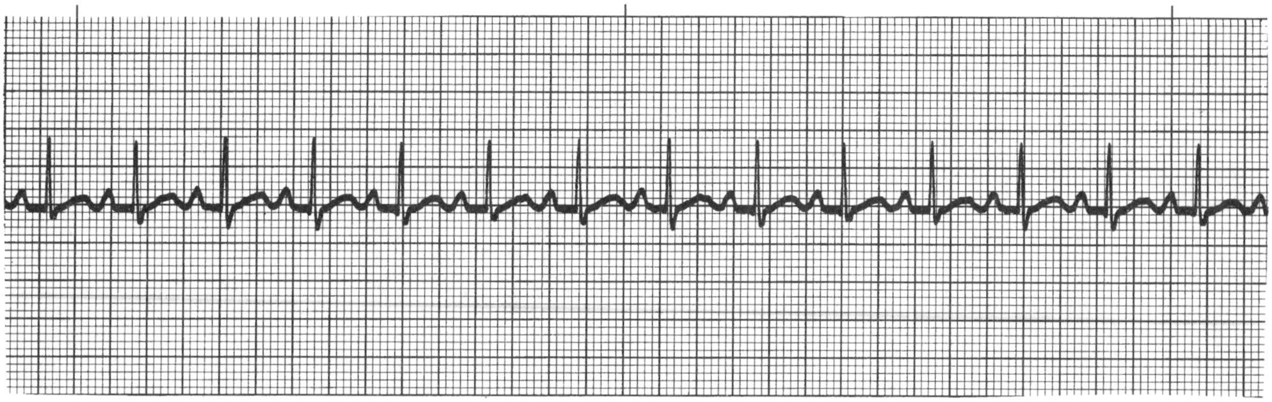

Strip 6-82. Rhythm:_____ Rate:_____ P wave:_____

PR interval:_____ QRS:_____

Rhythm interpretation:_____

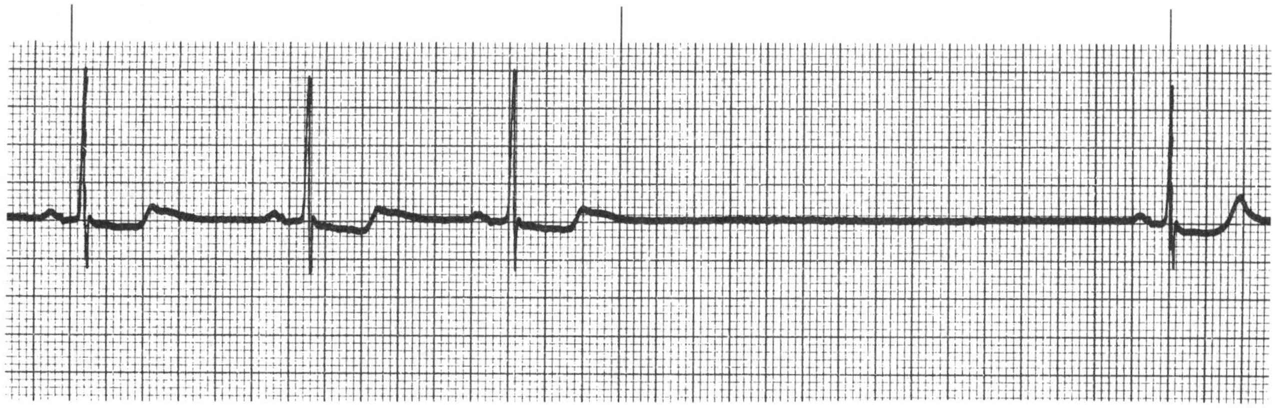

Strip 6-83. Rhythm:_____ Rate:_____ P wave:_____

PR interval:_____ QRS:_____

Rhythm interpretation:_____

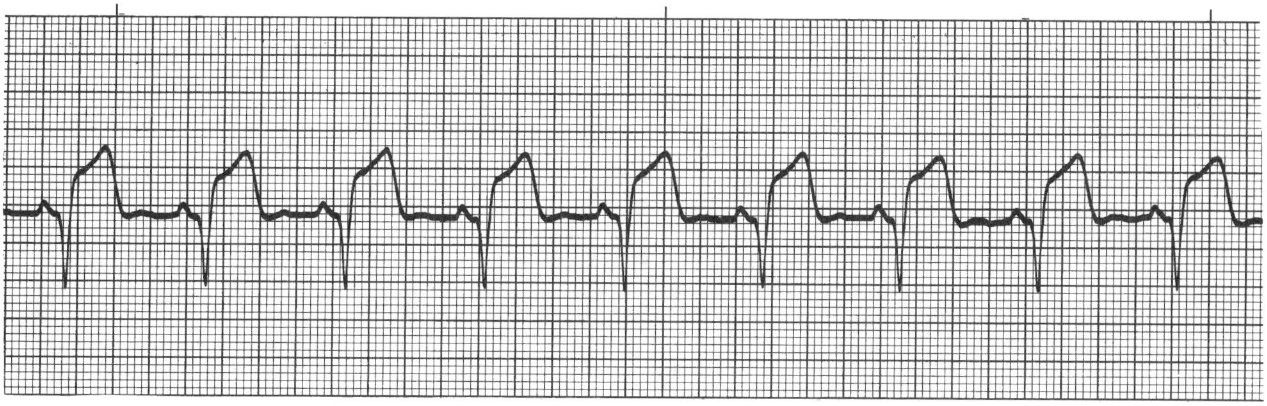

Strip 6-84. Rhythm:_____ Rate:_____ P wave:_____

PR interval:_____ QRS:_____

Rhythm interpretation:_____

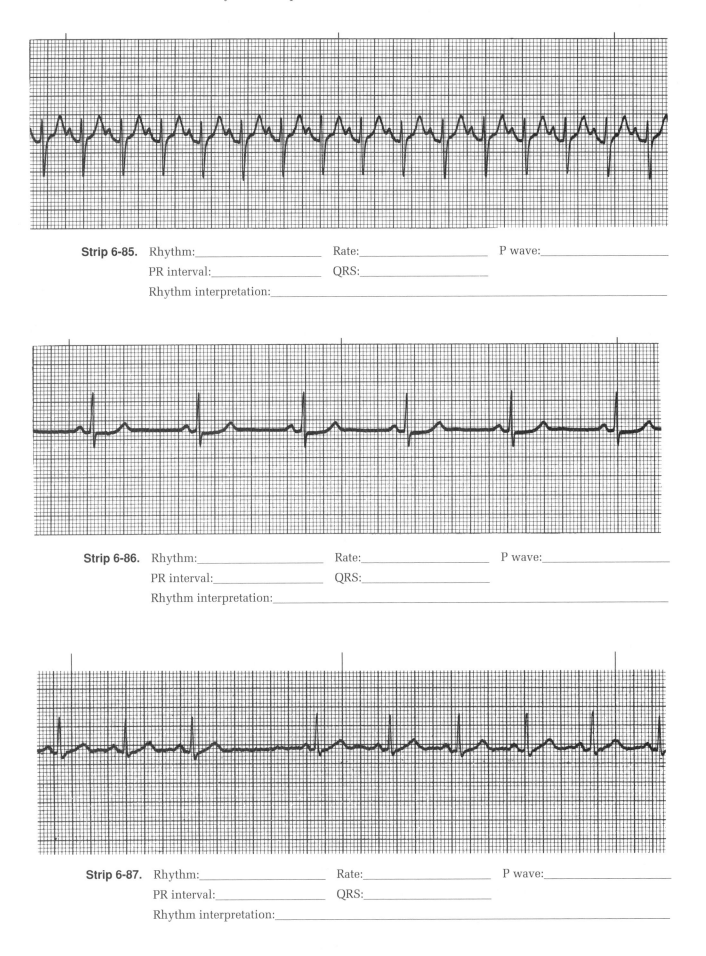

Strip 6-85. Rhythm:_____ Rate:_____ P wave:_____

PR interval:_____ QRS:_____

Rhythm interpretation:_____

Strip 6-86. Rhythm:_____ Rate:_____ P wave:_____

PR interval:_____ QRS:_____

Rhythm interpretation:_____

Strip 6-87. Rhythm:_____ Rate:_____ P wave:_____

PR interval:_____ QRS:_____

Rhythm arterpretation:_____

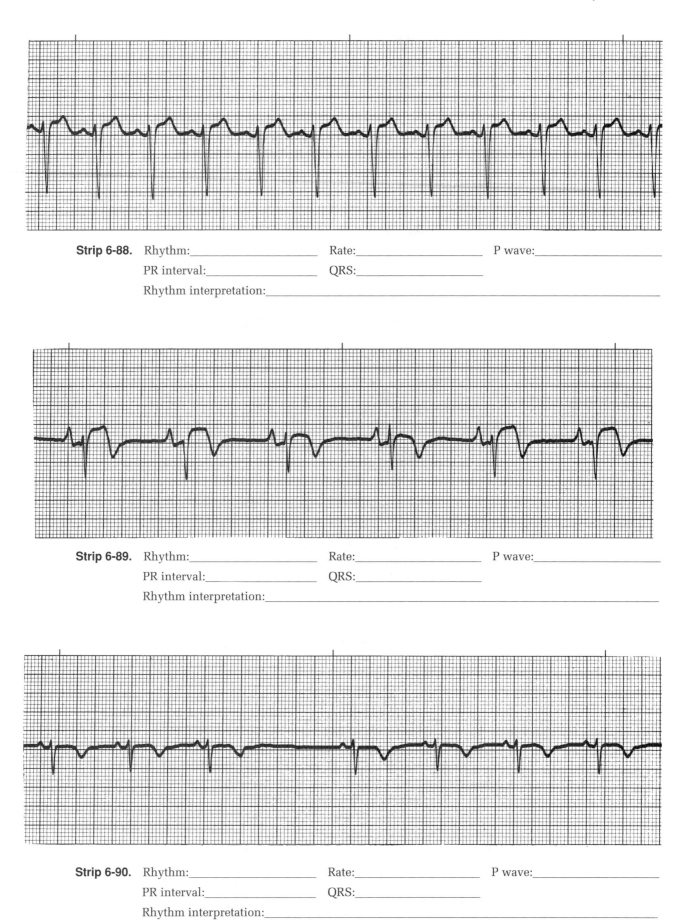

Strip 6-88. Rhythm:_____ Rate:_____ P wave:_____

PR interval:_____ QRS:_____

Rhythm interpretation:_____

Strip 6-89. Rhythm:_____ Rate:_____ P wave:_____

PR interval:_____ QRS:_____

Rhythm interpretation:_____

Strip 6-90. Rhythm:_____ Rate:_____ P wave:_____

PR interval:_____ QRS:_____

Rhythm interpretation:_____

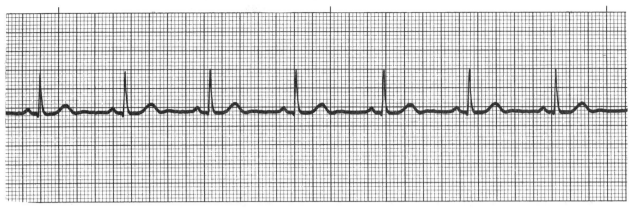

Strip 6-91. Rhythm:_____ Rate:_____ P wave:_____

PR interval:_____ QRS:_____

Rhythm interpretation:_____

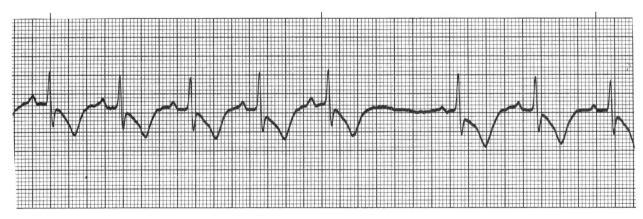

Strip 6-92. Rhythm:_____ Rate:_____ P wave:_____

PR interval:_____ QRS:_____

Rhythm interpretation:_____

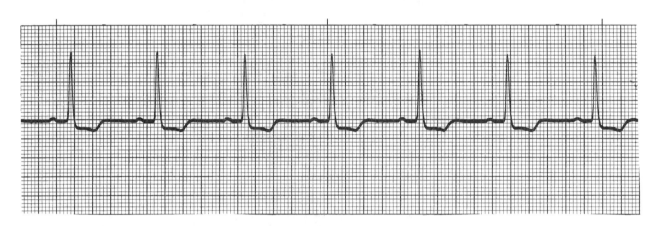

Strip 6-93. Rhythm:_____ Rate:_____ P wave:_____

PR interval:_____ QRS:_____

Rhythm interrpretation:_____

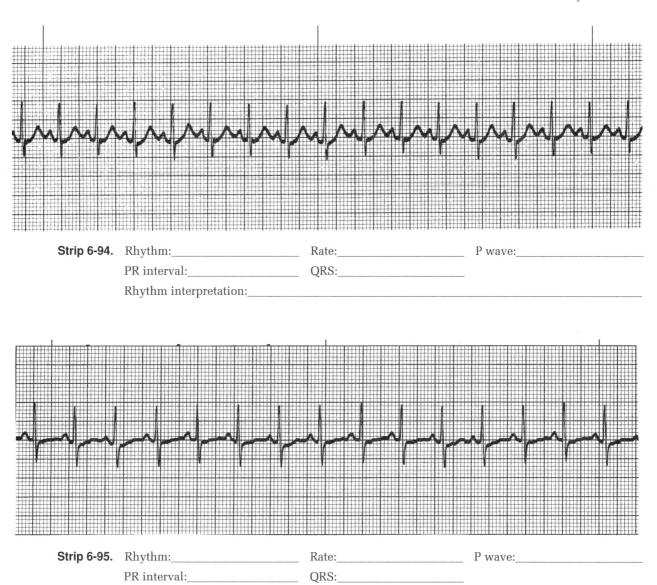

Strip 6-94. Rhythm:_____ Rate:_____ P wave:_____

PR interval:_____ QRS:_____

Rhythm interpretation:_____

Strip 6-95. Rhythm:_____ Rate:_____ P wave:_____

PR interval:_____ QRS:_____

Rhythm interpretation:_____

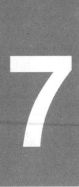

Atrial Arrhythmias

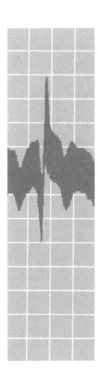

The intrinsic pacemaker of the heart is the sinus node, which normally initiates each heartbeat. However, electrical impulses can arise from other parts of the heart (the atria, the AV junction, or the ventricles) and assume pacemaker control for one beat, several beats, or continuously. The term "ectopic" is used to described these non-sinus arrhythmias.

Atrial arrhythmias (Figure 7-1) result from ectopic stimuli—that is, they arise outside the SA node in either the right or left atrium. Because of the ectopic origin of the impulse, the P-waves will be different in configuration (morphology) from the sinus P-waves. In slower atrial rhythms (rates less than 200 per minute), the P-wave is often visible as an upright (frequently pointed) or an inverted waveform in ECG lead II (Figure 7-2A). In faster atrial rhythms (rates greater than 200 per minute), the P-wave is superimposed on the preceding T-wave, hidden in the QRS complex, or appears as a sawtooth (Figure 7-2B) or wavy (Figure 7-2C) baseline.

The electrophysiological mechanisms most often responsible for atrial arrhythmias are enhanced automaticity or reentry. Both mechanisms are capable of causing the atrial muscles to fire quickly, producing rapid atrial rates often accompanied by rapid ventricular responses. With faster atrial rates, the AV node triages impulses (prevents some impulses from conducting to the ventricles). This results in a ventricular rate which is slower than the atrial rate (less QRS complexes than P-waves). With slower atrial rates, the AV node accepts and conducts each impulse to the ventricles. This results in a ventricular rate which is the same as the atrial rate (one P-wave to each QRS complex).

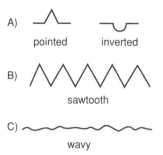

Figure 7-2. Atrial P-waves.

Younger patients and individuals without significant underlying heart disease may tolerate episodes of rapid heart rate with no serious problems. However, in patients with limited cardiac reserve, increased heart rates can have serious consequences. In atrial rhythms associated with rapid ventricular rates, the ventricles are unable to fill completely during diastole. This results in a significant reduction in cardiac output, which may produce hypotension or lead to heart failure. In addition, rapid ventricular rates increase myocardial oxygen demands, which can cause myocardial ischemia and even lead to myocardial infarction.

WANDERING ATRIAL PACEMAKER

A wandering atrial pacemaker (Figure 7-3) (Box 7-1) occurs when the pacemaker site shifts back and forth between the SA node and ectopic sites in the

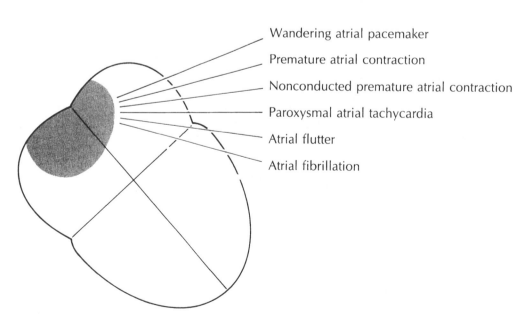

Figure 7-1. Atrial arrhythmias.

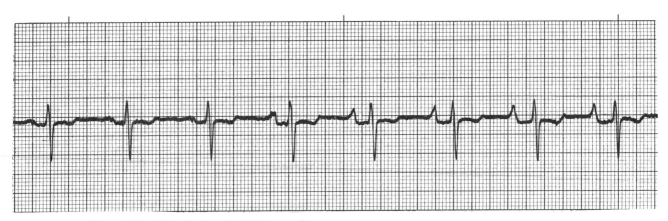

Figure 7-3. **Wandering Atrial Pacemaker**

Rhythm: Regular

Rate: 68

P waves: Vary in size, shape, direction across rhythm strip

PR interval: 0.20–0.22 seconds

QRS: 0.08–0.10 seconds

Comment: A biphasic T-wave is noted

atria or AV junction, producing P-waves of varying size, shape, and direction. The heart rate is usually 60–100 but may be slower. The rhythm may be regular or irregular. The PR interval may vary slightly depending on the changing pacemaker location. The QRS is normal in duration. The distinguishing feature of this rhythm is the changing P-wave morphology across the rhythm strip.

A wandering atrial pacemaker is caused, in most cases, by an increase in parasympathetic (vagal) tone on the SA node or AV junction. It occurs in normal individuals, particularly during sleep. It can also be seen in chronic lung disease, valvular heart disease, and with digitalis excess.

A wandering atrial pacemaker is usually not clinically significant and treatment is not indicated. If the heart rate is slow, medications should be reviewed and discontinued if necessary. Asking the patient to cough may decrease vagal tone and encourage the reappearance of a normal sinus rhythm.

Box 7-1.	**Wandering Atrial Pacemaker: Identifying ECG Features**
Rhythm:	Regular or irregular
Rate:	Usually normal (60–100) but may be slower
P-waves:	Vary in size, shape, and direction across rhythm strip
PR interval:	May vary slightly depending on the changing pacemaker location
QRS:	Normal (0.10 seconds or less)

PREMATURE ATRIAL CONTRACTIONS (PAC)

A premature atrial contraction (Figures 7-4, 7-5, 7-6, and 7-7) (Box 7-2) is an early beat that originates in an ectopic pacemaker in the atria and is usually caused by enhanced automaticity in the atrial tissue. It occurs in addition to the patient's underlying rhythm. PACs may originate from a single ectopic pacemaker site or from multiple sites in the atria. The early beat is characterized by an abnormal (occasionally normal appearing) P-wave, a QRS complex that is identical or very similar to the QRS complex of the normally conducted beats, and followed by a pause. An ectopic atrial P-wave followed by a QRS complex is considered a conducted PAC.

The shape of the P-wave depends on the location

Box 7-2.	**Premature Atrial Contraction (PAC): Identifying ECG Features**
Rhythm:	Underlying rhythm usually regular; irregular with PACs
Rate:	Heart rate is that of underlying rhythm
P-waves:	P-wave associated with PAC is premature and abnormal in size, shape, or direction (in lead II the P-wave is usually upright (often pointed), or it may be inverted); abnormal P-wave often found hidden in preceding T-wave distorting the T-wave contour.
PR:	Normal or prolonged—usually differs from that of underlying rhythm
QRS:	Normal (0.10 seconds or less)

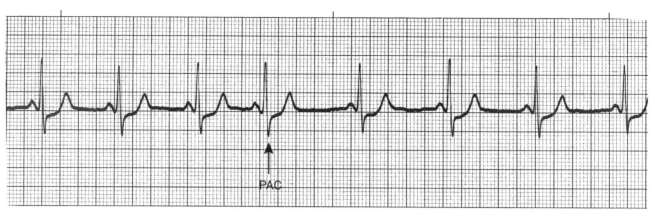

Figure 7-4. **Normal Sinus Rhythm with Premature Atrial Contraction**

Rhythm: Basic rhythm regular—irregular with PAC

Rate: Basic rhythm rate 72—rate slows to 60 following PAC (temporary rate suppression is common following a pause in the basic rhythm—after several cardiac cycles the rate usually returns to the basic rhythm rate).

P waves: Sinus P-waves with basic rhythm; P-wave associated with PAC is premature and closely resembles that of the sinus P-waves in the underlying rhythm—this indicates the ectopic atrial pacemaker site is close to the SA node

PR interval: 0.12 seconds (basic rhythm and PAC)

QRS: 0.08 seconds (basic rhythm and PAC)

of the ectopic pacemaker site. If the ectopic focus is in the vicinity of the SA node, the P-wave may closely resemble the sinus P-wave (Figure 7-4). Its sole distinguishing feature may be its prematurity. As a rule, however, the P-wave is usually different from the sinus P-waves. In ECG lead II it is generally

upright (often pointed), or it may be inverted if the pacemaker site is near the AV junction. If the premature beat occurs very early, the abnormal P-wave can be found hidden in the preceding T-wave, causing a distortion of the T-wave contour (Figure 7-5).

The PR intervals of the PACs may be normal in

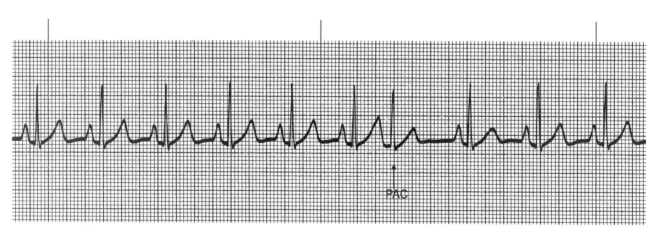

Figure 7-5. **Normal Sinus Rhythm with Premature Atrial Contraction**

Rhythm: Basic rhythm regular, irregular with PAC

Rate: Basic rhythm rate 84

P waves: Sinus P-waves with basic rhythm; premature, abnormal P-wave with PAC. The P-wave of the PAC is hidden in the preceding T-wave distorting the T-wave contour (T-wave is taller and more pointed.)

PR interval: 0.12 to 0.14 seconds (basic rhythm)

QRS: 0.06 to 0.08 seconds

duration but they usually differ from those of the underlying rhythm. Occasionally, the PR is prolonged if there is a delay in conduction. The PR interval will be unmeasurable if the abnormal P-wave is obscured in the preceding T-wave.

The QRS of the PAC usually resembles that of the underlying rhythm because the conduction of the electrical impulse through the bundle branches is unchanged. If, however, the ectopic atrial impulse is discharged very early, the bundle branches may not have repolarized sufficiently to conduct the impulse normally. This results in the impulse being conducted down one bundle branch (usually the left) and blocked in the right. The resulting QRS complex will be wide and bizarre and resemble a right bundle branch block. The term for such a PAC is premature atrial contraction with aberrant ventricular conduction (Figure 7-6). This wide complex must be differentiated from a premature ventricular contraction (PVC), especially if the abnormal P-wave associated with the PAC is obscured in the preceding T-wave. PVCs are discussed in Chapter 9.

The pause associated with the PAC is usually noncompensatory—that is, the measurement between the R-wave preceding the PAC to the R-wave following the PAC is less than two R-R cycles of the underlying regular rhythm (Figure 7-7). With the noncompensatory pause the SA node is depolarized by the PAC, causing the timing of the SA node to be reset. This results in the resumption of the underlying rhythm a little earlier than expected. Occasionally, the PAC will occur with a compensatory pause

(a pause that equals two R-R cycles), but this is usually seen with the PVC. With the compensatory pause the SA node is not depolarized by the PAC, the discharge timing remains unchanged, and the underlying rhythm resumes as expected. Rarely, the PAC may occur with a pause that is longer than compensatory.

PACs may appear as a single beat, every other beat (bigeminal PACs), every third beat (trigeminal PACs), every fourth beat (quadrigeminal PACs), in pairs (also called couplets), or in runs. When PACs occur in consecutive runs of three or more, atrial tachycardia is considered to be present. Frequent PACs may warn of or initiate more serious atrial arrhythmias such as paroxysmal atrial tachycardia, atrial flutter, or atrial fibrillation.

Premature atrial beats are very common. They can occur in individuals with a normal heart or in persons with heart disease. In normal subjects PACs are seen with emotional stress (which can increase sympathetic tone and catecholamine release) and excessive intake of alcohol, caffeine, or tobacco. Other causes include: electrolyte imbalance, hypoxia, digitalis toxicity, hyperthyroidism, chronic lung disease, dilated or hypertrophied atria, cardiovascular diseases (myocardial ischemia, coronary artery disease, heart failure, valvular disease) and the administration of sympathomimetic drugs (epinephrine, isoproterenol, and theophylline). PACs can also occur without apparent cause.

Infrequent PACs require no treatment. If treatment is needed, the best approach is to eliminate the

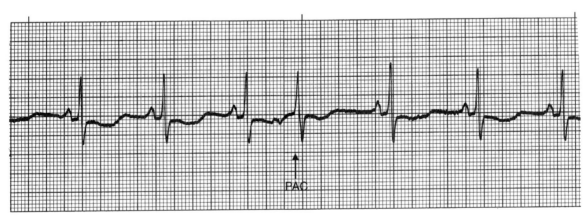

Figure 7-6. Normal Sinus Rhythm with 1 PAC with Aberrant Ventricular Conduction

Rhythm: Basic rhythm regular; irregular with PAC

Rate: Basic rhythm rate 68

P waves: Sinus in basic rhythm; premature, abnormal P-wave with PAC

PR interval: 0.16 to 0.18 seconds (basic rhythm)
                 0.24 seconds (PAC)

QRS: 0.08 to 0.10 seconds (basic rhythm)
                 0.12 seconds (PAC)

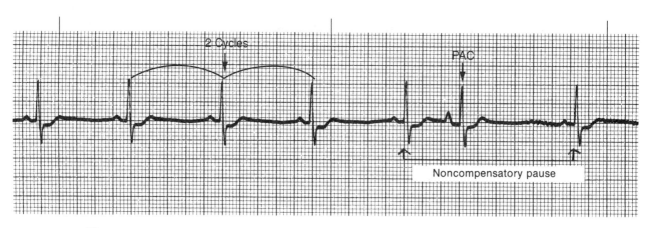

Figure 7-7. Normal Sinus Rhythm with Premature Atrial Contraction

Rhythm: Basic rhythm regular, irregular with PAC

Rate: Basic rhythm rate 60

P waves: Sinus P-waves with basic rhythm; premature, abnormal P-wave with PAC

PR interval: 0.12 to 0.16 seconds (basic rhythm)

QRS: 0.08 seconds

Comment: To determine the type of pause following premature beats, measure from the QRS preceding the premature beat to the QRS following the premature beat. If the measurement equals two RR intervals, the pause is compensatory. If the measurement is less than two RR intervals, the pause is noncompensatory. ST segment depression is present.

cause (e.g., caffeine, alcohol, tobacco, stress). If drug therapy is recommended, agents such as quinidine, procainamide, digitalis (if not a cause of the rhythm), or disopyramide may be used.

On some occasions an ectopic atrial beat will occur late instead of early. These beats are called atrial escape beats. Atrial escape beats are more likely to occur due to increased vagal effect on the SA node rather than enhanced automaticity as is associated with the premature beat. Atrial escape beats may occur following a pause in the underlying rhythm (e.g., sinus arrest, sinus block, non-conducted PAC, or type I second degree AV block). The morphologic characteristics of the late beat will be the same as the PAC. Escape beats require no treatment. It is important, however, to identify the cause of the initiating pause so that appropriate intervention can be started if necessary.

NONCONDUCTED PAC

A nonconducted PAC (Figures 7-8, 7-9, and 7-10) (Box 7-3) results when an ectopic atrial focus occurs so early that it finds the AV node refractory and the impulse is not conducted to the ventricles. This results in an ectopic P-wave not accompanied by a QRS complex, but followed by a pause (Figure 7-8).

Box 7-3.	Nonconducted PACs: Identifying ECG Features
Rhythm:	Underlying rhythm usually regular; irregular with nonconducted PACs
Rate:	Heart rate is that of underlying rhythm
P-waves:	P-wave associated with the nonconducted PAC is premature, and abnormal in size, shape, or direction; often found hidden in preceding T-wave, distorting the T-wave contour
PR:	Absent with nonconducted PAC
QRS:	Absent with nonconducted PAC

Like the conducted PAC, the P-wave associated with the nonconducted PAC will be premature and abnormal in size, shape, or direction. Again, the P-wave is often found hidden in the preceding T-waves, distorting the T-wave contour (Figure 7-9), and the pause that follows is usually noncompensatory. The nonconducted PAC is the most common cause of unexpected pauses in a regular sinus rhythm.

The nonconducted PAC can be confused with sinus arrest or block. All produce a sudden pause in the rhythm without QRS complexes. To differentiate between these rhythms, one must examine and com-

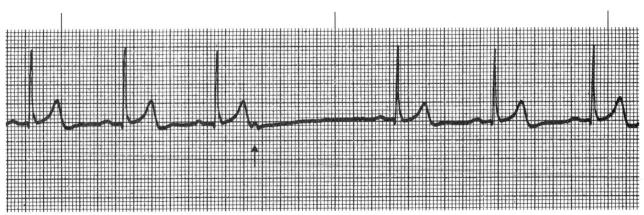

Figure 7-8. **Normal Sinus Rhythm with Nonconducted PAC**

Rhythm: Basic rhythm regular; irregular with nonconducted PAC

Rate: Basic rate 60; rate slows following nonconducted PAC; rate suppression can occur following a pause in the basic rhythm. After several cycles, the rate will return to the basic rhythm rate.

P waves: Sinus P-waves with basic rhythm; premature, abnormal P-wave with nonconducted PAC

PR interval: 0.20 seconds with basic rhythm

QRS: 0.06 to 0.08 seconds with basic rhythm

Comment: A U wave is present

pare T-wave contours (Figure 7-10). The early P-wave of the nonconducted PAC will distort the preceding T-wave. In sinus arrest or sinus block, there is no P-wave produced and the T-wave contour remains unchanged.

Nonconducted PACs have the same significance as conducted PACs and may be treated in the same manner.

PAROXYSMAL ATRIAL TACHYCARDIA

Atrial tachycardia (Figures 7-11 and 7-12) (Box 7-4) is an arrhythmia originating in an ectopic pacemaker site in the atria. It involves enhanced automaticity of atrial tissue or conduction of the ectopic impulse through a reentry circuit involving the atria

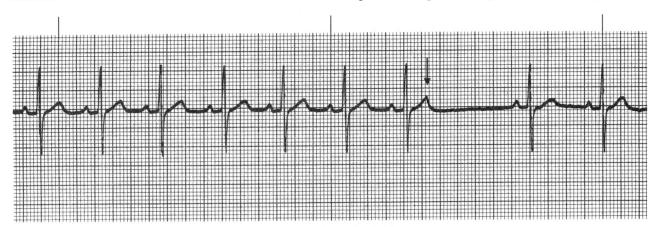

Figure 7-9. **Normal Sinus Rhythm with Nonconducted PAC**

Rhythm: Basic rhythm regular; irregular with nonconducted PACs

Rate: Basic rhythm rate 88

P waves: Sinus P-waves with basic rhythm; P-wave of nonconducted PAC is premature, abnormal, and hidden in the preceding T-wave (T-wave is taller and more pointed than those of underlying rhythm)

PR interval: 0.16 to 0.18 seconds (basic rhythm); not present with nonconducted PAC

QRS: 0.06 to 0.08 seconds (basic rhythm); not present with nonconducted PAC

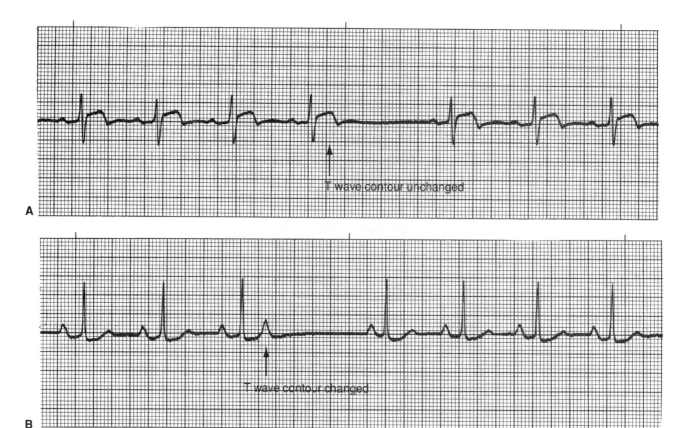

Figure 7-10. Differentiation of Sinus Arrest or Block from the Nonconducted PAC

A Sinus Arrest or Block
1. Sudden pause in the basic rhythm
2. No P-wave present
3. T-wave contour occurring during pause remains unchanged

B Nonconducted PAC
1. Sudden pause in the basic rhythm
2. Abnormal, premature P-wave present and often found hidden in T-wave
3. T-wave contour occurring during pause will be different from the contours of the basic rhythm

and AV node, or through an accessory pathway involving the atria and ventricles. Atrial tachycardia commonly starts and ends abruptly, occurring in paroxysms (thus the name "paroxysmal atrial tachycardia," or PAT). PAT is often initiated by a PAC. By definition, three or more consecutive PACs are considered to be atrial tachycardia (Figure 7-12).

Atrial tachycardia is a regular tachycardia with an atrial rate between 140–250 per minute. The ventricular rate will be the same as the atrial rate unless AV block is involved. The P-waves associated with atrial tachycardia will be abnormal but may be difficult to identify at times. If the tachycardia involves enhanced automaticity, the atrial rate is usually less than 200 per minute, with P-waves that are upright and pointed, precede the QRS, and often are superimposed on the preceding T-wave (in the same manner as PACs commonly occur). Both the reentry cir-

cuit and the accessory pathway involve two pathways in which the impulse is conducted to the ventricles in one and back to the atria in the other, depolarizing both atria and the ventricles simultane-

Box 7-4.	Atrial Tachycardia: Identifying ECG Features
Rhythm:	Regular
Rate:	Atrial: 140–250
	Ventricular: 140–250
P-waves:	Abnormal (often pointed); may precede the QRS, frequently obscured in preceding T-wave or may be hidden in QRS complex
PR interval:	Not measurable
QRS:	Normal (0.10 seconds or less)

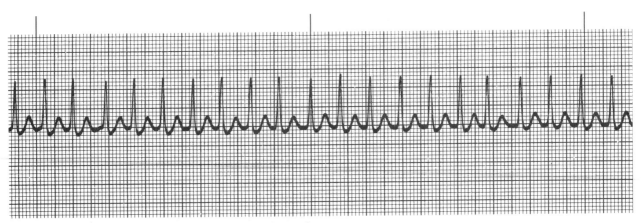

Figure 7-11. Paroxysmal Atrial Tachycardia

Rhythm: Regular

Rate: 188

P waves: Hidden

PR interval: Not measurable

QRS: 0.06 to 0.08 seconds

ously or almost simultaneously. A continuous cycle is perpetuated and rapid heart rates are attained (usually greater than 200 per minute). The P-waves associated with reentry and accessory pathway mechanisms are not easily identified, most often being hidden in the QRS complex. The acute management is the same for all types of PAT. Identification of the specific mechanism responsible for the tachycardia often requires electrophysiological testing, once the acute episode has resolved, since long-term management may be different.

The causes of atrial tachycardia are essentially the same as for premature atrial contractions. Like PACs, atrial tachycardia can occur in healthy hearts as well as in diseased hearts. Most often, atrial tachycardia occurs in patients with emotional stress, excessive intake of alcohol, caffeine, or tobacco, valvular heart disease (especially rheumatic), coronary artery disease, and digitalis toxicity.

The signs and symptoms of atrial tachycardia depend on the presence or absence of heart disease, the ventricular rate, and the duration of the tachycardia.

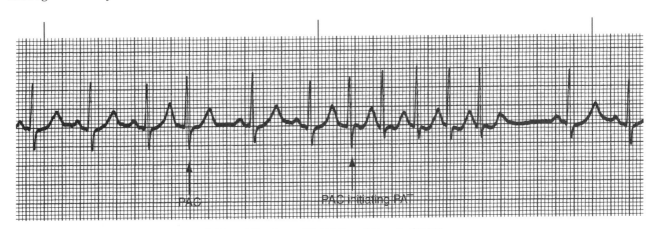

Figure 7-12. Normal Sinus Rhythm with PAC and Burst of PAT

Rhythm: Basic rhythm regular; irregular with PAC and burst of PAT

Rate: Basic rhythm rate 94; PAT rate (167)

P waves: Sinus P-waves with basic rhythm; premature, pointed P-waves with PAC and PAT (P-waves are superimposed on preceding T-waves)

PR interval: 0.16 seconds (basic rhythm)

QRS: 0.08 seconds

Comment: A run of three or more consecutive PACs is considered PAT

When the heart rate is very rapid the ventricles are unable to fill completely during diastole, causing a reduction in cardiac output and a decrease in perfusion to the brain and vital organs. In addition, rapid heart rates increase myocardial oxygen demands, resulting in an increased workload on the heart. Because of this, atrial tachycardia may increase myocardial ischemia, increase frequency and severity of chest pain, increase infarct size, cause heart failure, hypotension, and shock, or predispose the patient to more serious arrhythmias.

Priorities of treatment depend on the patient's tolerance of the rhythm. If the patient is hemodynamically stable (normotensive, normal level of consciousness, without chest pain, dyspnea, or heart failure), attempt vagal maneuvers (Valsalva maneuver, unilateral carotid massage, or having the patient take a deep breath while in a head-down tilt position). Immersing the patient's face in ice water ("diving reflex") may also be tried, but only if ischemic heart disease is not present or suspected. If vagal maneuvers fail, administer a 6 mg bolus of adenosine IV rapidly over 1–2 seconds, followed by a rapid 20 cc flush of saline or plain IV fluid. If the initial dose is ineffective after 1–2 minutes, administer a 12 mg bolus of adenosine IV rapidly over 1–2 seconds, followed by a rapid 20 cc flush of saline or plain IV fluid. If the second dose is ineffective after 1–2 minutes, repeat a 12 mg dose of adenosine in the same manner. Patients who fail to respond to adenosine can be treated with verapamil 5–10 mg IV slowly.

PAT unresponsive to drug therapy may be treated with synchronized countershock (cardioversion). Cardioversion is the initial treatment in patients who are hemodynamically unstable.

ATRIAL FLUTTER

Atrial flutter (Figures 7-13 and 7-14) (Box 7-5) is an arrhythmia arising from an ectopic pacemaker site in the atria discharging impulses at a rate of 250–400 per minute. The atrial muscles respond to this rapid stimulation by producing wave deflections called flutter (F) waves. The typical atrial flutter wave consists of an initial negative component followed by a positive component, producing V-shaped waveforms

Box 7-5.	Atrial Flutter: Identifying ECG Features
Rhythm:	Regular or irregular (depends on AV conduction ratios)
Rate:	Atrial rate: 250–400
	Ventricular rate: Varies with number of impulses conducted through AV node; will be less than the atrial rate
P-waves:	V-shaped (sawtooth) waveforms called flutter (F) waves
PR:	Not measurable
QRS:	Normal (0.10 seconds or less)

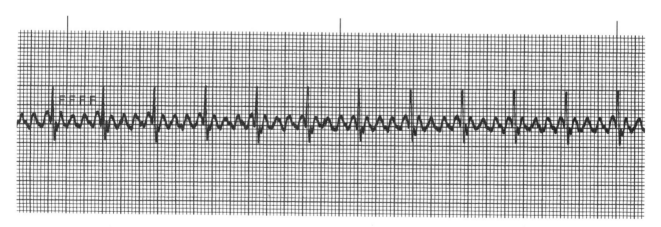

Figure 7-13. **Atrial Flutter with 4 : 1 AV Conduction**

Rhythm: Regular

Rate: Atrial: 428
Ventricular: 107
Note: If the ventricular rate is regular, multiply the number of flutter waves before each QRS × the ventricular rate to determine atrial rate.

P waves: Four flutter waves before each QRS (marked as F-waves above)

PR interval: Not measurable

QRS: 0.06 to 0.08 seconds

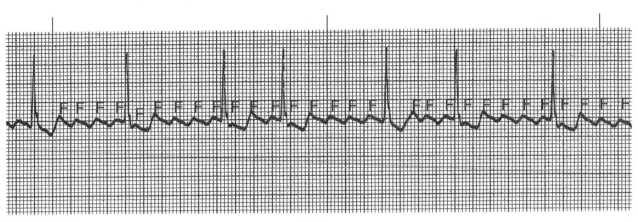

Figure 7-14 Atrial Flutter with Variable AV Conduction

Rhythm: Irregular

Rate: Atrial: 280
Ventricular: 60
Note: If the ventricular rate is irregular, count the number of flutter waves in a
6-second strip and multiply × 10 to obtain atrial rate.

P waves: Flutter waves before each QRS (varying ratios)

PR interval: Not measurable

QRS: 0.06 to 0.08 seconds

with a sawtooth appearance. The sawtooth waves affect the whole baseline to such a degree that there is no isoelectric line between the F waves, and the T-wave is completely or partially obscured by the flutter waves. Atrial flutter is primarily recognized by this sawtooth baseline. The QRS complexes are usually narrow as long as conduction in the ventricles is normal.

The AV node is bombarded by the rapid atrial impulses but will only conduct some of the impulses to the ventricles. The rest are not conducted. The AV node conducts the impulses in various ratios. For example, the AV node might allow every second impulse to travel through the AV junction to the ventricles, resulting in a 2:1 AV conduction ratio (a 2:1 conduction ratio indicates that for every two flutter waves, one is followed by a QRS). Even ratios (2:1, 4:1) are more common than odd ratios (3:1, 5:1). If the conduction ratio remains constant (e.g., 2:1), the ventricular rhythm will be regular, and the rhythm is described as atrial flutter with 2:1 AV conduction. If the conduction ratio varies (from 4:1 to 2:1 to 6:1, and so forth), the ventricular rhythm will be irregular, and the rhythm is described as atrial flutter with variable AV conduction. In atrial flutter the ventricular rate is slower than the atrial rate, with the rate depending on the number of impulses conducted through the AV node to the ventricles.

Atrial flutter is rarely seen in people with normal hearts. It can occur in patients with valvular (especially rheumatic) heart disease, coronary heart disease, hypertensive heart disease, cardiomyopathy, hyperthyroidism, hypoxia, heart failure, pericarditis, myocarditis, pulmonary disease, pulmonary emboli, and after cardiac surgery.

The signs, symptoms and clinical significance of atrial flutter with a rapid ventricular response are the same as those for atrial tachycardia. Pharmacologic therapy may include drugs to slow impulse conduction through the AV node (digitalis, beta-blockers, calcium-channel blockers) and, in some cases, the addition of antiarrhythmics in an attempt to convert the rhythm or to slow the firing rate of the ectopic atrial focus. In many patients atrial flutter will persist despite pharmacologic therapy and, for this reason, cardioversion is the initial treatment of choice. Cardioversion promptly and effectively restores sinus rhythm, often requiring relatively low energy levels (starting at 50 joules).

ATRIAL FIBRILLATION

Atrial fibrillation (Figures 7-15 and 7-16) (Box 7-6) is an arrhythmia arising from ectopic foci in the atrium discharging impulses at a rate of 400 or more. These impulses are so rapid that they cause the atria to quiver instead of contract regularly, producing irregular, wavy deflections of varying shapes, amplitudes, and directions. These wavy deflections are called fibrillatory (f) waves. If the waves are small they are called fine fibrillatory waves. If large, they

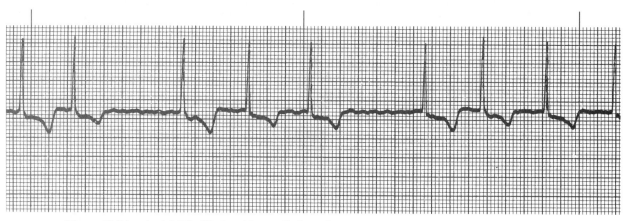

Figure 7-15. **Atrial Fibrillation (Controlled rate)**

Rhythm: Irregular

Rate: Ventricular rate 70

P waves: Fibrillatory waves present

PR interval: Not measurable

QRS: 0.04 to 0.06 seconds

Comment: ST segment depression and T wave inversion are present

are called coarse fibrillatory waves. Like atrial flutter, the wavy deflections seen in atrial fibrillation affect the whole baseline. Flutter waves are sometimes seen mixed with the fibrillatory waves. This mixed rhythm is often called atrial fib-flutter. The QRS complexes are usually narrow as long as conduction in the ventricles is normal.

As in atrial flutter the AV node is being bombarded by these rapid atrial impulses, but is refractory to most of the impulses and allows only a fraction to reach the ventricles. Characteristically, the ventricular rate is grossly irregular because the AV junction is being stimulated in an apparently random fashion by the rapidly fibrillating atria. The ventricular rate is slower than the atrial rate and will depend on the number of impulses conducted through the AV node to the ventricles. When the ventricular rate is less than 100 per minute, the rhythm is called controlled atrial fibrillation. When the ventricular rate is greater than 100 per minute, the rhythm is called uncontrolled atrial fibrillation, or atrial fibrillation with a rapid ventricular response. Atrial fibrillation is primarily recognized by the wavy baseline and the grossly irregular ventricular rhythm (unless the ventricular rate is very rapid, in which case the rhythm becomes more regular).

Atrial fibrillation can occur in normal individuals or in those with a variety of cardiac diseases. In normal individuals the rhythm is usually temporary, lasting only a few hours or days, and may be associated with emotional stress or excessive alcohol consumption. This type of atrial fib often spontaneously reverts to sinus rhythm or is easily converted with

Box 7-6.   Atrial Fibrillation: Identifying ECG Features

Rhythm:	Grossly irregular (unless the ventricular rate is very rapid, in which case the rhythm becomes more regular)
Rate:	Atrial rate: 400 or more—unmeasurable on surface ECG
	Ventricular rate: varies with number of impulses conducted through AV node to ventricles
P waves:	Wavy deflections called fibrillatory (f) waves which occur irregularly and are of varying shapes, amplitudes, and directions
PR:	Unmeasurable
QRS:	Normal (0.10 seconds or less)

pharmacologic therapy alone. In other individuals the rhythm is chronic and may persist indefinitely. Chronic atrial fibrillation is associated with valvular heart disease, hypertensive or coronary heart disease, cardiomyopathy, myocarditis, pericarditis, heart failure, hyperthyroidism, pulmonary disease, and following cardiac surgery.

The signs, symptoms, and clinical significance of atrial fibrillation with a rapid ventricular response are the same as those of atrial tachycardia. In addition, in atrial fibrillation, the atria can be visualized as quivering chambers which do not contract normally and fill the ventricles with blood during the last part of diastole, thus losing an important atrial

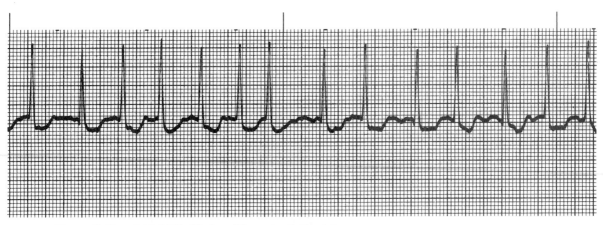

Figure 7-16. Atrial Fibrillation (Uncontrolled rate)

Rhythm: Irregular

Rate: Ventricular rate 130

P waves: Fibrillatory waves present

PR interval: Not measurable

QRS: 0.06 to 0.08 seconds

Comment: ST segment depression is present

contribution to cardiac output called the "atrial kick." Loss of the atrial kick causes a reduction in cardiac output by as much as 25%. Hemodynamically, the most significant effect of atrial fibrillation is decreased cardiac output. Decreased cardiac output in atrial fib is related to the rapid ventricular rate as well as to the loss of the atrial kick. The noncontracting atria also tend to pool blood in the atrial chambers, increasing the potential for thrombus formation and placing the patient at risk for systemic thromboembolism, particularly stroke.

Treatment of atrial fibrillation includes controlling the ventricular rate, returning the atria to a sinus rhythm, and providing anticoagulation for prophylaxis of systemic thromboembolism. Priorities of treatment depend on the patient's tolerance of the rhythm. For patients who are stable, the rhythm can be treated with

digitalis, beta-blockers, or calcium-channel blockers, all of which act by slowing conduction through the AV node. If sinus rhythm is not restored following rate slowing, an attempt to do so using antiarrhythmics or electrical cardioversion may be made. Cardioversion is the initial treatment of choice if the patient is hemodynamically unstable. Attempts to convert atrial fibrillation to sinus rhythm with either pharmacologic therapy or electrical countershock should not be made unless the patient is sufficiently anticoagulated. Restoration of normal atrial contraction can cause dislodgement of an atrial thrombus, resulting in systemic embolization. Patients with chronic atrial fibrillation (present for months or years) may not convert to sinus rhythm with any therapy. Treatment of these patients should be directed at controlling the ventricular rate and providing anticoagulation.

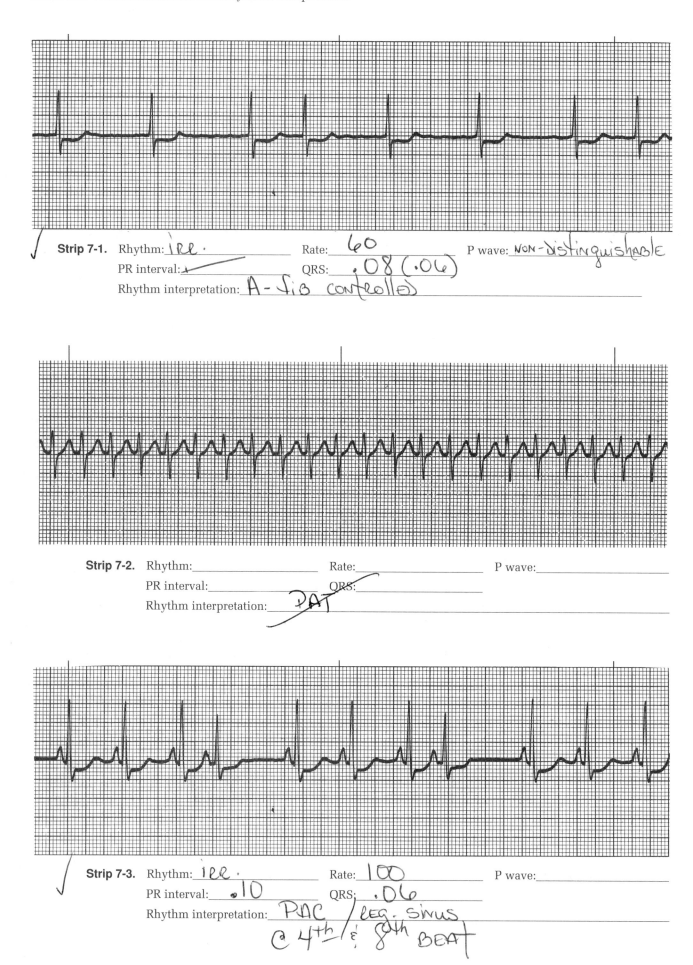

Strip 7-1. Rhythm: _irr._   Rate: _60_   P wave: _NON-distinguishable_

PR interval: _____   QRS: _.08 (.06)_

Rhythm interpretation: _A-fib controlled_

Strip 7-2. Rhythm: _____   Rate: _____   P wave: _____

PR interval: _____   QRS: _____

Rhythm interpretation: _PAT_

Strip 7-3. Rhythm: _irr._   Rate: _100_   P wave: _____

PR interval: _.10_   QRS: _.06_

Rhythm interpretation: _PAC / reg. sinus_
@ 4th & 8th beat

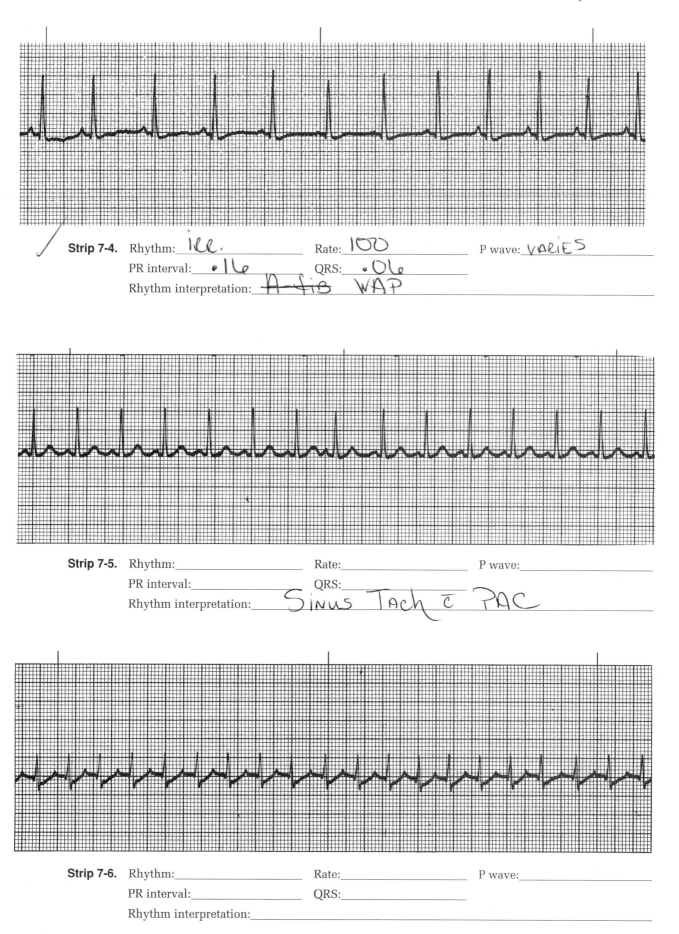

Strip 7-4. Rhythm: _irr._   Rate: _100_   P wave: _VARiES_

PR interval: _.16_   QRS: _.06_

Rhythm interpretation: _A-fib WAP_

Strip 7-5. Rhythm:_____   Rate:_____   P wave:_____

PR interval:_____   QRS:_____

Rhythm interpretation: _Sinus Tach c̄ PAC_

Strip 7-6. Rhythm:_____   Rate:_____   P wave:_____

PR interval:_____   QRS:_____

Rhythm interpretation:_____

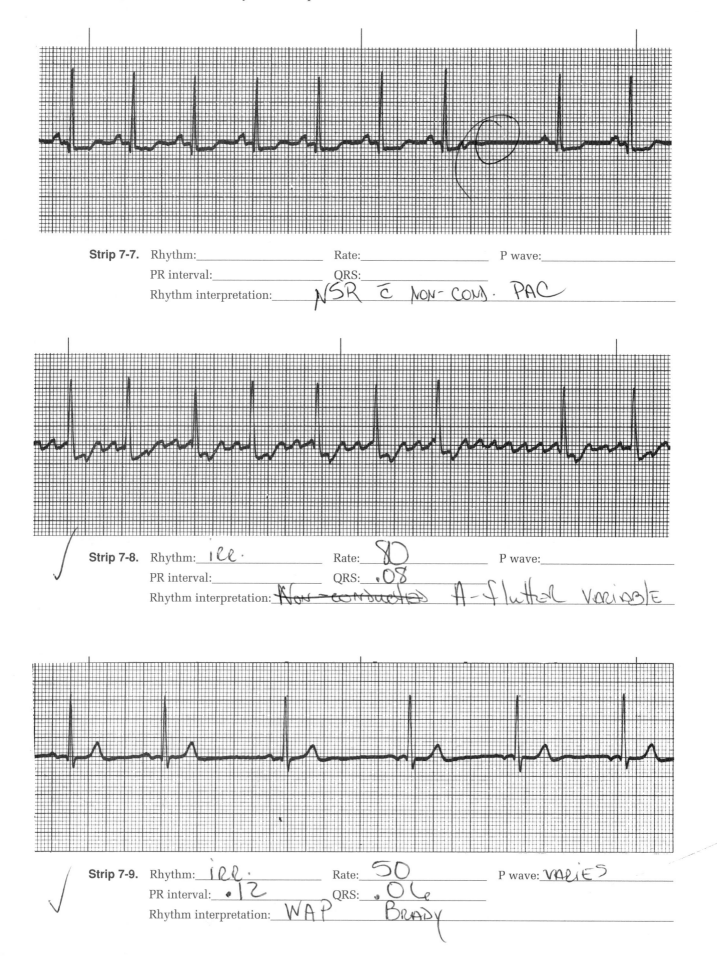

Strip 7-7. Rhythm:_____ Rate:_____ P wave:_____

PR interval:_____ QRS:_____

Rhythm interpretation:___ NSR c̄ NON-COND. PAC___

Strip 7-8. Rhythm:__iʀʀ.___ Rate:__80___ P wave:_____

PR interval:_____ QRS:__.08___

Rhythm interpretation:___Non-conducted A-flutter variable___

Strip 7-9. Rhythm:__iʀʀ.___ Rate:__50___ P wave: VARIES___

PR interval:__.12___ QRS:__.06___

Rhythm interpretation:___WAP   BRADY___

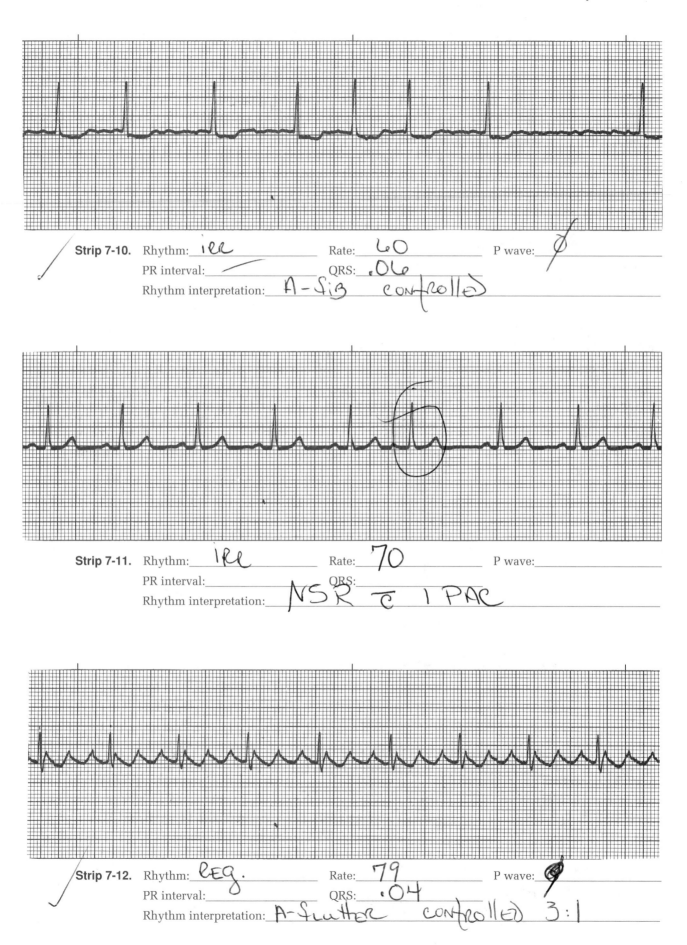

Strip 7-10. Rhythm: irr Rate: 60 P wave: Ø
PR interval: ___ QRS: .06
Rhythm interpretation: A-fib controlled

Strip 7-11. Rhythm: irr Rate: 70 P wave: ___
PR interval: ___ QRS: ___
Rhythm interpretation: NSR c̄ 1 PAC

Strip 7-12. Rhythm: Reg. Rate: 79 P wave: Ø
PR interval: ___ QRS: .04
Rhythm interpretation: A-flutter controlled 3:1

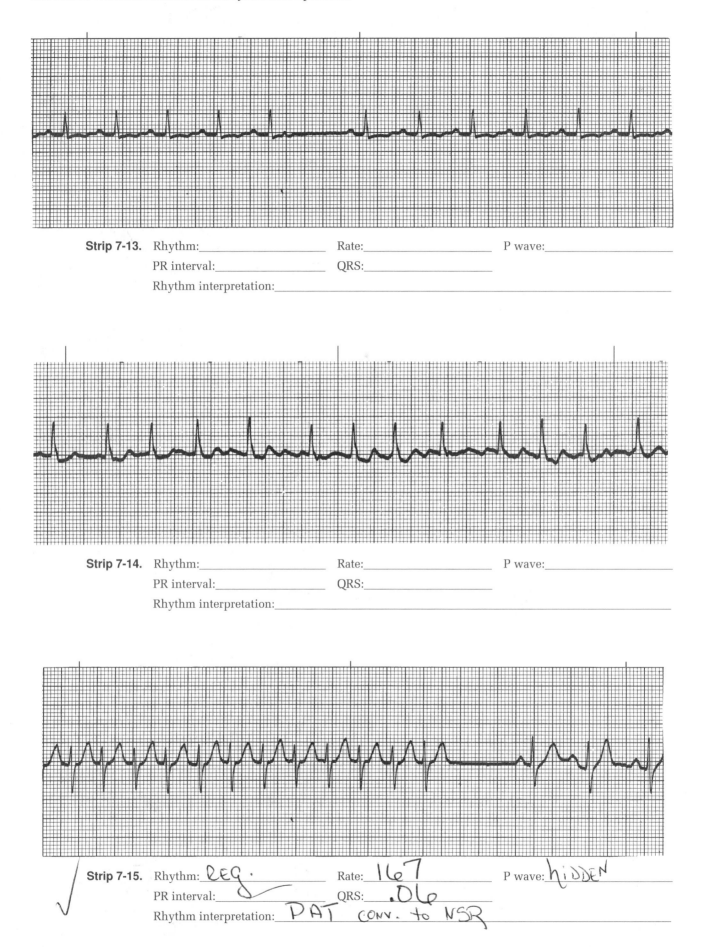

Strip 7-13. Rhythm:_____ Rate:_____ P wave:_____

PR interval:_____ QRS:_____

Rhythm interpretation:_____

Strip 7-14. Rhythm:_____ Rate:_____ P wave:_____

PR interval:_____ QRS:_____

Rhythm interpretation:_____

Strip 7-15. Rhythm: REG. Rate: 167 P wave: hiDDEN

PR interval: QRS: .06

Rhythm interpretation: PAT conv. to NSR

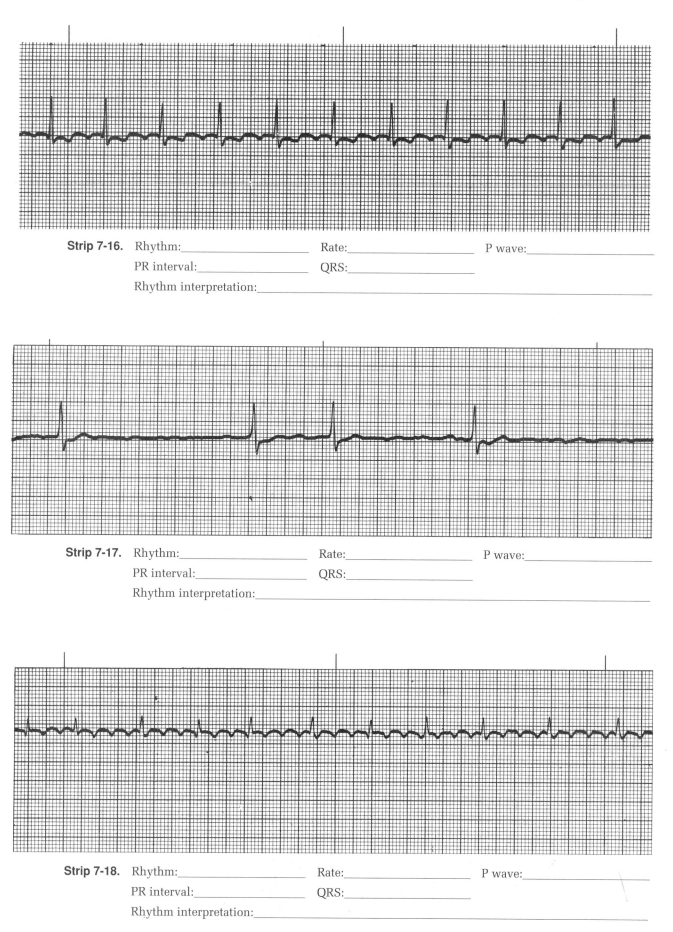

Strip 7-16. Rhythm:_____ Rate:_____ P wave:_____

PR interval:_____ QRS:_____

Rhythm interpretation:_____

Strip 7-17. Rhythm:_____ Rate:_____ P wave:_____

PR interval:_____ QRS:_____

Rhythm interpretation:_____

Strip 7-18. Rhythm:_____ Rate:_____ P wave:_____

PR interval:_____ QRS:_____

Rhythm interpretation:_____

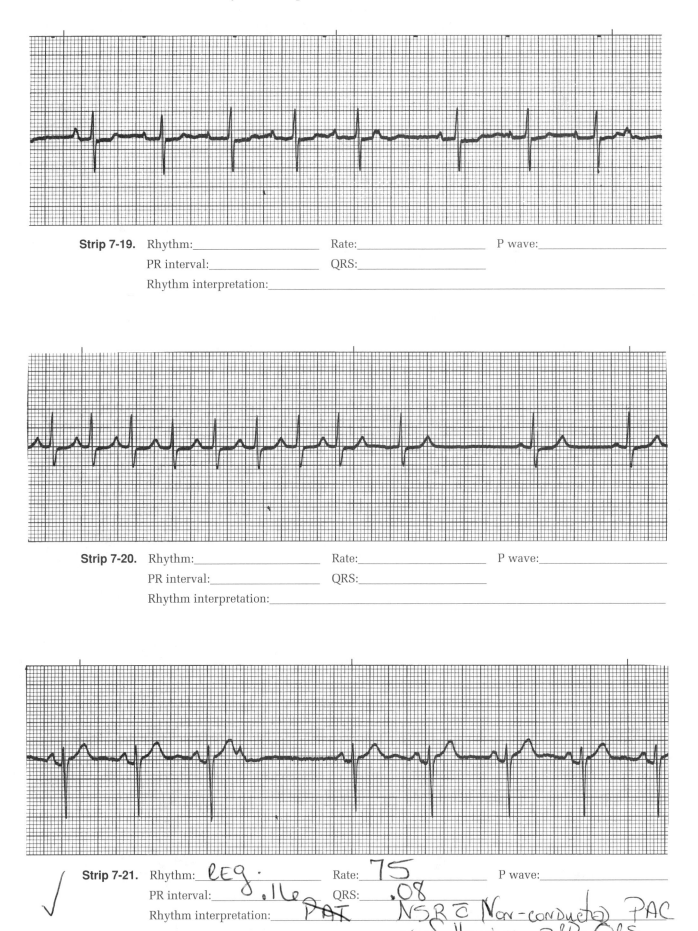

Strip 7-19. Rhythm:_____ Rate:_____ P wave:_____

PR interval:_____ QRS:_____

Rhythm interpretation:_____

Strip 7-20. Rhythm:_____ Rate:_____ P wave:_____

PR interval:_____ QRS:_____

Rhythm interpretation:_____

√ **Strip 7-21.** Rhythm: reg. Rate: 75 P wave:_____

PR interval: .16 QRS: .08

Rhythm interpretation: PAT NSR c̄ Non-conducted PAC following 3rd QRS

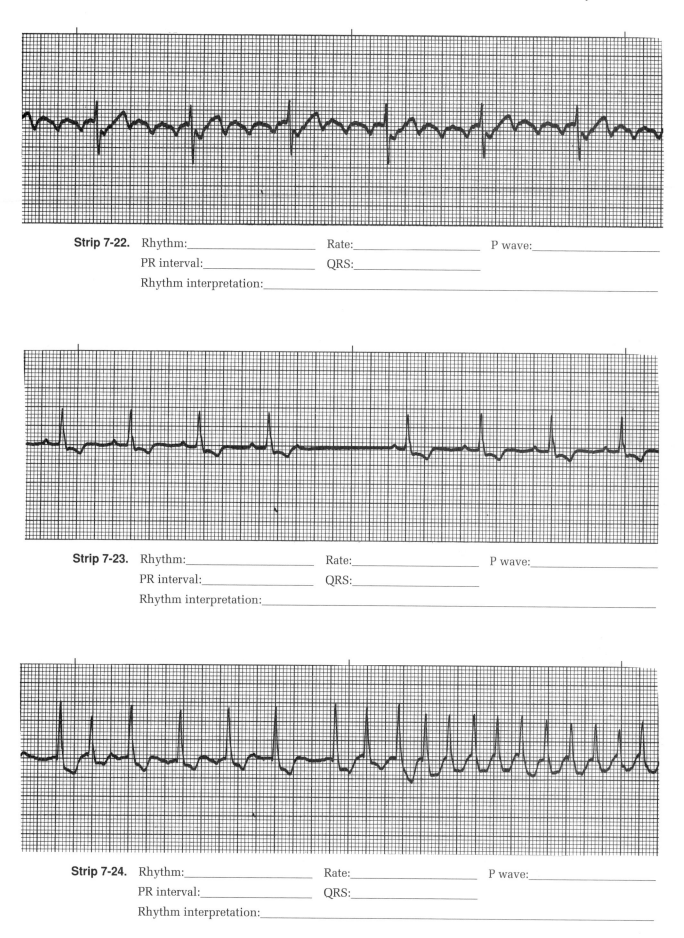

Strip 7-22. Rhythm:_____ Rate:_____ P wave:_____

PR interval:_____ QRS:_____

Rhythm interpretation:_____

Strip 7-23. Rhythm:_____ Rate:_____ P wave:_____

PR interval:_____ QRS:_____

Rhythm interpretation:_____

Strip 7-24. Rhythm:_____ Rate:_____ P wave:_____

PR interval:_____ QRS:_____

Rhythm interpretation:_____

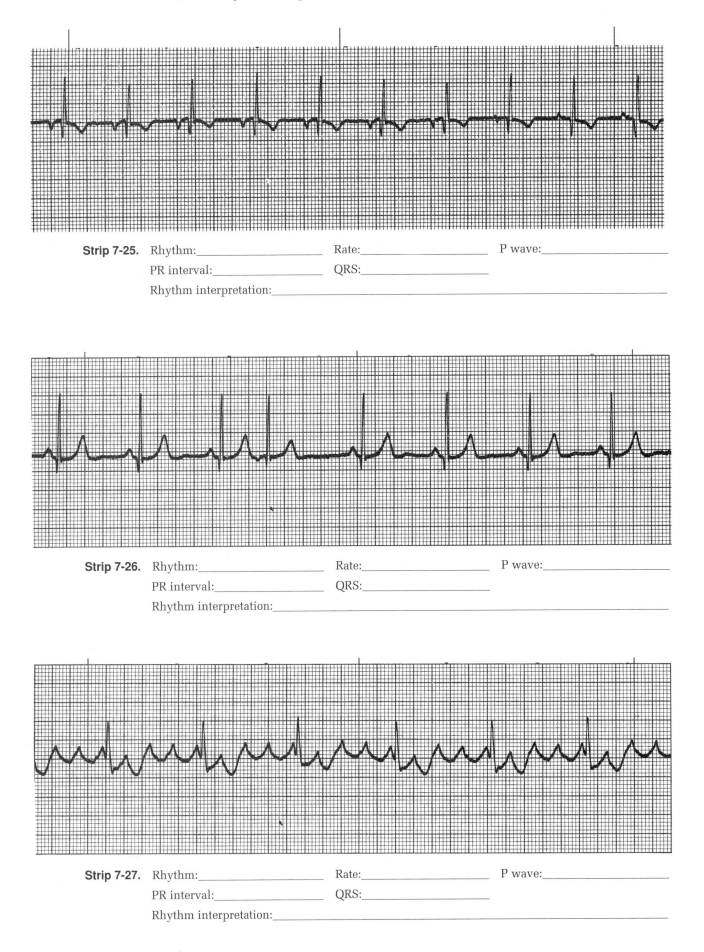

Strip 7-25. Rhythm:_____ Rate:_____ P wave:_____

PR interval:_____ QRS:_____

Rhythm interpretation:_____

Strip 7-26. Rhythm:_____ Rate:_____ P wave:_____

PR interval:_____ QRS:_____

Rhythm interpretation:_____

Strip 7-27. Rhythm:_____ Rate:_____ P wave:_____

PR interval:_____ QRS:_____

Rhythm interpretation:_____

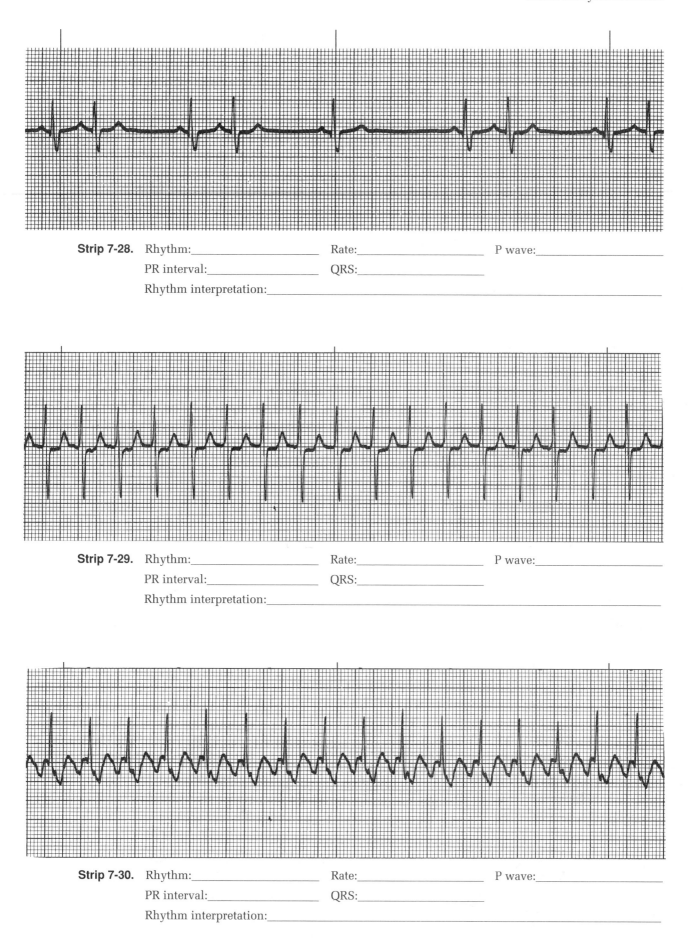

Strip 7-28. Rhythm:_____ Rate:_____ P wave:_____

PR interval:_____ QRS:_____

Rhythm interpretation:_____

Strip 7-29. Rhythm:_____ Rate:_____ P wave:_____

PR interval:_____ QRS:_____

Rhythm interpretation:_____

Strip 7-30. Rhythm:_____ Rate:_____ P wave:_____

PR interval:_____ QRS:_____

Rhythm interpretation:_____

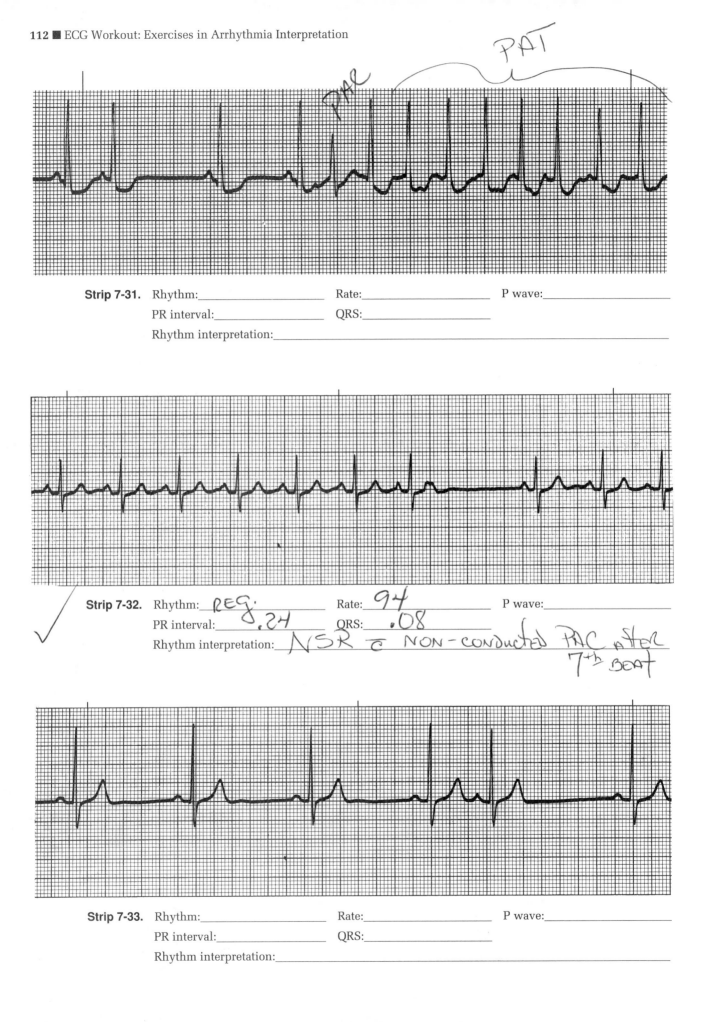

PAC

PAT

Strip 7-31. Rhythm:_____ Rate:_____ P wave:_____

PR interval:_____ QRS:_____

Rhythm interpretation:_____

Strip 7-32. Rhythm: _REG._ Rate: _94_ P wave:_____

PR interval: _0.24_ QRS: _.08_

Rhythm interpretation: _NSR c̄ NON-CONDUCTED PAC After 7th BEAT_

Strip 7-33. Rhythm:_____ Rate:_____ P wave:_____

PR interval:_____ QRS:_____

Rhythm interpretation:_____

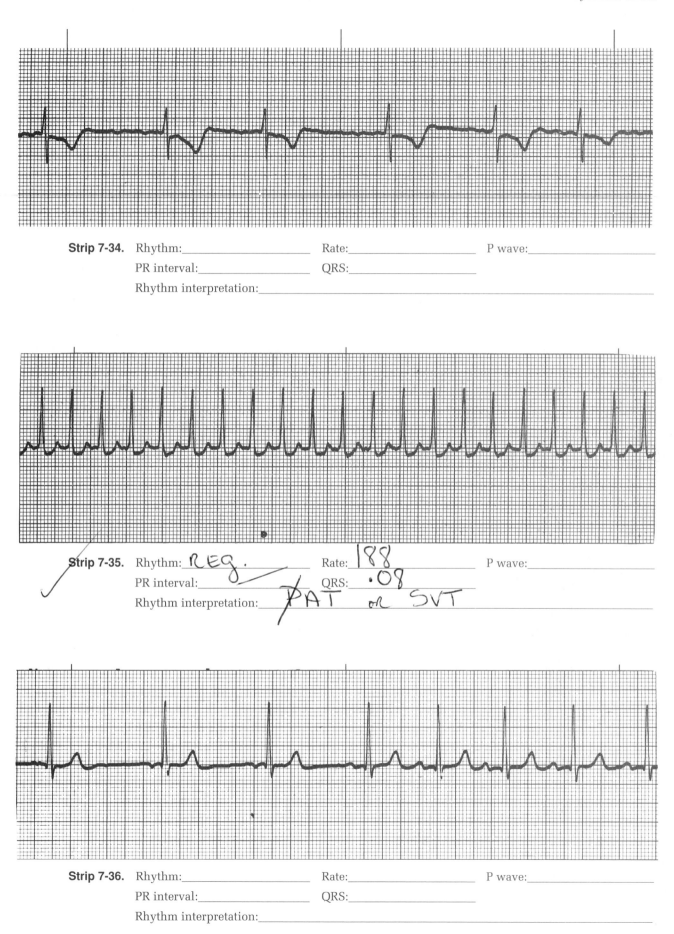

Strip 7-34. Rhythm:_____ Rate:_____ P wave:_____

PR interval:_____ QRS:_____

Rhythm interpretation:_____

Strip 7-35. Rhythm: REG._____ Rate: 188_____ P wave:_____

PR interval:_____0_____ QRS: .08_____

Rhythm interpretation: PAT or SVT_____

Strip 7-36. Rhythm:_____ Rate:_____ P wave:_____

PR interval:_____ QRS:_____

Rhythm interpretation:_____

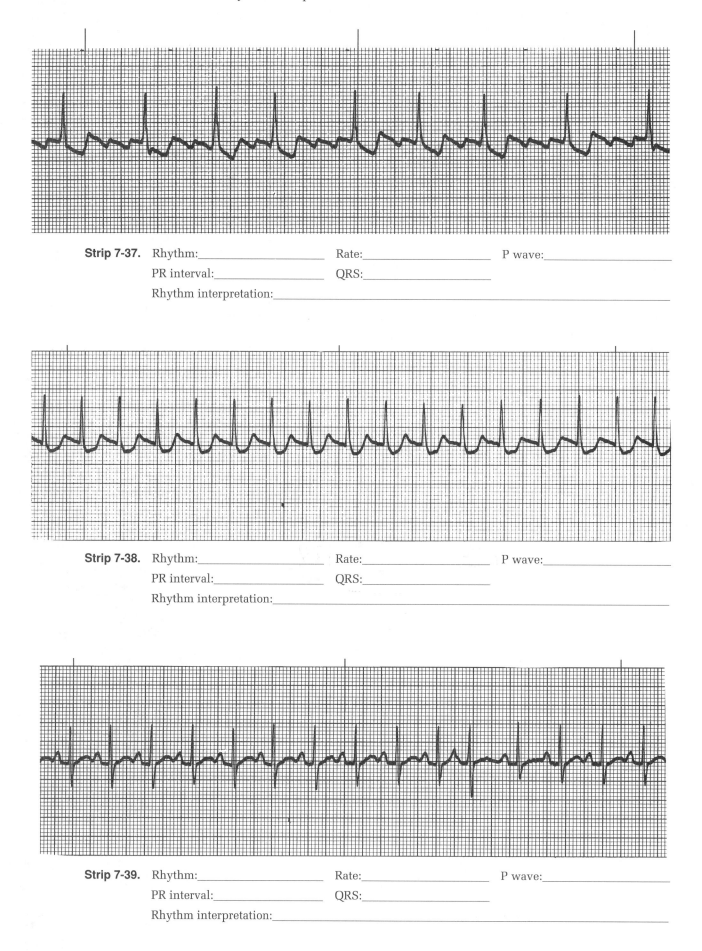

Strip 7-37. Rhythm:_____ Rate:_____ P wave:_____

PR interval:_____ QRS:_____

Rhythm interpretation:_____

Strip 7-38. Rhythm:_____ Rate:_____ P wave:_____

PR interval:_____ QRS:_____

Rhythm interpretation:_____

Strip 7-39. Rhythm:_____ Rate:_____ P wave:_____

PR interval:_____ QRS:_____

Rhythm interpretation:_____

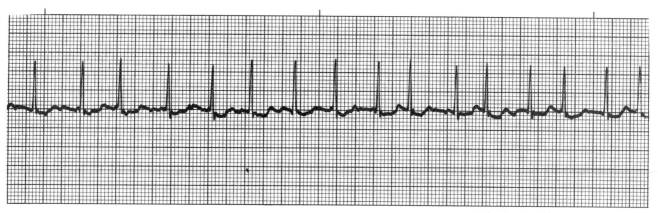

Strip 7-40. Rhythm:_____ Rate:_____ P wave:_____

PR interval:_____ QRS:_____

Rhythm interpretation:_____

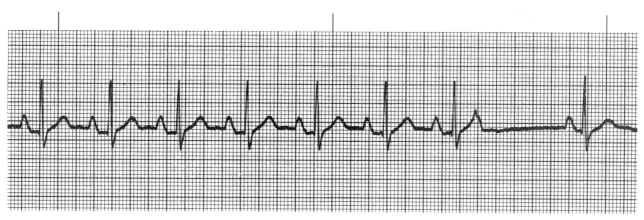

Strip 7-41. Rhythm:_____ Rate:_____ P wave:_____

PR interval:_____ QRS:_____

Rhythm interpretation:_____

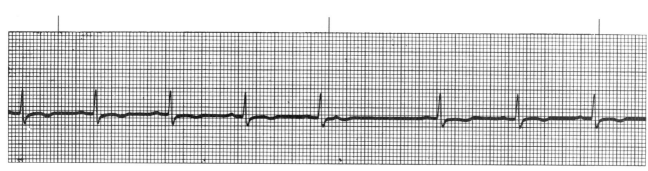

Strip 7-42. Rhythm:_____ Rate:_____ P wave:_____

PR interval:_____ QRS:_____

Rhythm interpretation:_____

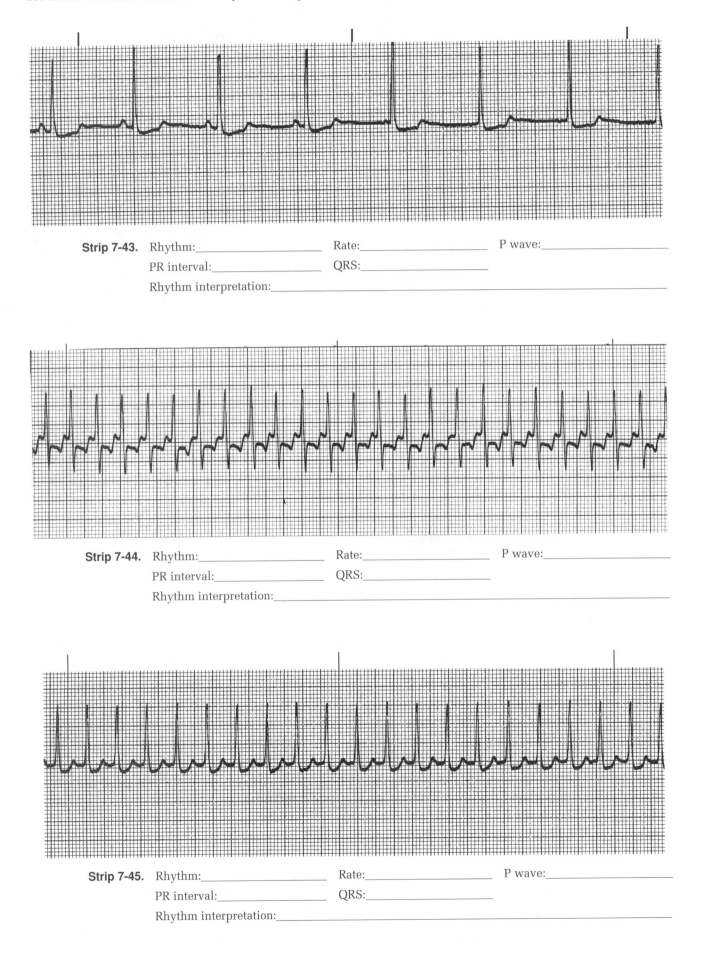

Strip 7-43. Rhythm:_____ Rate:_____ P wave:_____

PR interval:_____ QRS:_____

Rhythm interpretation:_____

Strip 7-44. Rhythm:_____ Rate:_____ P wave:_____

PR interval:_____ QRS:_____

Rhythm interpretation:_____

Strip 7-45. Rhythm:_____ Rate:_____ P wave:_____

PR interval:_____ QRS:_____

Rhythm interpretation:_____

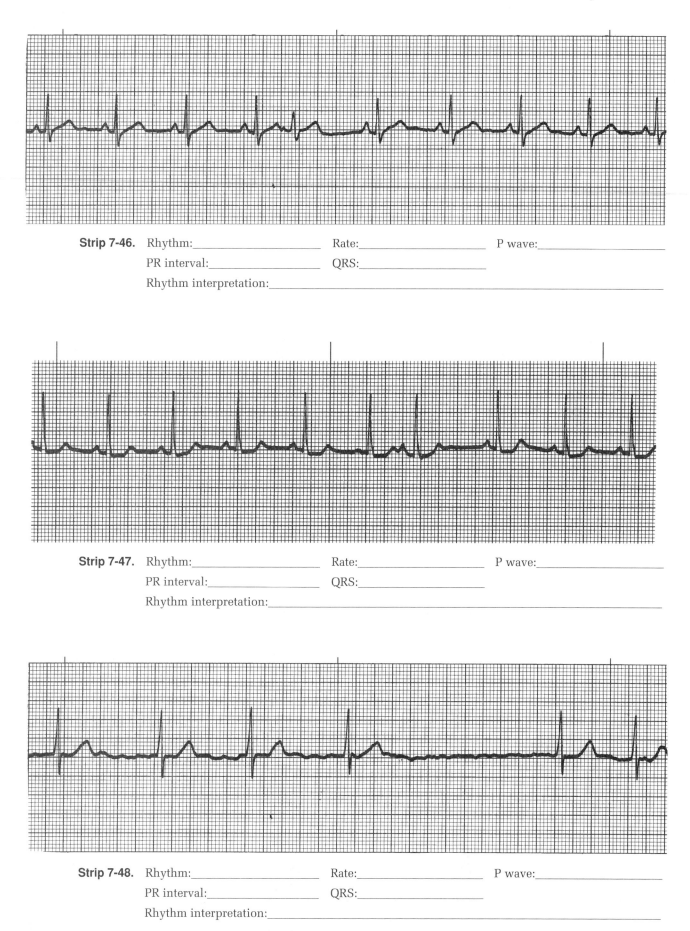

Strip 7-46. Rhythm:_____ Rate:_____ P wave:_____

PR interval:_____ QRS:_____

Rhythm interpretation:_____

Strip 7-47. Rhythm:_____ Rate:_____ P wave:_____

PR interval:_____ QRS:_____

Rhythm interpretation:_____

Strip 7-48. Rhythm:_____ Rate:_____ P wave:_____

PR interval:_____ QRS:_____

Rhythm interpretation:_____

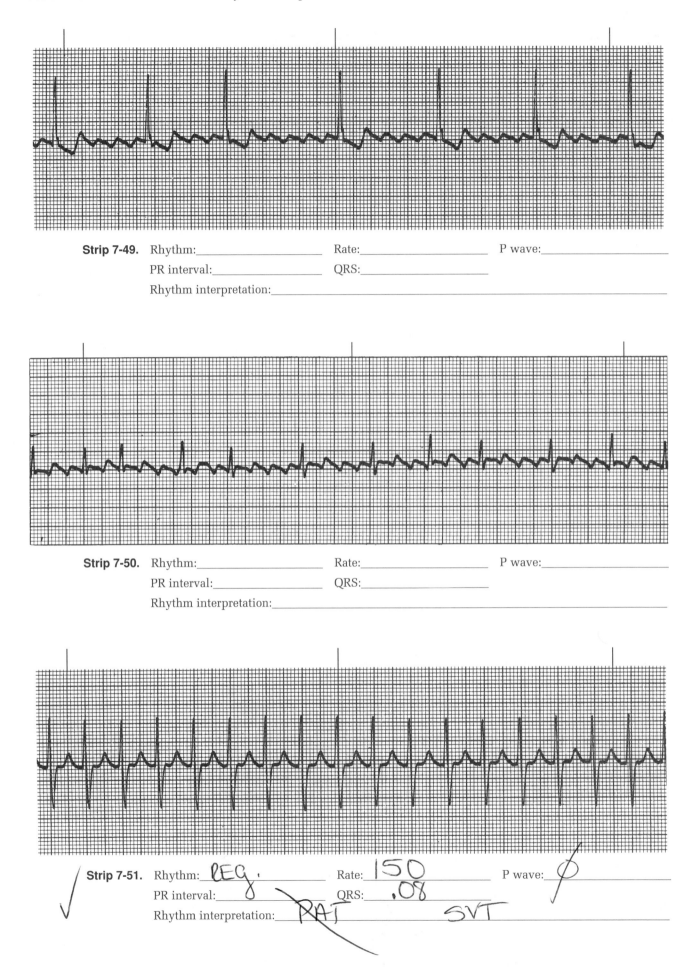

Strip 7-49. Rhythm:_____ Rate:_____ P wave:_____

PR interval:_____ QRS:_____

Rhythm interpretation:_____

Strip 7-50. Rhythm:_____ Rate:_____ P wave:_____

PR interval:_____ QRS:_____

Rhythm interpretation:_____

Strip 7-51. Rhythm: REG. Rate: 150 P wave: Ø

PR interval: Ø QRS: .08

Rhythm interpretation: PAT   SVT

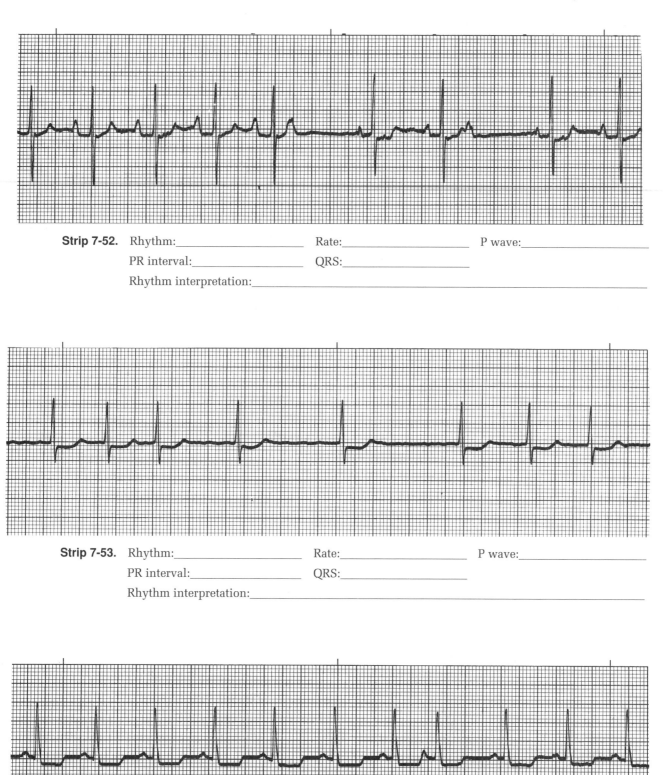

Strip 7-52. Rhythm:_____ Rate:_____ P wave:_____

PR interval:_____ QRS:_____

Rhythm interpretation:_____

Strip 7-53. Rhythm:_____ Rate:_____ P wave:_____

PR interval:_____ QRS:_____

Rhythm interpretation:_____

Strip 7-54. Rhythm:_____ Rate:_____ P wave:_____

PR interval:_____ QRS:_____

Rhythm interpretation:_____

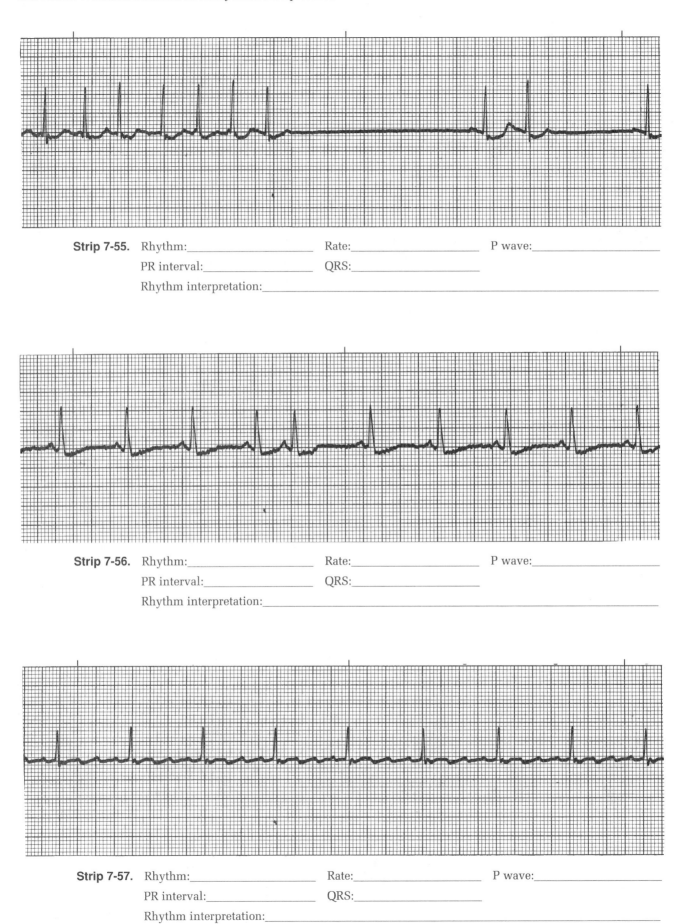

Strip 7-55. Rhythm:_____ Rate:_____ P wave:_____

PR interval:_____ QRS:_____

Rhythm interpretation:_____

Strip 7-56. Rhythm:_____ Rate:_____ P wave:_____

PR interval:_____ QRS:_____

Rhythm interpretation:_____

Strip 7-57. Rhythm:_____ Rate:_____ P wave:_____

PR interval:_____ QRS:_____

Rhythm interpretation:_____

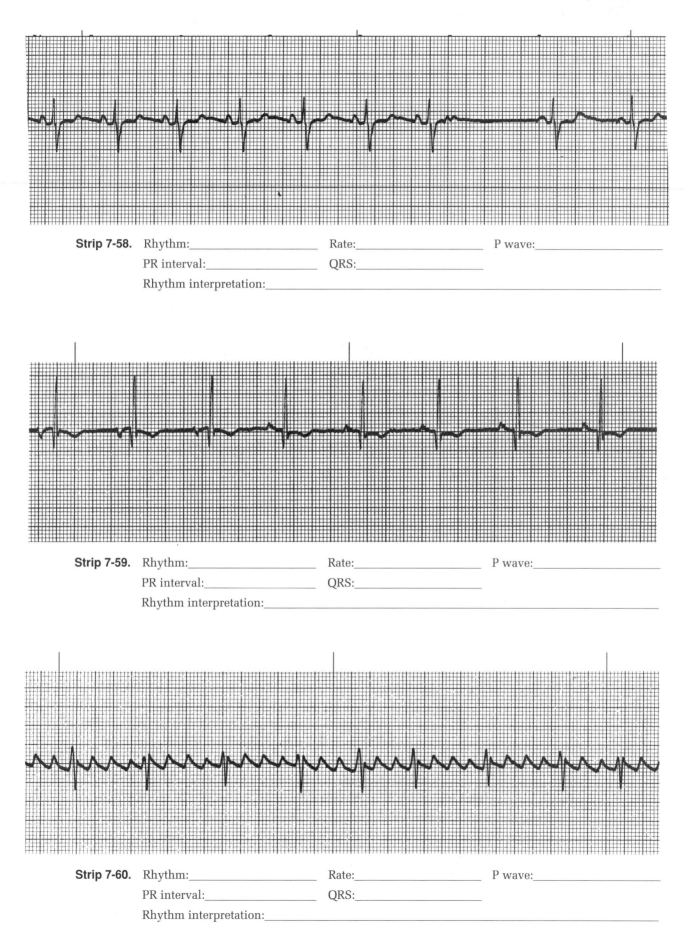

Strip 7-58. Rhythm:_____ Rate:_____ P wave:_____

PR interval:_____ QRS:_____

Rhythm interpretation:_____

Strip 7-59. Rhythm:_____ Rate:_____ P wave:_____

PR interval:_____ QRS:_____

Rhythm interpretation:_____

Strip 7-60. Rhythm:_____ Rate:_____ P wave:_____

PR interval:_____ QRS:_____

Rhythm interpretation:_____

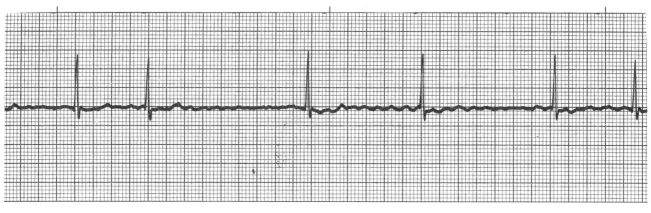

Strip 7-61. Rhythm:_____ Rate:_____ P wave:_____

PR interval:_____ QRS:_____

Rhythm interpretation:_____

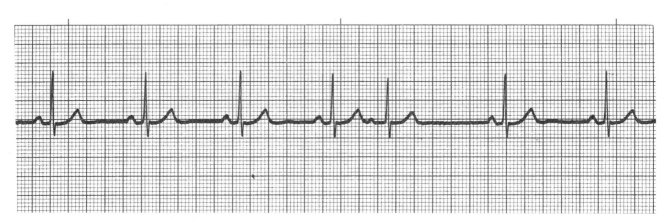

Strip 7-62. Rhythm:_____ Rate:_____ P wave:_____

PR interval:_____ QRS:_____

Rhythm interpretation:_____

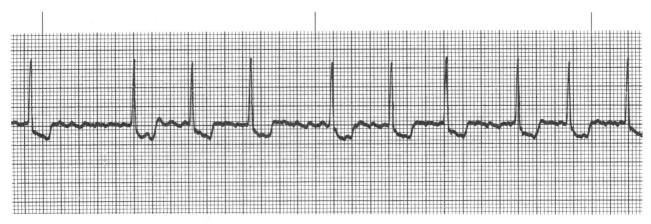

Strip 7-63. Rhythm:_____ Rate:_____ P wave:_____

PR interval:_____ QRS:_____

Rhythm interpretation:_____

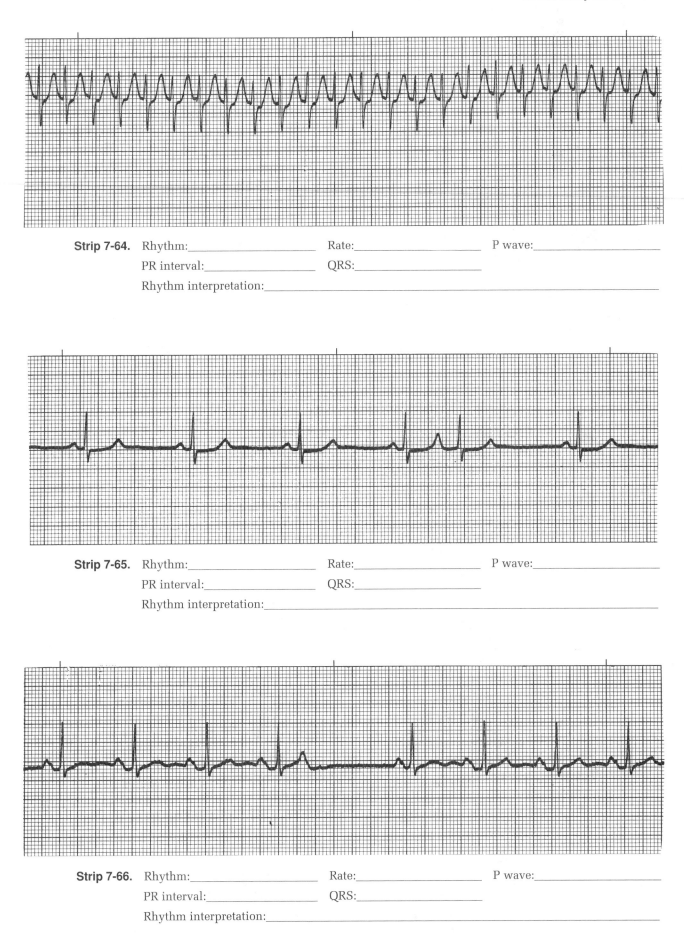

Strip 7-64. Rhythm:_____ Rate:_____ P wave:_____

PR interval:_____ QRS:_____

Rhythm interpretation:_____

Strip 7-65. Rhythm:_____ Rate:_____ P wave:_____

PR interval:_____ QRS:_____

Rhythm interpretation:_____

Strip 7-66. Rhythm:_____ Rate:_____ P wave:_____

PR interval:_____ QRS:_____

Rhythm interpretation:_____

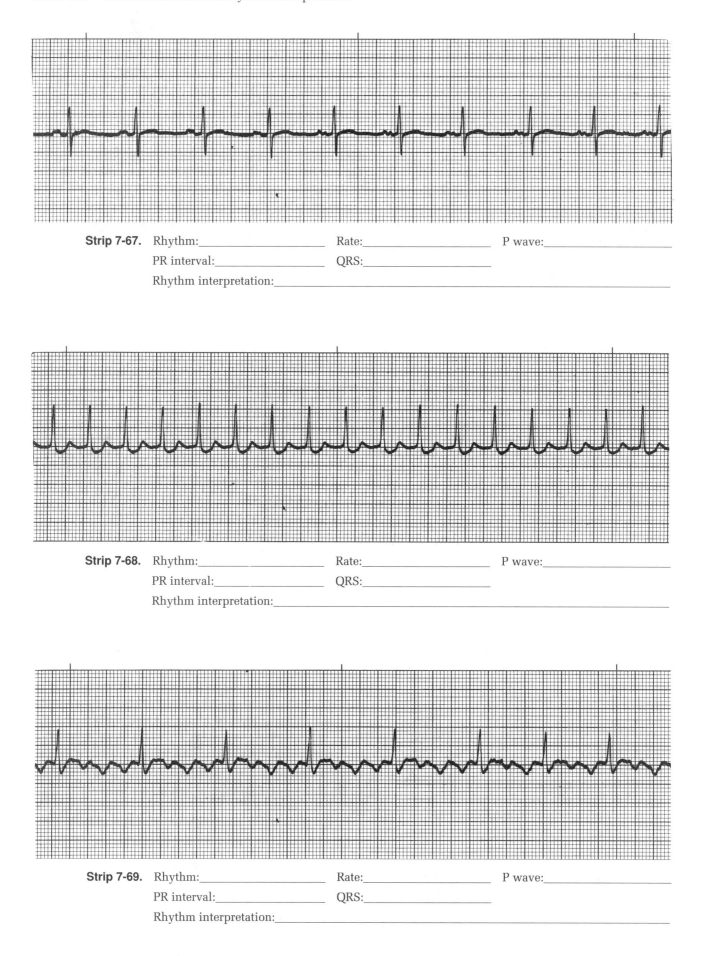

Strip 7-67. Rhythm:_____ Rate:_____ P wave:_____

PR interval:_____ QRS:_____

Rhythm interpretation:_____

Strip 7-68. Rhythm:_____ Rate:_____ P wave:_____

PR interval:_____ QRS:_____

Rhythm interpretation:_____

Strip 7-69. Rhythm:_____ Rate:_____ P wave:_____

PR interval:_____ QRS:_____

Rhythm interpretation:_____

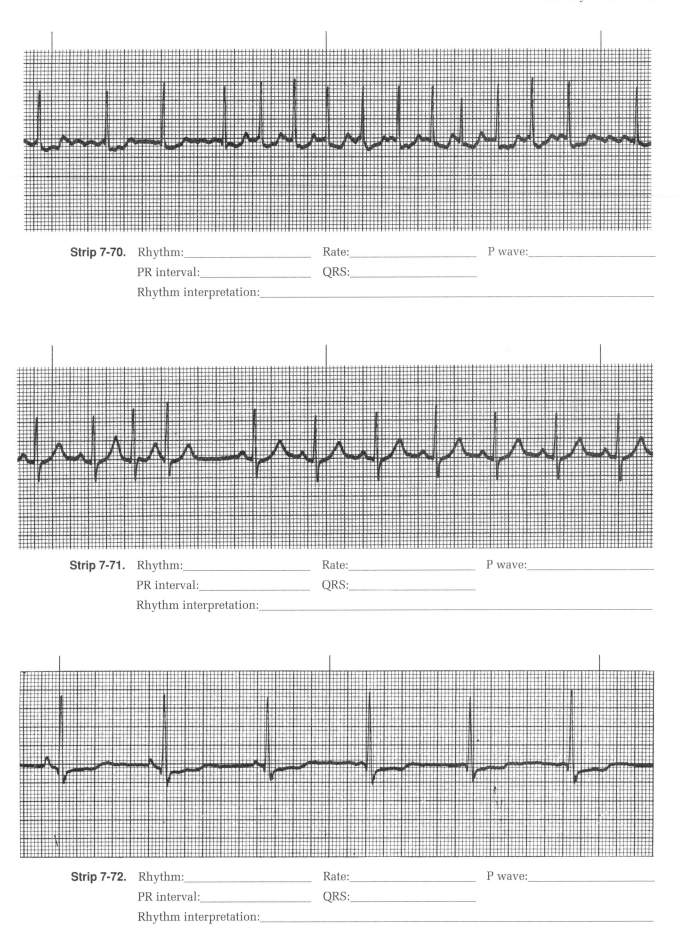

Strip 7-70. Rhythm:_____ Rate:_____ P wave:_____

PR interval:_____ QRS:_____

Rhythm interpretation:_____

Strip 7-71. Rhythm:_____ Rate:_____ P wave:_____

PR interval:_____ QRS:_____

Rhythm interpretation:_____

Strip 7-72. Rhythm:_____ Rate:_____ P wave:_____

PR interval:_____ QRS:_____

Rhythm interpretation:_____

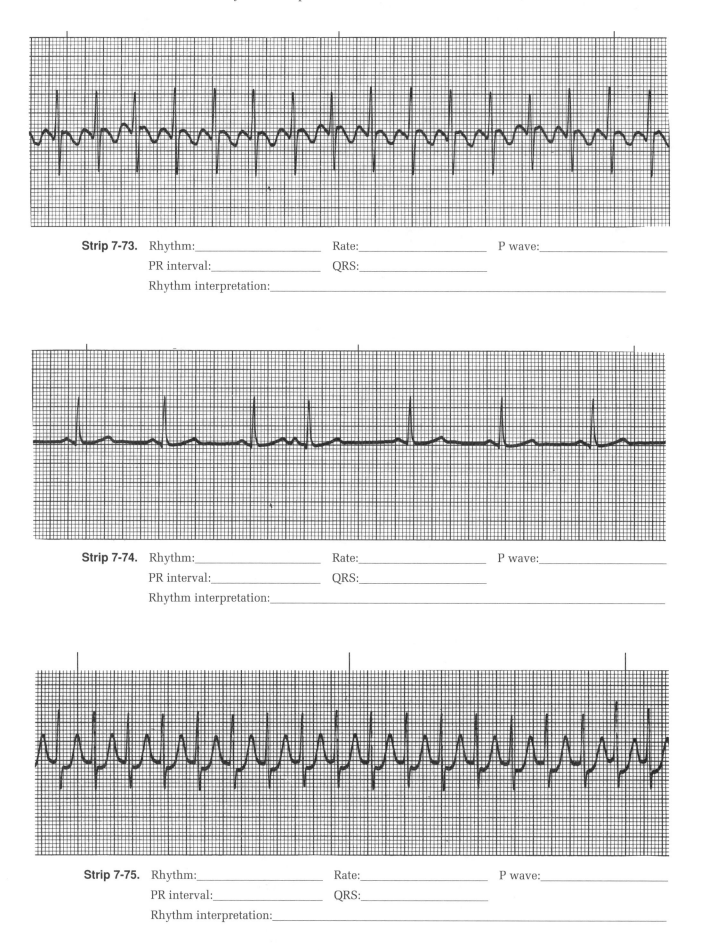

Strip 7-73. Rhythm:_____ Rate:_____ P wave:_____

PR interval:_____ QRS:_____

Rhythm interpretation:_____

Strip 7-74. Rhythm:_____ Rate:_____ P wave:_____

PR interval:_____ QRS:_____

Rhythm interpretation:_____

Strip 7-75. Rhythm:_____ Rate:_____ P wave:_____

PR interval:_____ QRS:_____

Rhythm interpretation:_____

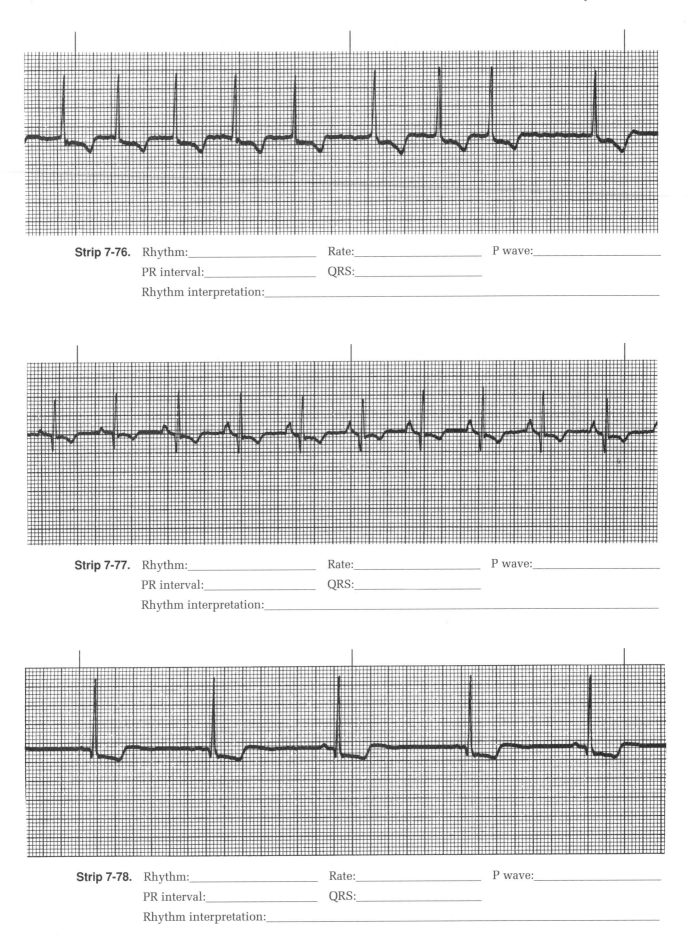

Strip 7-76. Rhythm:_____ Rate:_____ P wave:_____

PR interval:_____ QRS:_____

Rhythm interpretation:_____

Strip 7-77. Rhythm:_____ Rate:_____ P wave:_____

PR interval:_____ QRS:_____

Rhythm interpretation:_____

Strip 7-78. Rhythm:_____ Rate:_____ P wave:_____

PR interval:_____ QRS:_____

Rhythm interpretation:_____

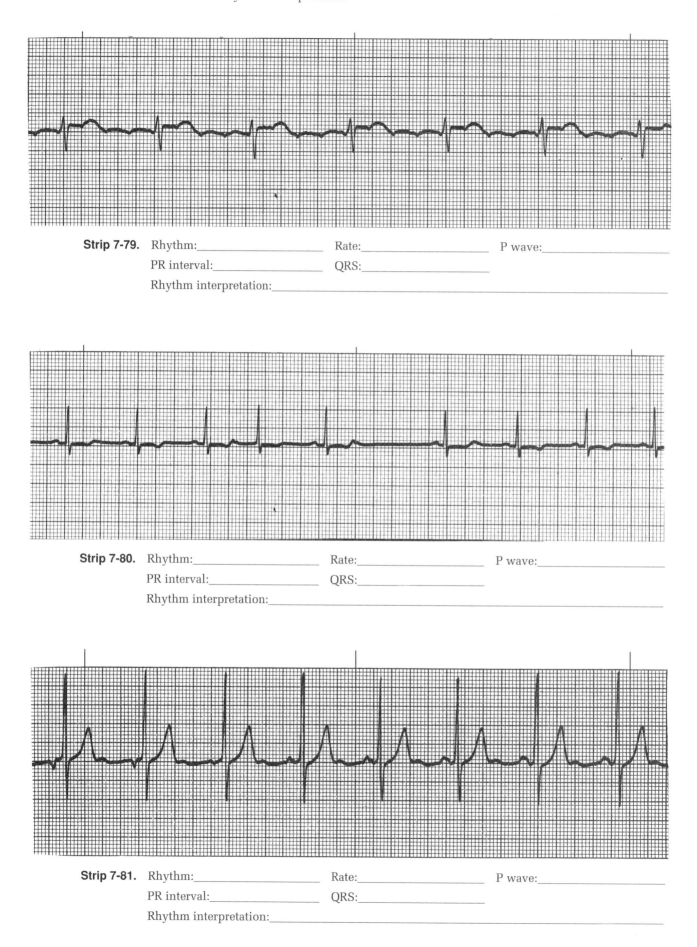

Strip 7-79. Rhythm:_____ Rate:_____ P wave:_____

PR interval:_____ QRS:_____

Rhythm interpretation:_____

Strip 7-80. Rhythm:_____ Rate:_____ P wave:_____

PR interval:_____ QRS:_____

Rhythm interpretation:_____

Strip 7-81. Rhythm:_____ Rate:_____ P wave:_____

PR interval:_____ QRS:_____

Rhythm interpretation:_____

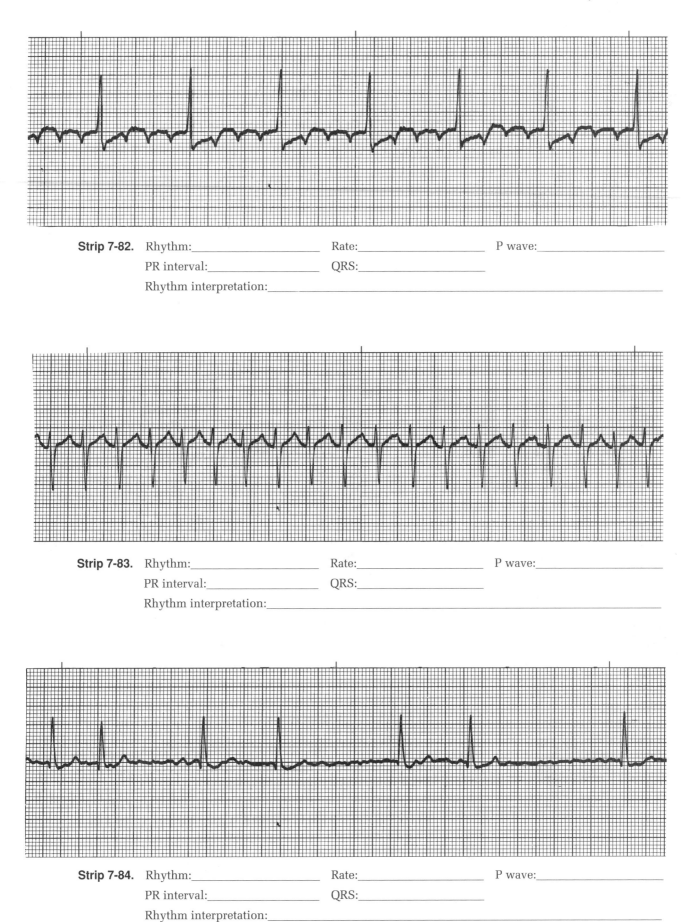

Strip 7-82. Rhythm:_____ Rate:_____ P wave:_____

PR interval:_____ QRS:_____

Rhythm interpretation:_____

Strip 7-83. Rhythm:_____ Rate:_____ P wave:_____

PR interval:_____ QRS:_____

Rhythm interpretation:_____

Strip 7-84. Rhythm:_____ Rate:_____ P wave:_____

PR interval:_____ QRS:_____

Rhythm interpretation:_____

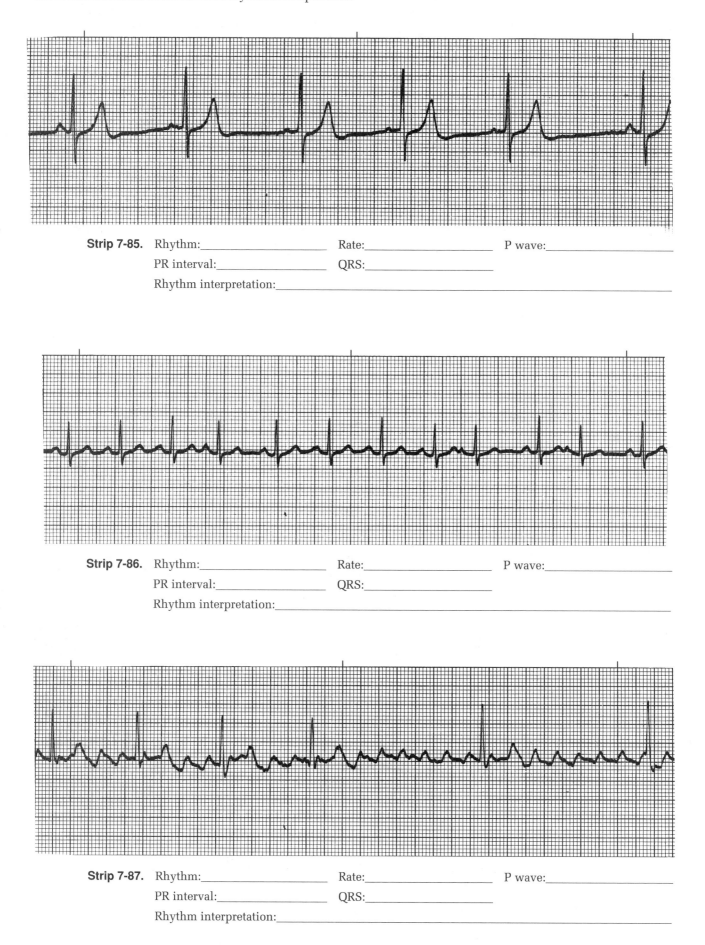

Strip 7-85. Rhythm:_____ Rate:_____ P wave:_____

PR interval:_____ QRS:_____

Rhythm interpretation:_____

Strip 7-86. Rhythm:_____ Rate:_____ P wave:_____

PR interval:_____ QRS:_____

Rhythm interpretation:_____

Strip 7-87. Rhythm:_____ Rate:_____ P wave:_____

PR interval:_____ QRS:_____

Rhythm interpretation:_____

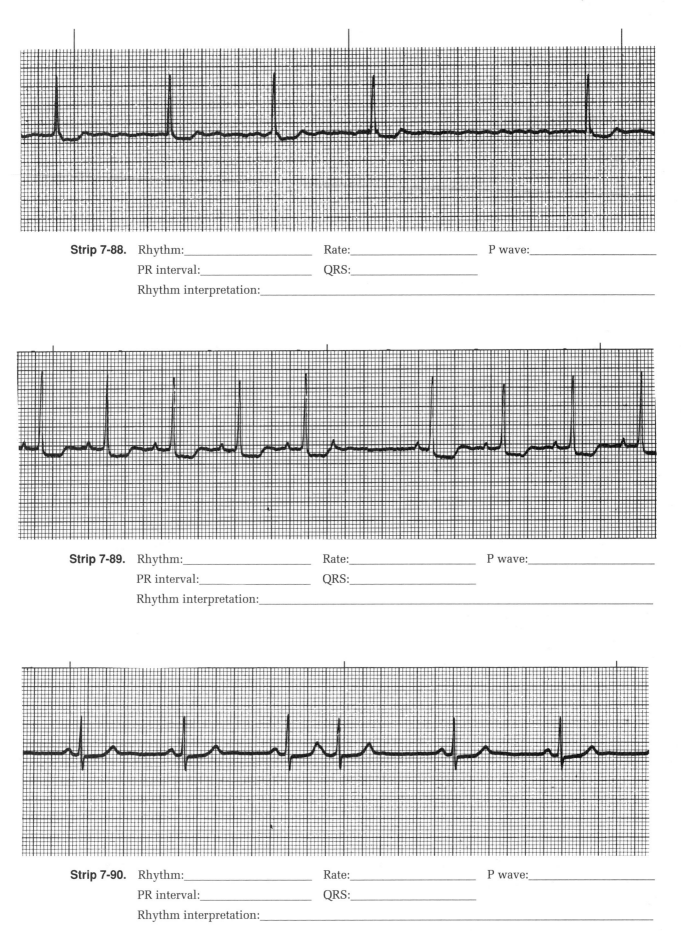

Strip 7-88. Rhythm:_____ Rate:_____ P wave:_____

PR interval:_____ QRS:_____

Rhythm interpretation:_____

Strip 7-89. Rhythm:_____ Rate:_____ P wave:_____

PR interval:_____ QRS:_____

Rhythm interpretation:_____

Strip 7-90. Rhythm:_____ Rate:_____ P wave:_____

PR interval:_____ QRS:_____

Rhythm interpretation:_____

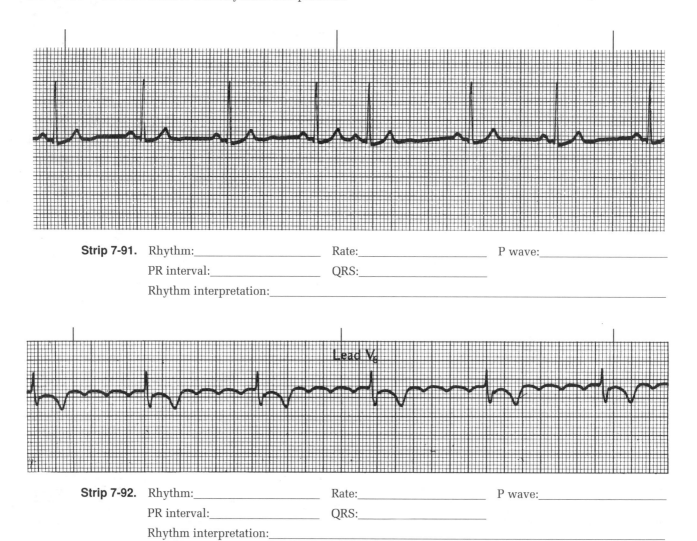

Strip 7-91. Rhythm:_____ Rate:_____ P wave:_____

PR interval:_____ QRS:_____

Rhythm interpretation:_____

Strip 7-92. Rhythm:_____ Rate:_____ P wave:_____

PR interval:_____ QRS:_____

Rhythm interpretation:_____

8

AV Junctional Arrhythmias and AV Blocks

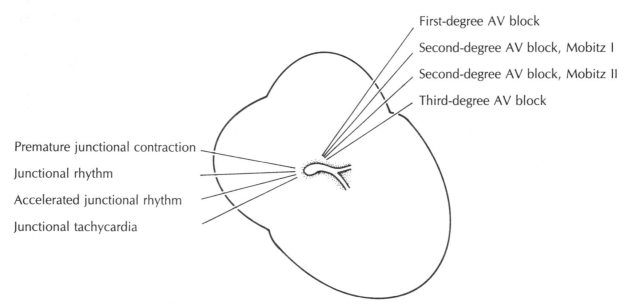

Figure 8-1. AV junctional arrhythmias and AV blocks.

AV JUNCTIONAL ARRHYTHMIAS

AV junctional arrhythmias (Figure 8-1) originate from the area in and around the AV node. The AV node contains specialized pacemaker cells and can serve as a secondary pacemaker site if the SA node fails to function properly as the primary (or dominant) pacemaker, or if conduction of the electrical impulses is blocked for some reason. The inherent firing rate of the junctional pacemaker cells is 40–60 per minute. A rhythm occurring at this rate is called a junctional rhythm. On some occasions enhanced automaticity may accelerate the rate beyond the inherent firing rate. Three arrhythmias may result from this increased activity: premature junctional contractions, accelerated junctional rhythm, and junctional tachycardia.

When the AV node is functioning as the pacemaker of the heart, the electrical impulse leaves the AV junction and is conducted backward (retrograde) to depolarize the atria, and forward (antegrade) to depolarize the ventricles. The location of the P-wave relative to the QRS will depend on the speed of antegrade and retrograde conduction:

1. If the electrical impulse from the AV junction depolarizes the atria first and then depolarizes the ventricles, the P-wave will be in front of the QRS.
2. If the electrical impulse from the AV junction depolarizes the ventricles first and then depolarizes the atria, the P-wave will be after the QRS.
3. If the electrical impulse from the AV junction depolarizes both the atria and the ventricles simultaneously, the P-wave will be hidden in the QRS.

Retrograde stimulation of the atria is just opposite the direction of atrial depolarization when normal sinus rhythm is present, and will produce negative P-waves (instead of upright) in Lead II. The PR interval will be short (0.10 seconds or less). The ventricles will be depolarized normally, resulting in a narrow QRS. Identifying features of AV junctional rhythms are shown in Figure 8-2.

Figure 8-2. Identifying features of junctional rhythms.
1. P waves inverted in Lead II
2. P waves will occur in one of three patterns:
   a. immediately before the QRS
   b. immediately after the QRS
   c. hidden within the QRS complex
3. PR interval will be short (0.10 seconds or less)
4. QRS will be normal (0.10 seconds or less)

Lead II	Lead II	Lead II
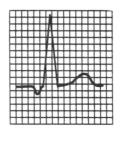	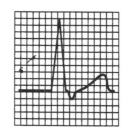	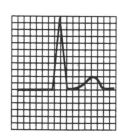
P wave before QRS	P wave after QRS	P wave hidden in QRS

Lead II

Figure 8-3. Premature junctional contractions will appear as a single beat in any of the above three patterns.

PREMATURE JUNCTIONAL CONTRACTION (PJC)

A premature junctional contraction (PJC) (Figure 8-3 and 8-4) (Box 8-1) is an early beat that originates in an ectopic pacemaker site in the AV junction and is usually caused by enhanced automaticity of the junctional tissue. Like the PAC, the premature junctional beat is characterized by an abnormal P-wave, a QRS complex that is identical or very similar to the QRS complex of the normally conducted beats, and is followed by a pause that is usually noncompensatory. Some differences do exist, however. Since atrial depolarization occurs in a retrograde fashion with the PJC, the P-waves associated with the premature beat will be negative (inverted) in Lead II and will occur immediately before the QRS (with a short PR interval of 0.10 seconds or less), immediately after the QRS, or will be hidden within the QRS. Inverted P-waves in Lead II may also occur with PACs arising from the lower atria, but the associated PR interval will be within normal limits. If difficulty is encountered in differentiating PJCs from PACs, keep the following in mind—PACs are much more common than PJCs. As a result, narrow complex premature beats should probably not be interpreted as

PJCs unless P-waves are definitely absent or the P-wave is inverted in Lead II with a short PR interval.

PJCs occur in addition to the underlying rhythm. They occur in the same patterns as PACs: as a single beat; in bigeminal, trigeminal, or quadrigeminal patterns; or in pairs. A series of 3 or more consecutive junctional beats is considered a rhythm (i.e. junctional rhythm, accelerated junctional rhythm, or junctional tachycardia). Differentiation of the rhythm will depend on the heart rate.

Enhanced automaticity of the junctional tissue is felt to be the primary cause of PJCs and may be related to ischemia. Other causes include: stress, caffeine, alcohol, heart failure, pericarditis, valvular heart disease, coronary heart disease, chronic lung disease, hyperthyroidism, electrolyte imbalances, and digitalis toxicity.

Isolated PJCs are not treated. If PJCs increase in frequency the best approach is to eliminate the

---

Box 8-1. Premature Junctional Contraction: Identifying ECG Features

Rhythm:	Underlying rhythm usually regular; irregular with PJC
Rate:	Rate is that of underlying rhythm
P waves:	P-wave associated with the PJC will be inverted in lead II and occur immediately before the QRS, immediately after the QRS, or will be hidden within the QRS complex
PR:	Short (0.10 seconds or less)
QRS:	Normal (0.10 seconds or less)

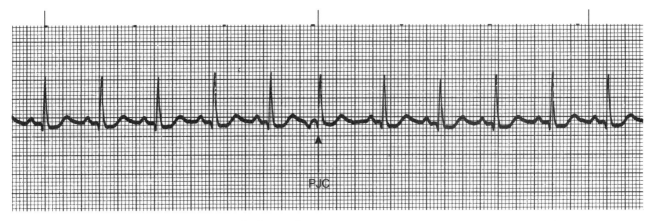

Figure 8-4. Normal Sinus Rhythm with One PJC

Rhythm:	Basic rhythm regular; irregular with PJC
Rate:	Basic rhythm rate 94
P waves:	Sinus P waves with basic rhythm; inverted P wave with PJC
PR:	0.14 to 0.16 seconds (basic rhythm) 0.08 seconds (PJC)
QRS:	0.08 seconds
Comment:	ST segment depression is present.

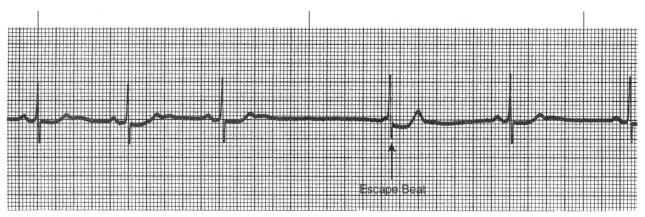

Figure 8-5. **Normal Sinus Rhythm with a Junctional Escape Beat**

Rhythm: Basic rhythm regular; irregular with escape beat

Rate: Basic rhythm 60; rate slows to 45 after escape beat. Rate suppression can occur following a premature or escape beat. After several cycles the rate will return to the basic rate.

P waves: Sinus P waves with basic rhythm; hidden P wave with escape beat

PR: 0.16 seconds

QRS: 0.06 seconds

Comment: ST segment depression and a U wave are present.

cause. Frequent PJCs may warn of or initiate more serious junctional arrhythmias.

Occasionally an ectopic junctional beat will occur late instead of early—these are called junctional escape beats (Figure 8-5). Escape beats are more likely to occur due to increased vagal effect on the SA node rather than to enhanced automaticity, as is associated with the premature beat. Junctional escape beats are common following a pause in the underlying rhythm (e.g., sinus arrest or block, nonconducted PACs, type I second degree AV block). The morphologic characteristics of the late beat are the same as the PJC. Escape beats require no treatment. It is important, however, to identify the cause of the initiating pause so that appropriate intervention can be started if necessary.

JUNCTIONAL RHYTHM

Junctional rhythm (Figures 8-6, 8-7, and 8-8) (Box 8-2) is an arrhythmia originating in the AV junction, with a rate between 40–60 beats per minute. This rhythm is often referred to as junctional escape rhythm because it usually only appears secondary to depression of the higher pacing centers of the heart (SA node).

Junctional escape rhythm is the normal response of the AV junction when:

1. The rate of the dominant pacemaker (usually SA node) becomes less than the rate of the AV node, or

2. The electrical impulses of the dominant pacemaker fail to reach the AV node, as in sinus arrest, sinus block, and the nonconducted PAC.

Retrograde stimulation of the atria by the AV node impulse produces a rhythm with the following characteristics:

1. Negative P-waves in Lead II that occur immediately before the QRS, immediately after the QRS, or are hidden within the QRS

2. A short PR interval of 0.10 seconds or less

3. A QRS complex that is identical or very similar to the normally conducted beats.

Junctional rhythm is a continuous rhythm, usually transient in nature, with the same ECG characteristics as accelerated junctional rhythm and junctional tachycardia. This rhythm is differentiated from the other junctional rhythms by the heart rate (40–60).

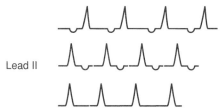

Lead II

Figure 8-6. Junctional rhythm will appear as a continuous rhythm at a rate of 40–60 beats per minute in either of the above three patterns.

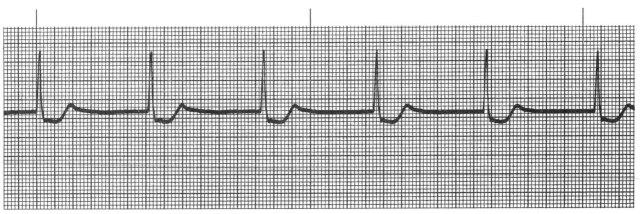

Figure 8-7. **Junctional Rhythm**

Rhythm: Regular

Rate: 50

P waves: Hidden in QRS complexes

PR: Not measurable

QRS: 0.06 to 0.08 seconds

Comment: ST segment depression is present.

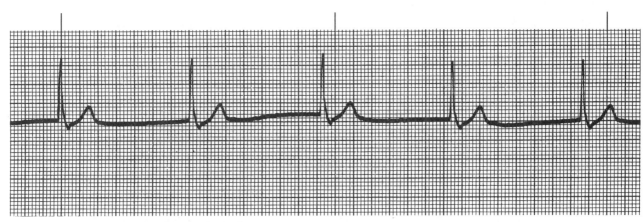

Figure 8-8. **Junctional Rhythm**

Rhythm: Regular

Rate: 42

P waves: Inverted after QRS

PR: 0.04 seconds

QRS: 0.08 seconds

Box 8-2. Junctional Rhythm: Identifying ECG Features

Rhythm: Regular

Rate: 40–60

P waves: Inverted in lead II and occurs immediately before the QRS, immediately after the QRS, or is hidden within the QRS complex

PR: Short (0.10 seconds or less)

QRS: Normal (0.10 seconds or less)

Junctional rhythm can be seen in a number of clinical settings. It may be caused by drug effects (digitalis, beta-blockers, calcium-channel blockers), damage to the AV node secondary to acute inferior wall myocardial infarction, hypoxia, electrolyte disturbances, heart failure, valvular heart disease, cardiomyopathy, and myocarditis.

Junctional rhythm, like other slow rhythms (e.g., sinus bradycardia), may cause hypotension, with a reduction in cardiac output and a decreased perfusion of the brain and other vital organs. A reduction

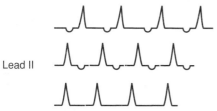

Lead II

Figure 8-9. Accelerated junctional rhythm will appear as a continuous rhythm at a rate of 60–100 beats per minute in any of the above three patterns.

in cardiac output may also occur due to retrograde activation of the atria associated with this rhythm. When the atria are stimulated (depolarized) simultaneously with or after the ventricles, the atrial contribution (atrial kick) is lost, resulting in incomplete filling of the ventricles and a reduction in cardiac output.

Treatment for symptomatic junctional rhythm includes increasing the heart rate (atropine, transcutaneous pacing or transvenous pacing) and reversing the consequences of reduced cardiac output. Treatment should also involve identifying and correcting the underlying cause, if possible.

ACCELERATED JUNCTIONAL RHYTHM

Accelerated junctional rhythm (Figures 8-9 and 8-10) (Box 8-3)is an arrhythmia originating in the AV junction, with a rate between 60–100. The term "accelerated" denotes a rhythm that occurs at a rate that exceeds the inherent junctional escape rate of 40–60, but is not fast enough to be junctional tachycardia. This rhythm is usually caused by enhanced automaticity of the AV junctional tissue.

Retrograde stimulation of the atria by the AV node impulse produces a rhythm with the following characteristics:

1. Negative P-waves in Lead II that occur immediately before the QRS, immediately after the QRS, or are hidden within the QRS complex

2. A short PR interval of 0.10 seconds or less

3. A QRS complex that is identical or very similar to the normally conducted beats

Accelerated junctional rhythm is a continuous rhythm, usually transient in nature, with the same ECG characteristics as junctional rhythm and junctional tachycardia. This rhythm is differentiated from the other junctional rhythms by the heart rate (60–100).

Box 8-3. Accelerated Junctional Rhythm: Identifying ECG Features

Rhythm:	Regular
Rate:	60–100
P waves:	Inverted in lead II and occurs immediately before the QRS, immediately after the QRS, or is hidden within the QRS complex
PR:	Short (0.10 seconds or less)
QRS:	Normal (0.10 seconds or less)

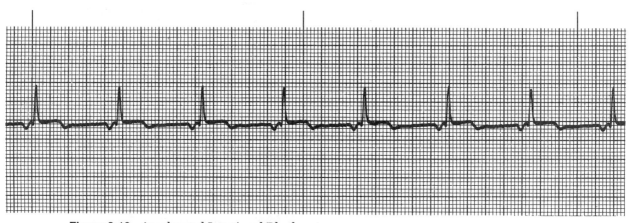

Figure 8-10. Accelerated Junctional Rhythm

Rhythm:	Regular
Rate:	65
P waves:	Inverted before each QRS
PR:	0.08 to 0.10 seconds
QRS:	0.08 seconds
Comment:	ST segment elevation and T wave inversion are present.

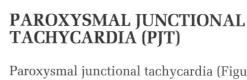

Lead II

Figure 8-11. Paroxysmal junctional tachycardia will appear as a continuous rhythm at a rate exceeding 100 per minute in any of the above three patterns.

Accelerated junctional rhythm is commonly a result of digitalis toxicity. Other causes include: damage to the AV node secondary to acute inferior wall MI, heart failure, acute rheumatic fever, valvular heart disease, following cardiac surgery, and myocarditis.

As a rule, the heart rate associated with accelerated junctional rhythm is not a problem since it corresponds to that of the sinus node (60–100). Problems arise clinically due to the retrograde activation of the atria. When the atria are stimulated simultaneously with the ventricles or after the ventricles, the atrial contribution (atrial kick) is lost, resulting in incomplete filling of the ventricles and a reduction in cardiac output.

In general, treatment should be directed at identifying the underlying cause and correcting it if possible (e.g., discontinue digitalis if the patient is dig toxic). If the patient is symptomatic, treatment must also be directed at reversing the consequences of reduced cardiac output.

PAROXYSMAL JUNCTIONAL TACHYCARDIA (PJT)

Paroxysmal junctional tachycardia (Figures 8-11 and 8-12) (Box 8-4) is an arrhythmia originating in the AV junction, with a heart rate that exceeds 100 beats per minute. The mechanism responsible for this rhythm is felt to be enhanced automaticity of the junctional tissue or conduction of the ectopic impulse through a reentry circuit involving the AV node and atria. Like PAT, junctional tachycardia is regular, and commonly starts and ends abruptly in a paroxysmal manner.

Retrograde stimulation of the atria by the AV node impulse produces a rhythm with the following characteristics:

1. Negative P-waves in Lead II that occur immediately before the QRS, immediately after the QRS, or are hidden within the QRS complex

---

Box 8-4. Paroxysmal Junctional Tachycardia: Identifying ECG Features

Rhythm:	Regular
Rate:	Over 100 per minute
P waves:	Inverted in lead II and occurs immediately before the QRS, immediately after the QRS, or is hidden within the QRS complex
PR:	Short (0.10 seconds or less)
QRS:	Normal (0.10 seconds or less)

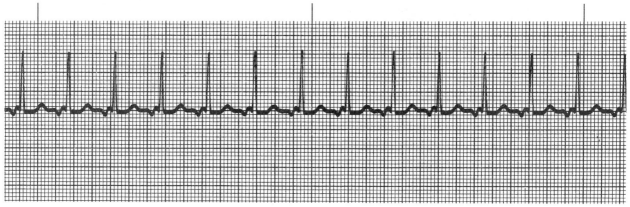

Figure 8-12. Paroxysmal Junctional Tachycardia

Rhythm:	Regular
Rate:	115
P waves:	Inverted before each QRS
PR:	0.08 seconds
QRS:	0.06 to 0.08 seconds

2. A short PR interval of 0.10 seconds or less

3. A QRS complex that is identical or very similar to the normally conducted beats

Junctional tachycardia has the same ECG characteristics as junctional rhythm and accelerated junctional rhythm. This rhythm is differentiated from the other junctional rhythms by the heart rate (greater than 100 per minute).

It is often impossible to distinguish PJT from PAT electrocardiographically. The ectopic P-waves are often hidden in the QRS complex in both these rhythms. If a differentiation cannot be made between the two, the term paroxysmal supraventricular tachycardia (PSVT) is used. This term implies that the tachycardia is paroxysmal in nature (either PAT or PJT) and has a supraventricular origin (above the level of the His bundle with a narrow QRS complex). The term "PSVT" should not be confused with the general term "superventricular," which refers to any rhythm above the level of the His bundle.

Paroxysmal junctional tachycardia is commonly a result of digitalis toxicity. Other causes include: damage to the AV node secondary to acute inferior MI, heart failure, acute rheumatic fever, valvular heart disease and after cardiac surgery (especially valve surgery), myocarditis, and electrolyte imbalance.

Acute treatment of PJT is managed in the same manner as PAT:

1. If the patient is stable, vagal maneuvers, adenosine IV, or verapamil IV should be attempted first.

2. If the rhythm fails to convert or if the patient is symptomatic, synchronized shock should be performed. Treatment should also involve reversing the consequences of reduced cardiac output as well as identifying and correcting the underlying cause if possible.

AV HEART BLOCKS

Heart block is the general term used to describe disturbances in atrioventricular (AV) conduction. Normally the AV node acts as a bridge between the atria and the ventricles. An AV block is a failure or delay in conduction across the bridge. The PR interval (normally 0.12–0.20 seconds in duration) measures the time between the initial depolarization of the atria (P-wave) and the initial depolarization of the ventricles (QRS). The greatest part of the PR interval is indicative of conduction time through the AV node (across the bridge).

AV heart blocks are classified into first-degree, second-degree (type I and type II), and third-degree. The classification system is based on the site of the block and the severity of the conduction disturbance. In first-degree AV block (the mildest form) the electrical impulses are delayed in the AV node longer than normal, but all impulses are conducted to the ventricles. In second-degree AV block, some impulses are conducted to the ventricles and some are blocked. The most extreme form of heart block is third-degree AV block, in which no impulses are conducted from the atria to the ventricles.

The ability to accurately diagnose AV blocks depends on the use of a systematic approach. The following steps are suggested:

1. Assess regularity of the rhythm (both atrial and ventricular)

2. Identify the P-wave

3. Assess QRS width (narrow or wide?)

4. Assess relationship of the P-wave to the QRS complexes. (Is the PR interval consistent or does it vary?)

FIRST-DEGREE AV BLOCK

In first-degree AV block (Figure 8-13) (Box 8-5) the sinus impulse is conducted normally to the AV node, where it is delayed longer than usual before being conducted to the ventricles. This delay in the AV node results in a prolonged PR interval (greater than 0.20 seconds in duration). This rhythm is reflected on the ECG by a regular rhythm (both atrial and ventricular); one P-wave preceding each QRS complex; a consistent but prolonged PR interval; and a narrow QRS. Anatomically, this conduction disorder is located at the level of the AV node (thus the narrow QRS complex) and is not a serious form of heart block. First-degree heart block is simply a normal sinus rhythm with a prolonged PR interval.

There are numerous causes of first-degree AV block, most of which are associated with second-degree and third-degree AV block also. Causes include: drugs (quinidine, procainamide, digitalis, beta-blockers, calcium-channel blockers), acute inferior wall myocardial infarction, increased vagal tone, hyperkalemia, rheumatic fever, and congenital abnormality.

First-degree AV block produces no symptoms and requires no treatment. Because first-degree heart block can progress to a higher degree of AV block, the rhythm should continue to be monitored until the block resolves or stabilizes.

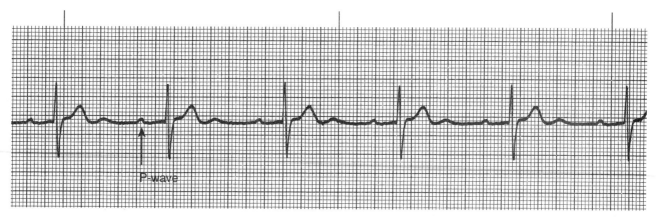

Figure 8-13. **Sinus Bradycardia with First Degree AV Block**

Rhythm: Regular

Rate: 48

P waves: Sinus P waves present; one P wave to each QRS

PR: 0.28 to 0.32 seconds (remains constant).

QRS: 0.08 to 0.10 seconds.

Note: A U wave is present.

Box 8-5. First-Degree AV Block: Identifying ECG Features

Rhythm: Regular

Rate: Heart rate is that of underlying rhythm (usually sinus); both atrial and ventricular rates will be the same

P waves: Sinus

PR: Prolonged (greater than 0.20 seconds); remains constant

QRS: Normal (0.10 seconds or less)

SECOND-DEGREE AV BLOCK, TYPE I (MOBITZ I OR WENCKEBACH)

Second-degree AV block, type I (commonly known as Mobitz I or Wenckebach) (Figure 8-14) (Box 8-6) is characterized by a failure of some of the sinus impulses to be conducted to the ventricles. In this rhythm the sinus impulse is conducted normally to the AV node but each successive impulse has more and more difficulty passing through the AV node, until finally an impulse does not pass through (i.e., it is blocked or not conducted). This rhythm is reflected on the ECG by regularly occurring P-waves and progressively lengthening PR intervals until a P-wave appears that is not followed by a QRS; instead, it is followed by a pause. The dropped QRS causes the ventricular rhythm to be irregular. The cycle then repeats itself. This repetitive cycle is called group beating and is a hallmark of Mobitz I. Escape beats (atrial, junctional, or ventricular) are common during the pause in the ventricular rhythm. The location of the conduction disturbance is at the level of the AV node; as a result, the QRS complex will be narrow.

Mobitz I can be confused with the nonconducted PAC (Figure 8-15). Both rhythms have P-waves not followed by a QRS, but followed by a pause. To differentiate between the two rhythms one must examine the configuration of the P-waves and measure the P-P regularity. The nonconducted PAC will have an abnormal P-wave and will occur prematurely. In Mobitz I the P-wave configuration remains the same as the sinus beats and the P-wave will occur on schedule, not prematurely.

Mobitz I is common following acute inferior wall MI, but it is usually a temporary rhythm, often spontaneously resolving. Other causes include drugs (digitalis, beta-blockers, calcium-channel blockers), acute infections (rheumatic fever and myocarditis), excessive vagal tone, and as a normal variant (especially in athletes).

Mobitz I is usually transient and reversible and seldom a serious form of heart block, although infrequently it can progress to a higher degree of AV block. Clinically, patients with Mobitz I AV block are usually without symptoms unless the ventricular

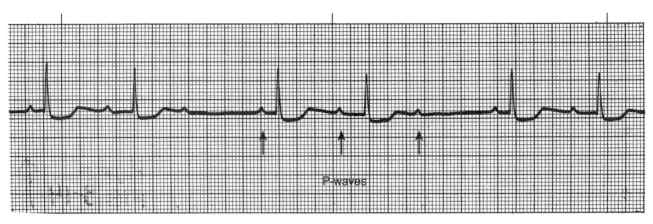

Figure 8-14. Second-Degree AV Block, Mobitz I

Rhythm:	Regular atrial rhythm; irregular ventricular rhythm
Rate:	Atrial: 72 Ventricular: 50
P waves:	Sinus P waves are present
PR:	Progressively lengthens from 0.20 to 0.30 seconds
QRS:	0.06–0.08 seconds
Note:	ST segment depression is present

rate is very slow. If hemodynamic status is compromised due to bradycardia, atropine will often be effective in improving AV conduction. Pacemaker therapy is rarely needed.

SECOND-DEGREE AV BLOCK, TYPE II (MOBITZ II)

Like Mobitz I, second-degree AV block Mobitz II (Figures 8-16 and 8-17) (Box 8-7) is characterized by a failure of some of the sinus impulses to be conducted to the ventricles. There are some differences, however, in the anatomical location and severity of the conduction disturbance, as well as in ECG features. In Mobitz II every 2nd, 3rd, or 4th sinus impulse is blocked and is not conducted to the ventri-

Box 8-6. Second-Degree AV Block (Mobitz I): Identifying ECG Features

Rhythm:	Atrial: regular Ventricular: irregular
Rate:	Atrial: rate is that of underlying rhythm (usually sinus) Ventricular: rate will depend on number of impulses conducted through AV node—will be less than the atrial rate
P waves:	Sinus
PR:	PR varies—PR progressively lengthens until a P-wave occurs without a QRS. A pause follows the dropped QRS.
QRS:	Normal (0.10 seconds or less)

cles. The ECG will show two, three or four P-waves (sometimes more) before each QRS, in a constant relationship (i.e., PR of the conducted beat remains constant). The atrial rhythm (P-P interval) will be regular, with the ventricular (R-R interval) usually regular unless the conduction ratio varies (alternating between 2 : 1, 3 : 1, 4 : 1, and so forth). The location of the conduction disturbance is below the AV node in the bundle of His or bundle branches. As a result the QRS may be narrow (if located in the bundle of His) or wide (if located in the bundle branches). The most common location is the bundle branches.

Mobitz II is usually associated with acute anterior or anteroseptal MI. Other causes include cardiomyopathy, rheumatic heart disease, severe coronary artery disease, drugs (digitalis, beta-blockers, calcium-channel blockers) and degeneration of the electrical conduction system, which is usually age-related.

Mobitz II is less common but more serious than Mobitz I. Since the anatomical location of the block is lower in the conduction system, Mobitz II has the potential to progress suddenly to third-degree AV block or ventricular standstill, with little or no warning. Due to the unpredictable nature of this rhythm, a temporary transvenous pacemaker should be inserted as soon as the rhythm is recognized. If the patient is symptomatic and a transvenous pacemaker is not readily available, a transcutaneous pacemaker may be used in the interim. Atropine, which increases the sinus rate and conduction through the AV node, has little or no effect on blocks below the

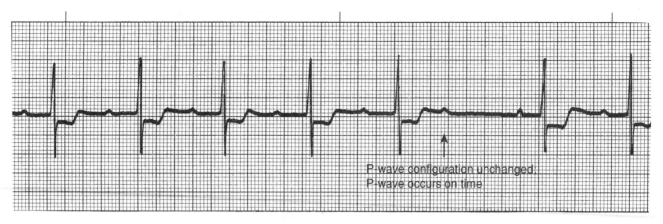

P-wave configuration unchanged;
P-wave occurs on time

MOBITZ I
1. Pause in basic ventricular rhythm
2. P-P regularity unchanged (P wave occurs on time)
3. P wave configuration same as sinus beats
4. PR interval of basic rhythm varies

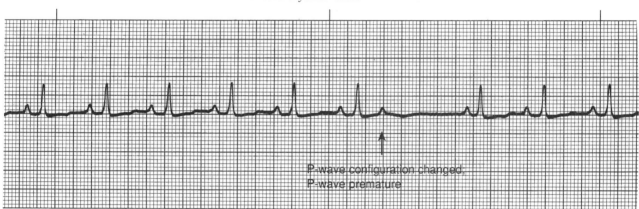

P-wave configuration changed;
P-wave premature

Nonconducted
PAC
1. Pause in basic ventricular rhythm
2. P-P regularity interrupted (P wave occurs prematurely)
3. P wave configuration different from sinus beats
4. PR interval of basic rhythm remains constant

Figure 8-15. Differentiation of the nonconducted PAC from Mobitz I.

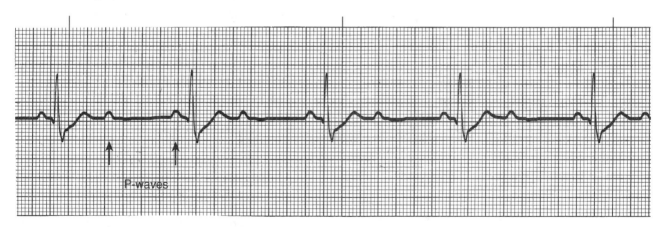

P-waves

Figure 8-16. Second-Degree AV Block, Mobitz II

Rhythm: Regular atrial and ventricular rhythm

Rate: Atrial: 82   Ventricular: 41

P waves: 2 sinus P waves to each QRS

PR: 0.16 seconds (remains constant)

QRS: 0.14 seconds

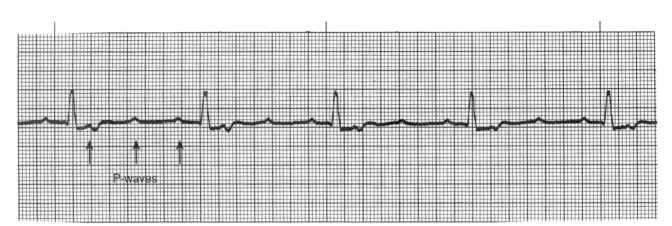

Figure 8-17. Second-Degree AV Block, Mobitz II

Rhythm:	Regular atrial and ventricular rhythm
Rate:	Atrial: 123 Ventricular: 41
P waves:	3 sinus P waves to each QRS
PR:	0.24–0.26 seconds (remains constant)
QRS:	0.12 seconds

AV node, so it is rarely used with this type of block. If the rhythm doesn't resolve, permanent pacing may be necessary.

THIRD-DEGREE AV BLOCK (COMPLETE HEART BLOCK)

With third-degree AV block (Figure 8-18) (Box 8-8) there is no conduction of stimuli from the atria to the ventricles. Instead, the atria and ventricles beat independently of each other. The atria generally continue to be paced by the sinus node while the ventricles are paced by an escape pacemaker located in the

AV node or in the ventricles. Even though independent beating between the atria and the ventricles is occurring, both the atrial rhythm and the ventricular rhythm will usually be regular. There is no relationship between atrial activity (P-waves) and ventricular activity (QRS complexes), resulting in P-waves which march through QRS complexes (hiding at times inside the QRS and within the T-wave) and PR intervals which vary greatly. Both the QRS width and the ventricular rate reflect the location of the blockage. If the block is at the level of the AV node or bundle of His, the QRS will be narrow and the heart rate between 40–60. If the blockage is in the bundle branches, the QRS will be wide and the heart rate much slower (30–40).

Complete heart block may be transient or permanent and may occur for a number of reasons. It is seen in both acute inferior and anterior MI, drug toxicity (digitalis, beta-blockers, calcium-channel blockers), excessive vagal tone, myocarditis, endocarditis, following cardiac surgery, and congenital abnormality. It is most commonly seen in older patients with chronic degeneration of their electrical conduction system.

Regardless of its cause, complete heart block is a serious and potentially life-threatening arrhythmia. Like Mobitz II, complete heart block can progress to ventricular standstill suddenly with little or no warning. If complete heart block occurs gradually, as seen in age-related degeneration of the electrical conduction system, the patient may have no significant symptoms and may only require cardiac monitoring with a transcutaneous pacemaker on standby until a permanent pacemaker is implanted. However, in the

---

Box 8-7. Second-Degree AV Block (Mobitz II): Identifying ECG Features

Rhythm:	Atrial: regular
	Ventricular: will be regular unless the AV conduction ratio varies
Rate:	Atrial: rate is that of underlying rhythm (usually sinus)
	Ventricular: rate will depend on number of impulses conducted through AV node—will be less than the atrial rate
P waves:	Sinus
PR:	May be normal or prolonged—remains constant
QRS:	Normal (if block located in bundle of His)
	Wide (if block located in bundle branches)

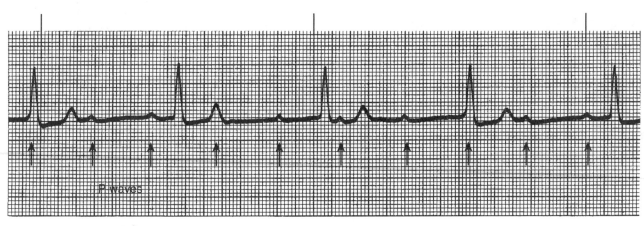

Figure 8-18. Third-Degree AV block

Rhythm: Regular atrial and ventricular rhythm

Rate: Atrial: 88   Ventricular: 38

P waves: Sinus P waves present; bear no relationship to QRS (found hidden in QRS and T waves)

PR: Varies greatly

QRS: 0.08 to 0.10 seconds.

acute setting (usually seen as a complication of my-ocardial infarction), the rhythm occurs suddenly and is often accompanied by signs and symptoms of he-modynamic compromise (dyspnea, heart failure, hy-potension, chest pain, fainting). Fainting spells asso-ciated with complete heart block are related to the low ventricular rate and reduced cardiac output and are called Stokes-Adams attacks or Stokes-Adams syncope. In the acute setting, once the rhythm is rec-ognized, a transcutaneous pacemaker should be ap-plied while preparations are made for insertion of a temporary transvenous pacemaker. Atropine may be effective on narrow complex third-degree AV block (AV node level), but has little or no effect on wide complex third-degree AV block (bundle branch level). Unresolved third-degree AV block will re-quire a permanent pacemaker.

Table 8-1 compares the ECG characteristics of each type of AV block and will assist in interpreta-tions of the heart block rhythms.

Box 8-8. Third-Degree AV Block (Complete Heart Block): Identifying ECG Features

Rhythm: Atrial: regular
          Ventricular: regular

Rate: Atrial: rate is that of underlying rhythm (usually sinus)
          Ventricular: rate is between 40–60 if paced by AV node
          rate is between 30–40 if paced by ventricles

P waves: Sinus

PR: Varies greatly—no constant relation-ship between P-waves and QRS. (P-waves can be seen marching through QRS complexes and T-waves.)

QRS: Normal (if block located at level of AV node or bundle of His) Wide (if block located at level of bundle branches)

Table 8-1. AV Block Comparisons

PR Constant *(First-degree)*	PR Varies *(Second-degree, Mobitz I)*
PR constant	PR varies
PR prolonged 1 P-wave to each QRS	PR progressively gets longer until a QRS is dropped
Regular atrial rhythm; regular ventricular rhythm	Regular atrial rhythm; irregular ventricular rhythm

(Second-degree, Mobitz II)	*(Third-degree)*
PR constant	PR varies
PR normal or prolonged 2, 3, 4 P-waves (or more) to each QRS	P waves have no constant relationship to QRS (found hidden in QRS complexes and T-waves)
Regular atrial rhythm; regular ventricular rhythm (unless conduction ratios vary)	Regular atrial rhythm; regular ventricular rhythm

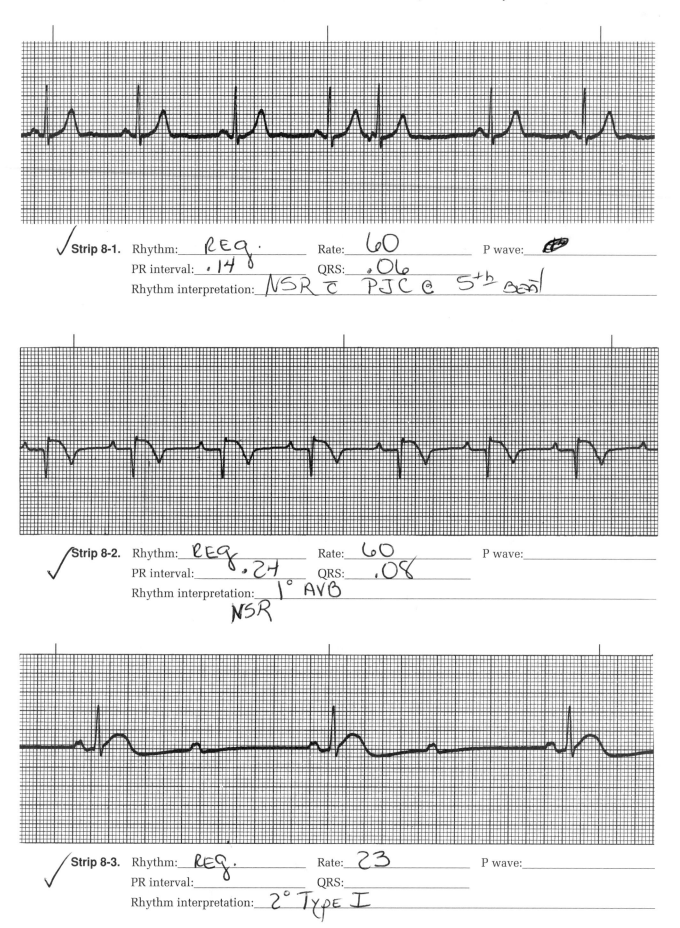

✓ **Strip 8-1.** Rhythm: _REg._ Rate: _60_ P wave: _⊕_

PR interval: _.14_ QRS: _.06_

Rhythm interpretation: _NSR c̄ PJC @ 5ᵗʰ beat_

✓ **Strip 8-2.** Rhythm: _REg_ Rate: _60_ P wave: _____

PR interval: _.24_ QRS: _.08_

Rhythm interpretation: _1° AVB_
NSR

✓ **Strip 8-3.** Rhythm: _REg._ Rate: _23_ P wave: _____

PR interval: _____ QRS: _____

Rhythm interpretation: _2° Type I_

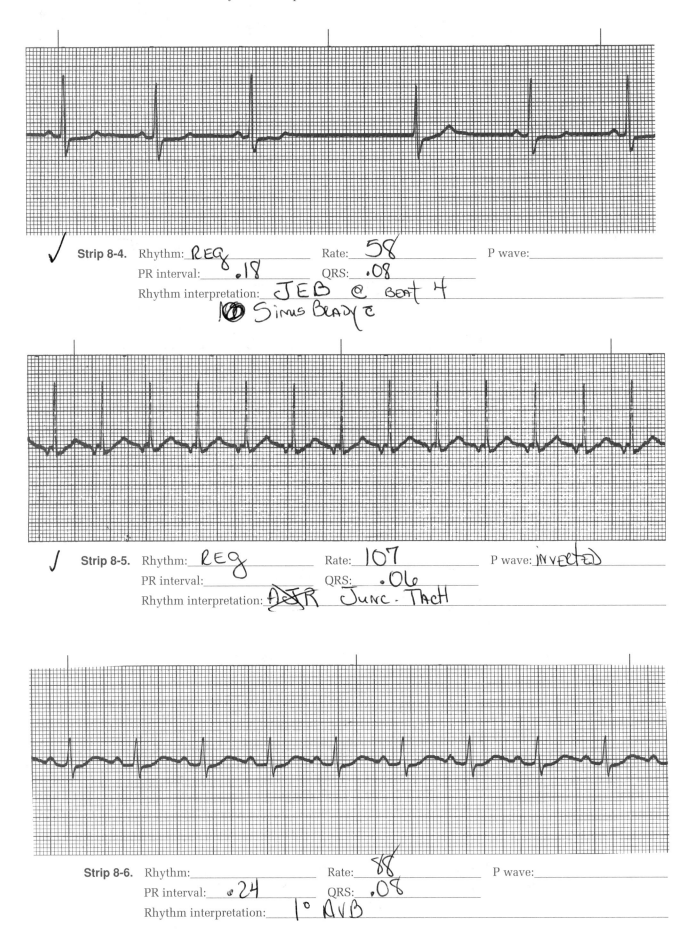

✓ **Strip 8-4.** Rhythm: REG   Rate: 58   P wave: _____

PR interval: .18   QRS: .08

Rhythm interpretation: JEB @ BEAT 4

100 Sinus Brady c̄

✓ **Strip 8-5.** Rhythm: REg   Rate: 107   P wave: INVERTED

PR interval: ___   QRS: .06

Rhythm interpretation: ASTR Junc. Tach

Strip 8-6. Rhythm: _____   Rate: 88   P wave: _____

PR interval: .24   QRS: .08

Rhythm interpretation: 1° AVB

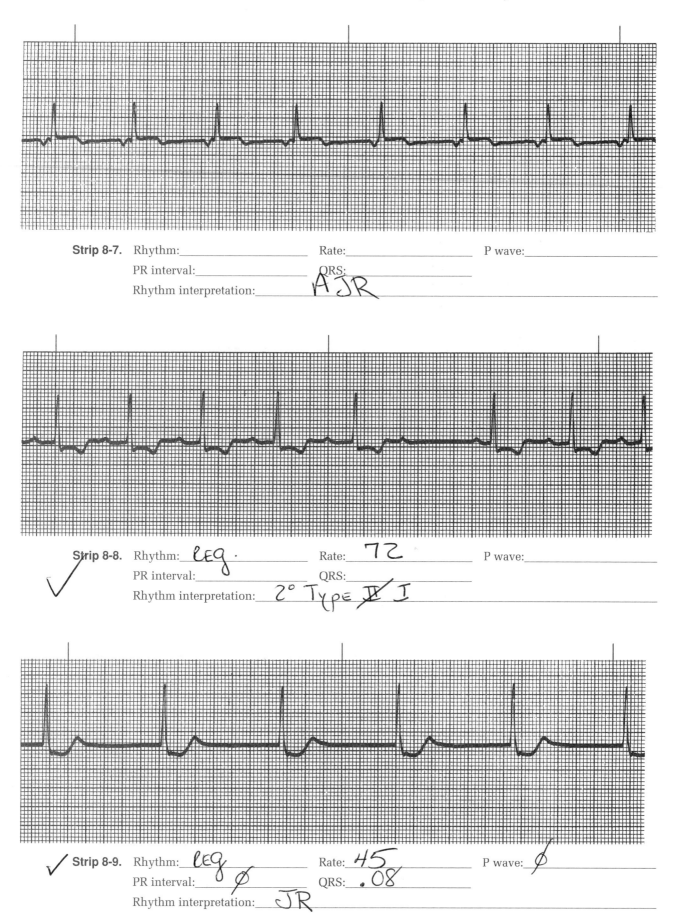

Strip 8-7. Rhythm:_____ Rate:_____ P wave:_____

PR interval:_____ QRS:_____

Rhythm interpretation:_____ AJR _____

Strip 8-8. Rhythm: REg . Rate: 72 P wave:_____

PR interval:_____ QRS:_____

Rhythm interpretation: 2° Type II I _____

✓

Strip 8-9. Rhythm: REg Rate: 45 P wave: Ø

PR interval: Ø QRS: .08

Rhythm interpretation: JR

✓

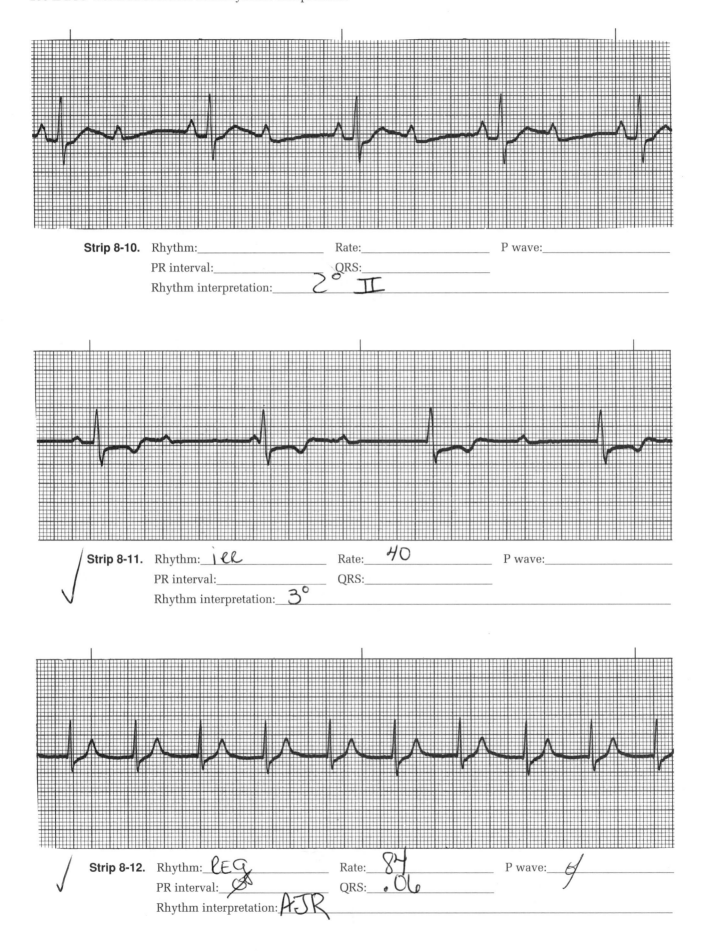

Strip 8-10. Rhythm:_____ Rate:_____ P wave:_____

PR interval:_____ QRS:_____

Rhythm interpretation:____2° II____

Strip 8-11. Rhythm:__irr____ Rate:__40____ P wave:_____

PR interval:_____ QRS:_____

Rhythm interpretation:__3°____

Strip 8-12. Rhythm:__REG__ Rate:__84__ P wave:__Ø__

PR interval:__Ø__ QRS:__.06__

Rhythm interpretation:__AJR__

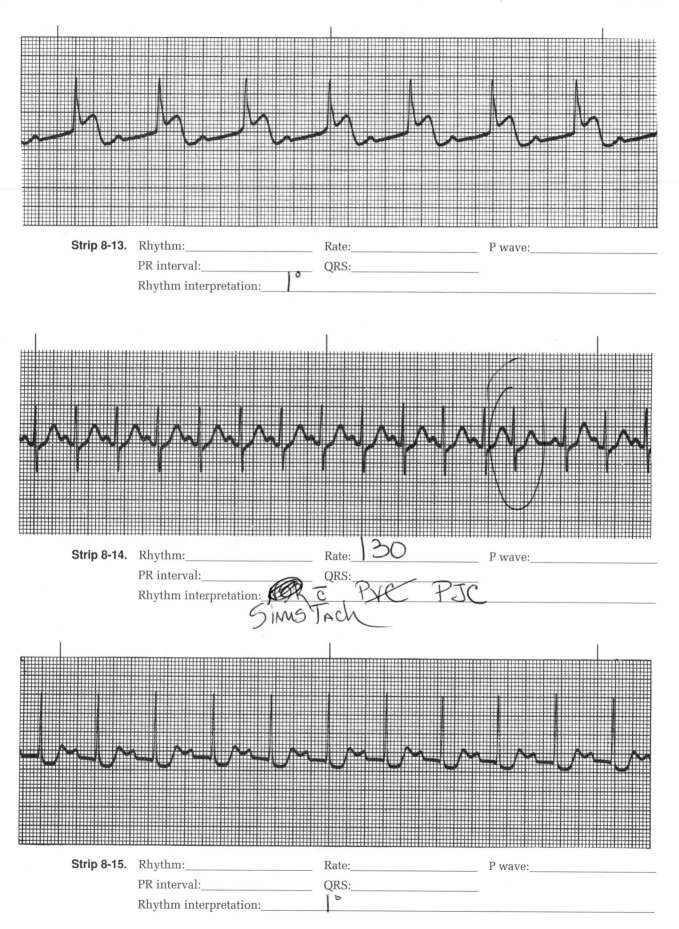

Strip 8-13. Rhythm:_____ Rate:_____ P wave:_____

PR interval:_____ QRS:_____

Rhythm interpretation:_____

Strip 8-14. Rhythm:_____ Rate: 130 P wave:_____

PR interval:_____ QRS:_____

Rhythm interpretation: QRS c̄ PVC PJC

Sinus Tach

Strip 8-15. Rhythm:_____ Rate:_____ P wave:_____

PR interval:_____ QRS:_____

Rhythm interpretation:_____

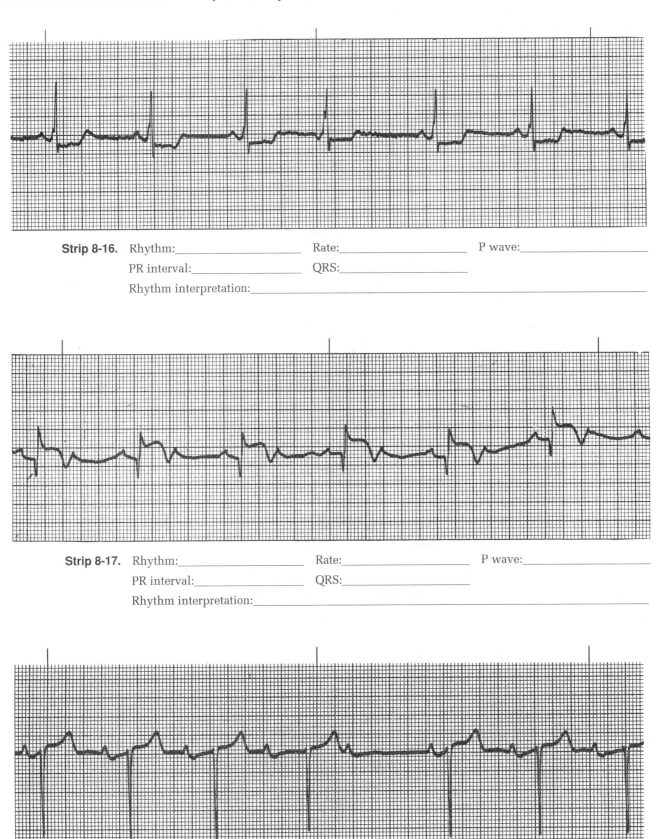

Strip 8-16. Rhythm:_____ Rate:_____ P wave:_____

PR interval:_____ QRS:_____

Rhythm interpretation:_____

Strip 8-17. Rhythm:_____ Rate:_____ P wave:_____

PR interval:_____ QRS:_____

Rhythm interpretation:_____

Strip 8-18. Rhythm:_____ Rate:_____ P wave:_____

PR interval:_____ QRS:_____

Rhythm interpretation:_____

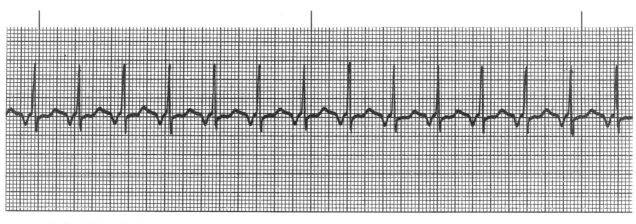

Strip 8-19. Rhythm:_____ Rate:_____ P wave:_____

PR interval:_____ QRS:_____

Rhythm interpretation:_____

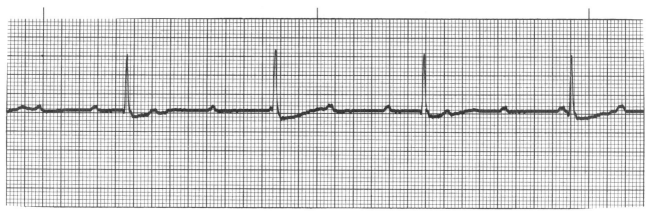

Strip 8-20. Rhythm:_____ Rate:_____ P wave:_____

PR interval:_____ QRS:_____

Rhythm interpretation:_____

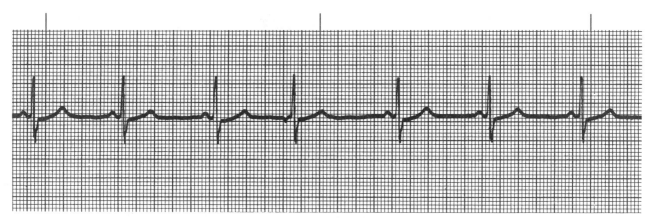

Strip 8-21. Rhythm:_____ Rate:_____ P wave:_____

PR interval:_____ QRS:_____

Rhythm interpretation:_____

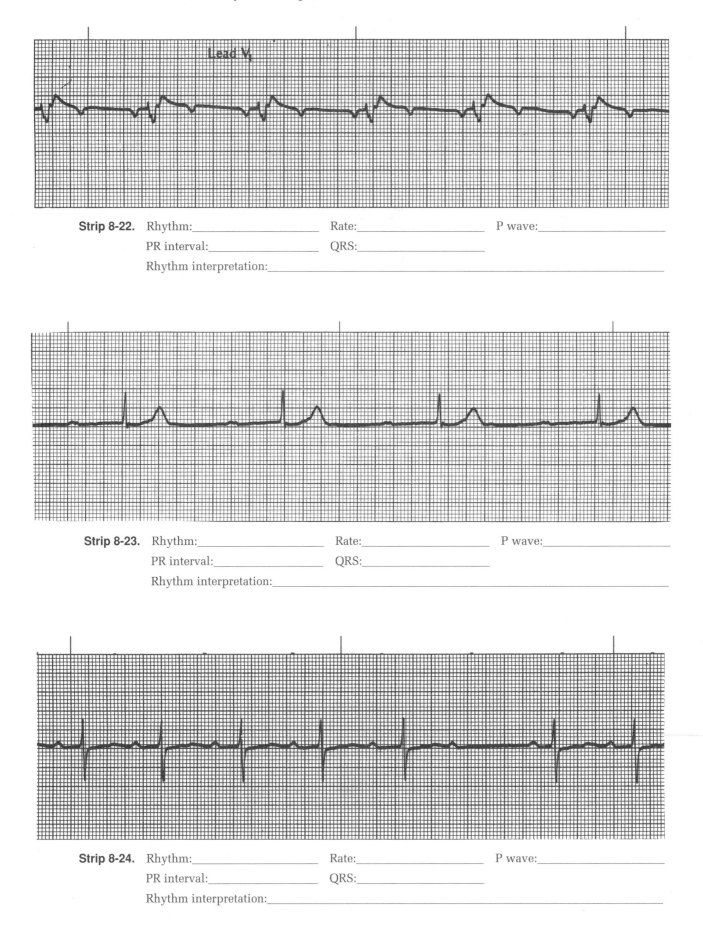

Lead V₁

Strip 8-22. Rhythm:_____ Rate:_____ P wave:_____

PR interval:_____ QRS:_____

Rhythm interpretation:_____

Strip 8-23. Rhythm:_____ Rate:_____ P wave:_____

PR interval:_____ QRS:_____

Rhythm interpretation:_____

Strip 8-24. Rhythm:_____ Rate:_____ P wave:_____

PR interval:_____ QRS:_____

Rhythm interpretation:_____

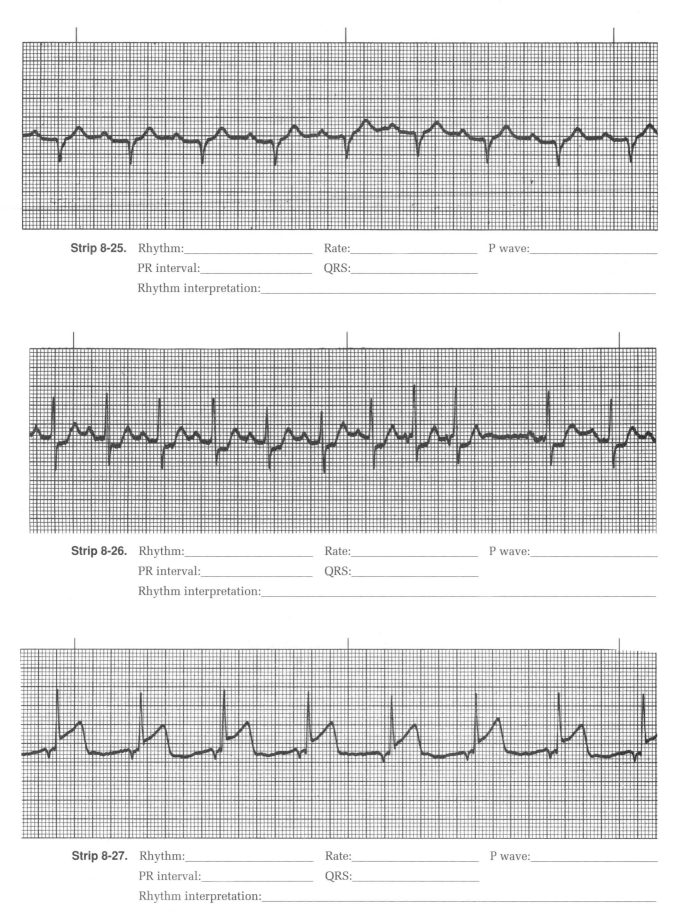

Strip 8-25. Rhythm:_____ Rate:_____ P wave:_____

PR interval:_____ QRS:_____

Rhythm interpretation:_____

Strip 8-26. Rhythm:_____ Rate:_____ P wave:_____

PR interval:_____ QRS:_____

Rhythm interpretation:_____

Strip 8-27. Rhythm:_____ Rate:_____ P wave:_____

PR interval:_____ QRS:_____

Rhythm interpretation:_____

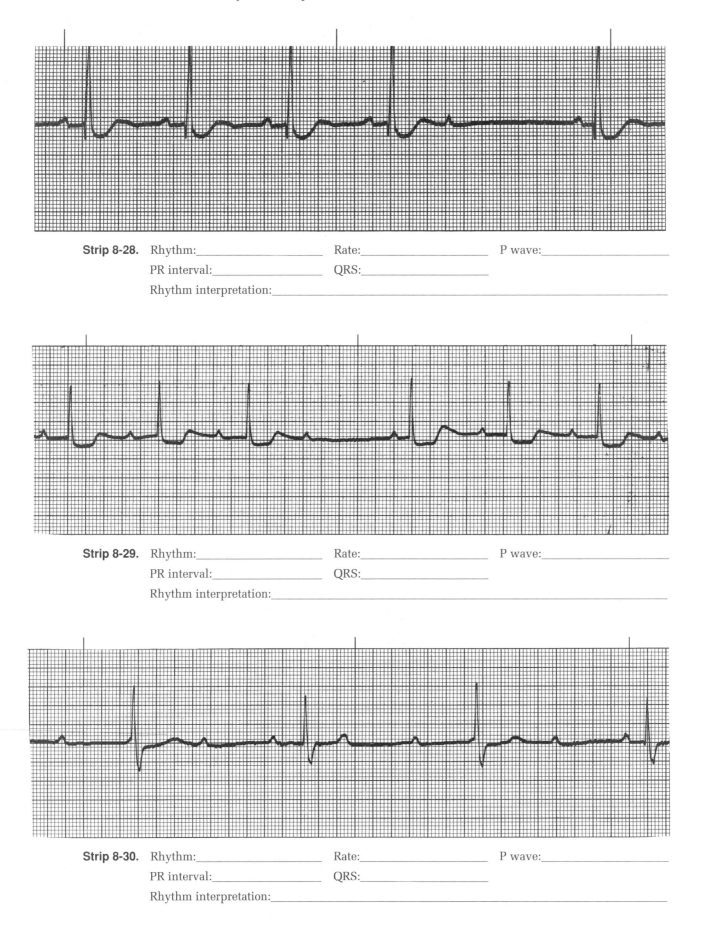

Strip 8-28. Rhythm:_____ Rate:_____ P wave:_____

PR interval:_____ QRS:_____

Rhythm interpretation:_____

Strip 8-29. Rhythm:_____ Rate:_____ P wave:_____

PR interval:_____ QRS:_____

Rhythm interpretation:_____

Strip 8-30. Rhythm:_____ Rate:_____ P wave:_____

PR interval:_____ QRS:_____

Rhythm interpretation:_____

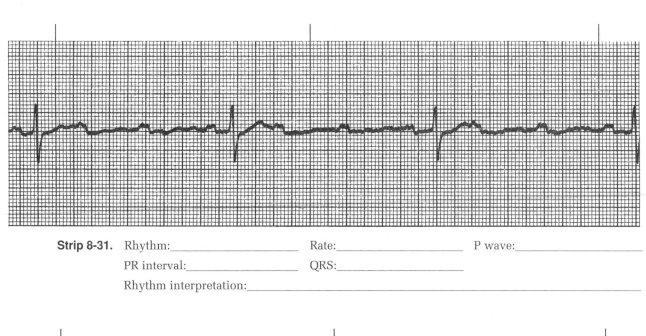

Strip 8-31. Rhythm:_____ Rate:_____ P wave:_____

PR interval:_____ QRS:_____

Rhythm interpretation:_____

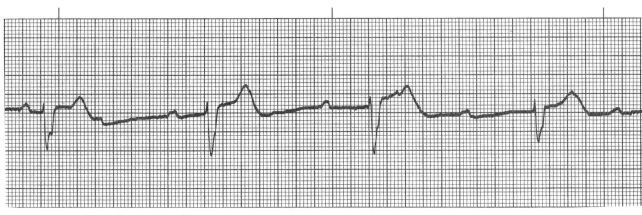

Strip 8-32. Rhythm:_____ Rate:_____ P wave:_____

PR interval:_____ QRS:_____

Rhythm interpretation:_____

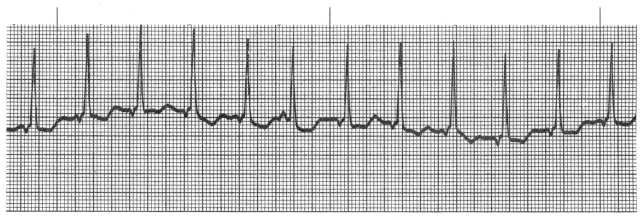

Strip 8-33. Rhythm:_____ Rate:_____ P wave:_____

PR interval:_____ QRS:_____

Rhythm interpretation:_____

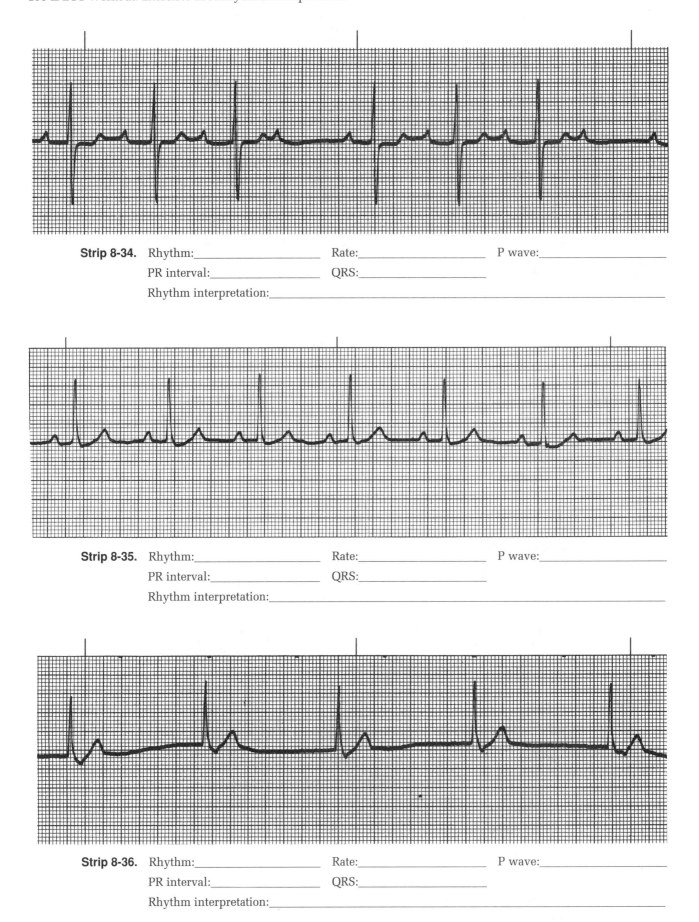

Strip 8-34. Rhythm:_____ Rate:_____ P wave:_____

PR interval:_____ QRS:_____

Rhythm interpretation:_____

Strip 8-35. Rhythm:_____ Rate:_____ P wave:_____

PR interval:_____ QRS:_____

Rhythm interpretation:_____

Strip 8-36. Rhythm:_____ Rate:_____ P wave:_____

PR interval:_____ QRS:_____

Rhythm interpretation:_____

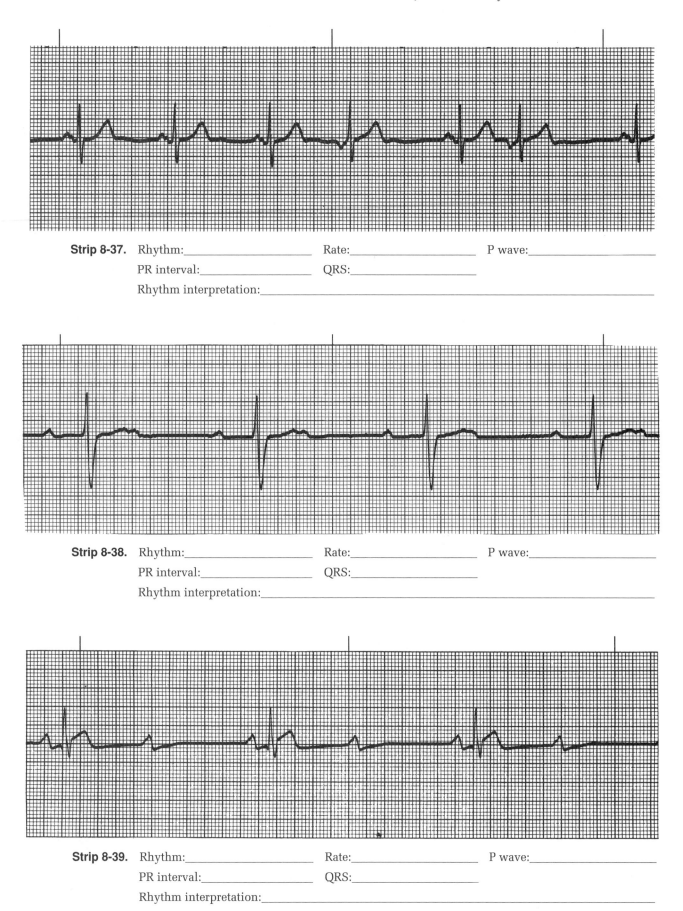

Strip 8-37. Rhythm:_____ Rate:_____ P wave:_____

PR interval:_____ QRS:_____

Rhythm interpretation:_____

Strip 8-38. Rhythm:_____ Rate:_____ P wave:_____

PR interval:_____ QRS:_____

Rhythm interpretation:_____

Strip 8-39. Rhythm:_____ Rate:_____ P wave:_____

PR interval:_____ QRS:_____

Rhythm interpretation:_____

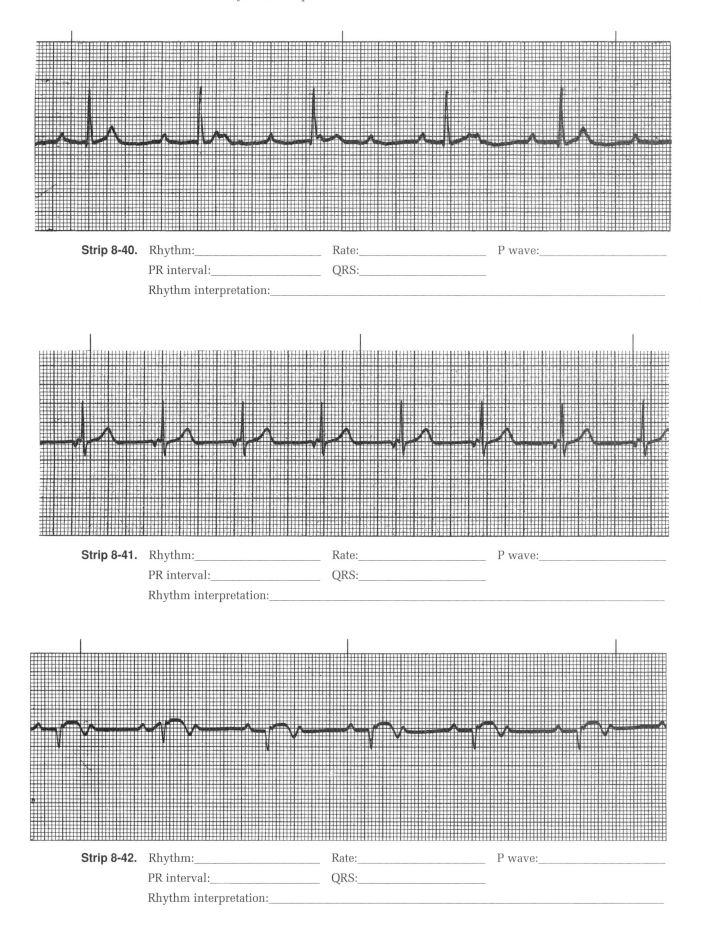

Strip 8-40. Rhythm:_____ Rate:_____ P wave:_____

PR interval:_____ QRS:_____

Rhythm interpretation:_____

Strip 8-41. Rhythm:_____ Rate:_____ P wave:_____

PR interval:_____ QRS:_____

Rhythm interpretation:_____

Strip 8-42. Rhythm:_____ Rate:_____ P wave:_____

PR interval:_____ QRS:_____

Rhythm interpretation:_____

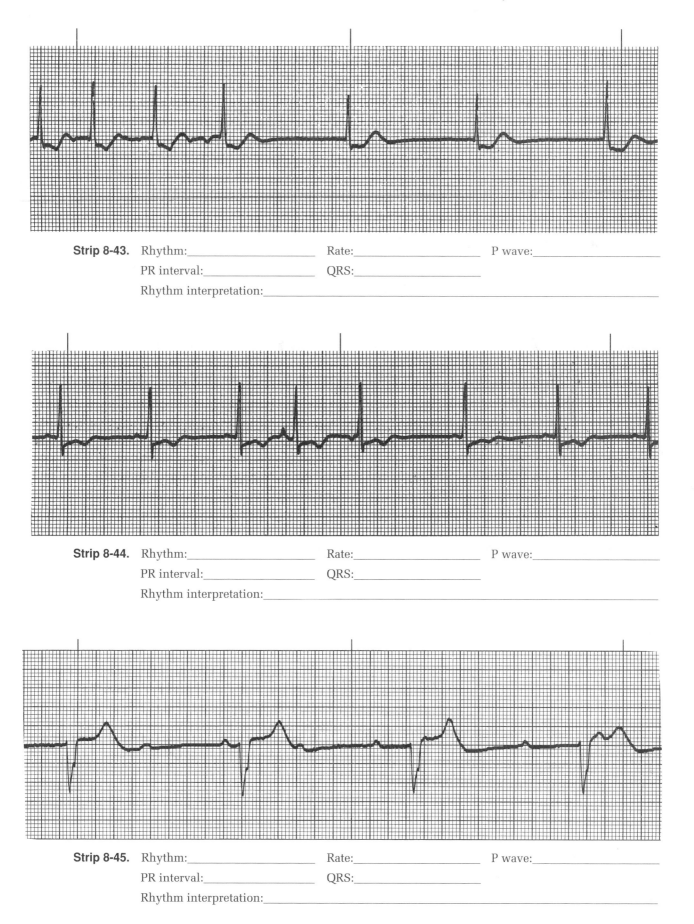

Strip 8-43. Rhythm:_____ Rate:_____ P wave:_____

PR interval:_____ QRS:_____

Rhythm interpretation:_____

Strip 8-44. Rhythm:_____ Rate:_____ P wave:_____

PR interval:_____ QRS:_____

Rhythm interpretation:_____

Strip 8-45. Rhythm:_____ Rate:_____ P wave:_____

PR interval:_____ QRS:_____

Rhythm interpretation:_____

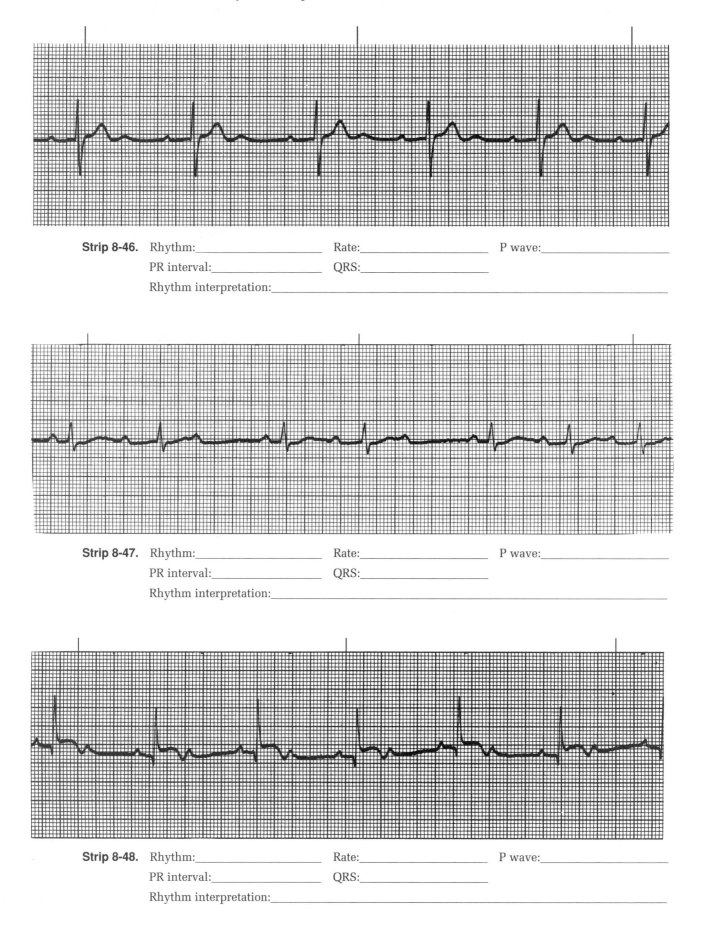

Strip 8-46. Rhythm:_____ Rate:_____ P wave:_____

PR interval:_____ QRS:_____

Rhythm interpretation:_____

Strip 8-47. Rhythm:_____ Rate:_____ P wave:_____

PR interval:_____ QRS:_____

Rhythm interpretation:_____

Strip 8-48. Rhythm:_____ Rate:_____ P wave:_____

PR interval:_____ QRS:_____

Rhythm interpretation:_____

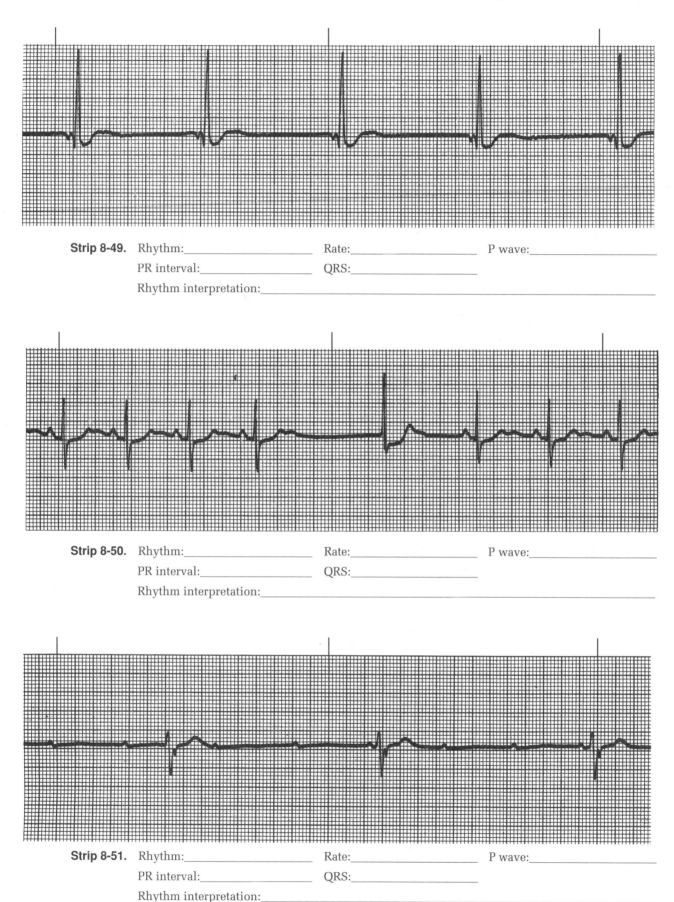

Strip 8-49. Rhythm:_____ Rate:_____ P wave:_____

PR interval:_____ QRS:_____

Rhythm interpretation:_____

Strip 8-50. Rhythm:_____ Rate:_____ P wave:_____

PR interval:_____ QRS:_____

Rhythm interpretation:_____

Strip 8-51. Rhythm:_____ Rate:_____ P wave:_____

PR interval:_____ QRS:_____

Rhythm interpretation:_____

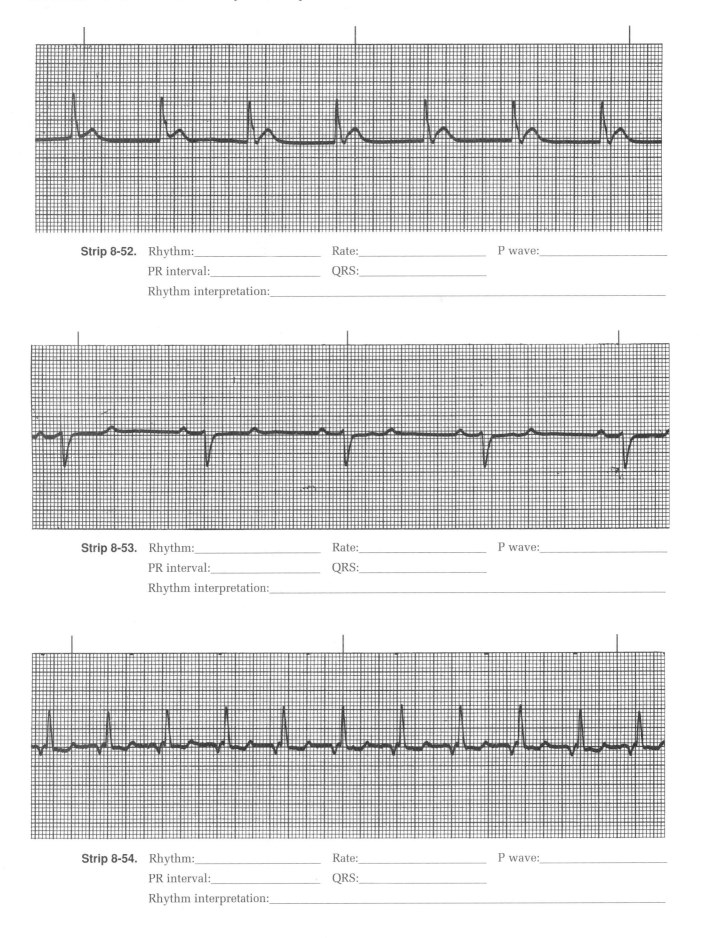

Strip 8-52. Rhythm:_____ Rate:_____ P wave:_____

PR interval:_____ QRS:_____

Rhythm interpretation:_____

Strip 8-53. Rhythm:_____ Rate:_____ P wave:_____

PR interval:_____ QRS:_____

Rhythm interpretation:_____

Strip 8-54. Rhythm:_____ Rate:_____ P wave:_____

PR interval:_____ QRS:_____

Rhythm interpretation:_____

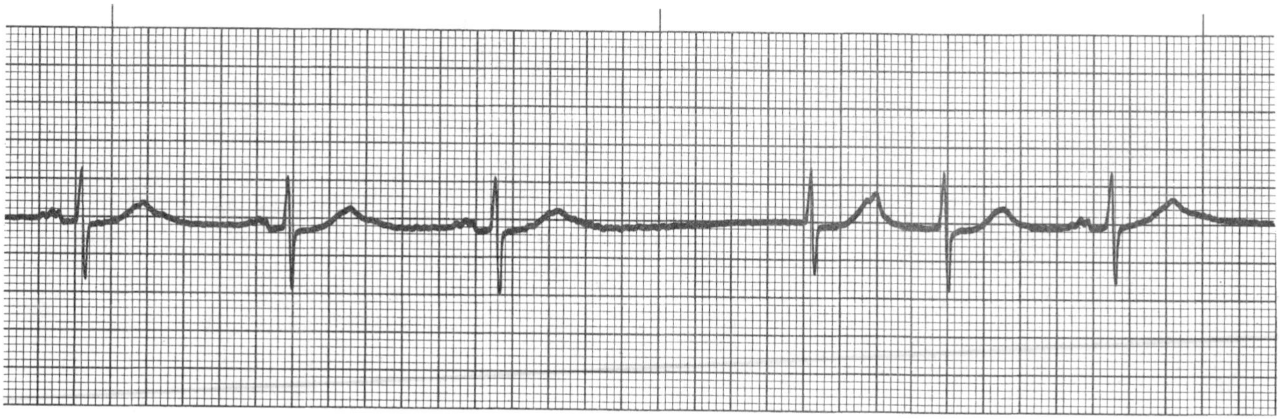

Strip 8-55. Rhythm:_____ Rate:_____ P wave:_____

PR interval:_____ QRS:_____

Rhythm interpretation:_____

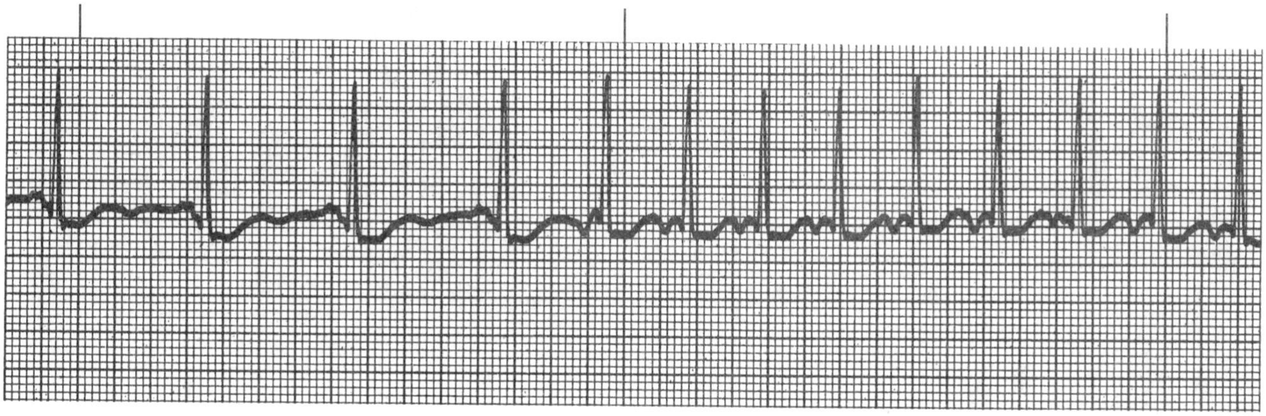

Strip 8-56. Rhythm:_____ Rate:_____ P wave:_____

PR interval:_____ QRS:_____

Rhythm interpretation:_____

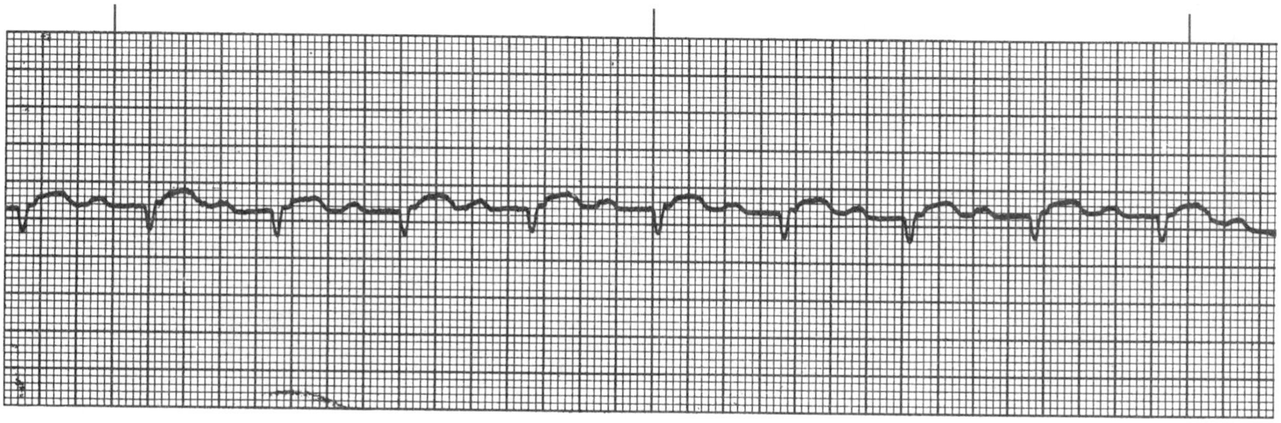

Strip 8-57. Rhythm:_____ Rate:_____ P wave:_____

PR interval:_____ QRS:_____

Rhythm interpretation:_____

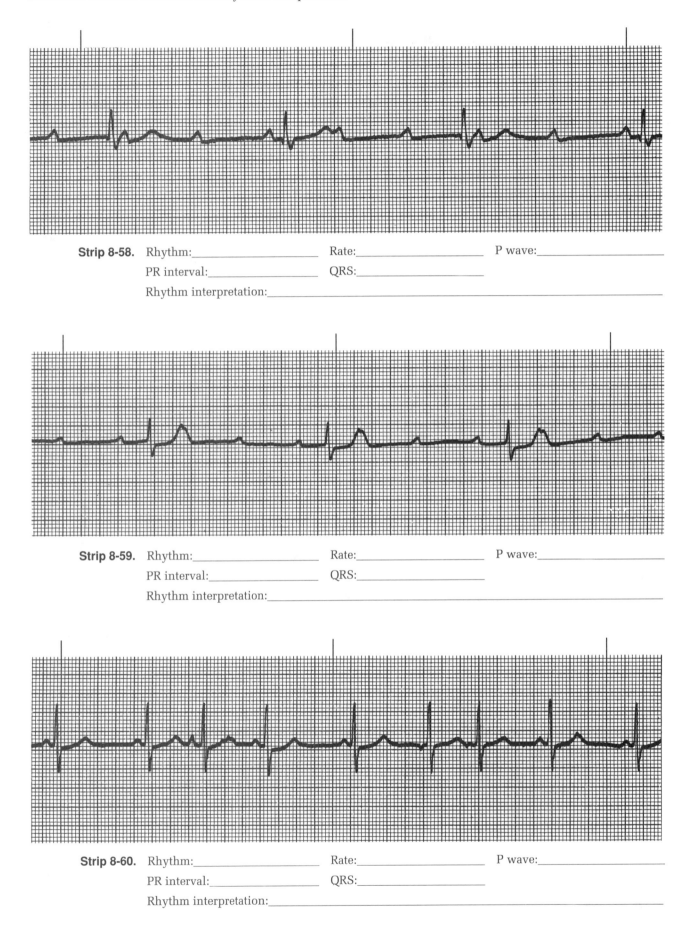

Strip 8-58. Rhythm:_____ Rate:_____ P wave:_____

PR interval:_____ QRS:_____

Rhythm interpretation:_____

Strip 8-59. Rhythm:_____ Rate:_____ P wave:_____

PR interval:_____ QRS:_____

Rhythm interpretation:_____

Strip 8-60. Rhythm:_____ Rate:_____ P wave:_____

PR interval:_____ QRS:_____

Rhythm interpretation:_____

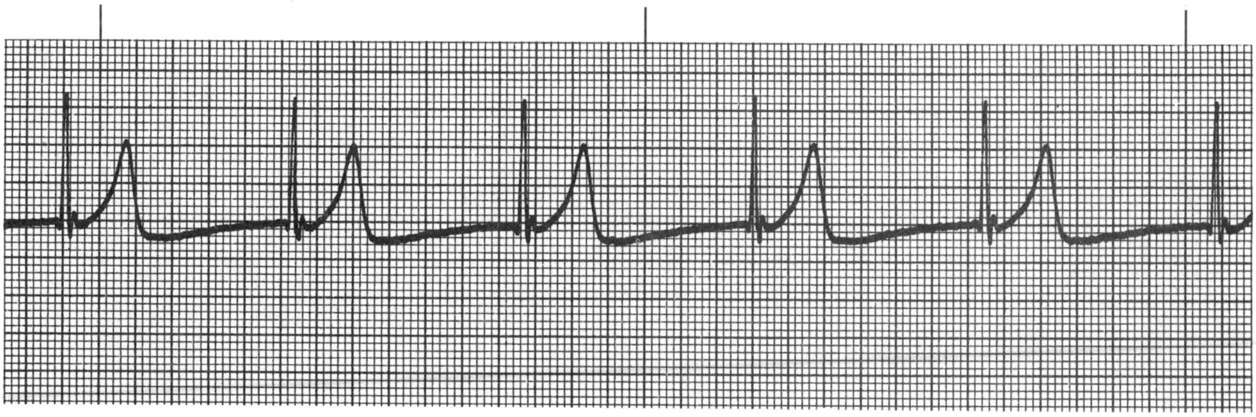

Strip 8-61. Rhythm:_____ Rate:_____ P wave:_____

PR interval:_____ QRS:_____

Rhythm interpretation:_____

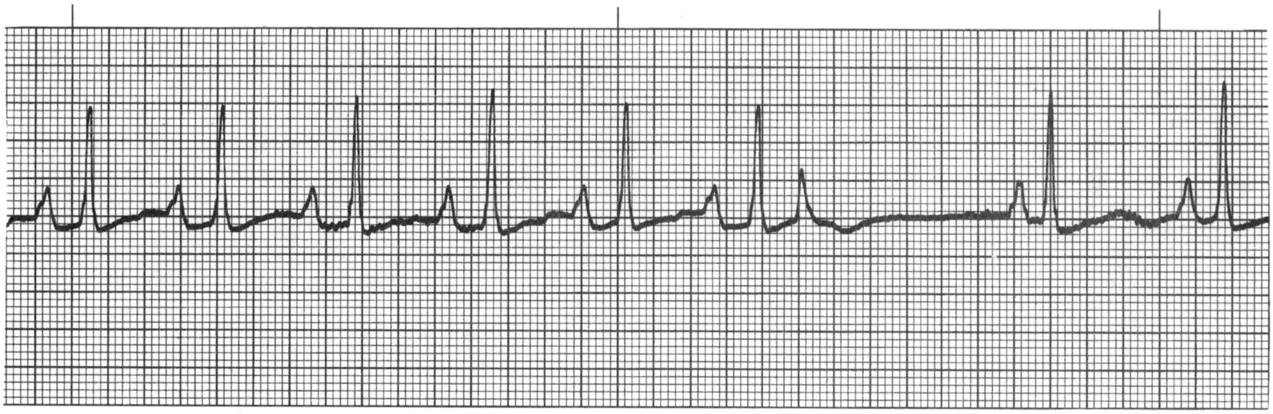

Strip 8-62. Rhythm:_____ Rate:_____ P wave:_____

PR interval:_____ QRS:_____

Rhythm interpretation:_____

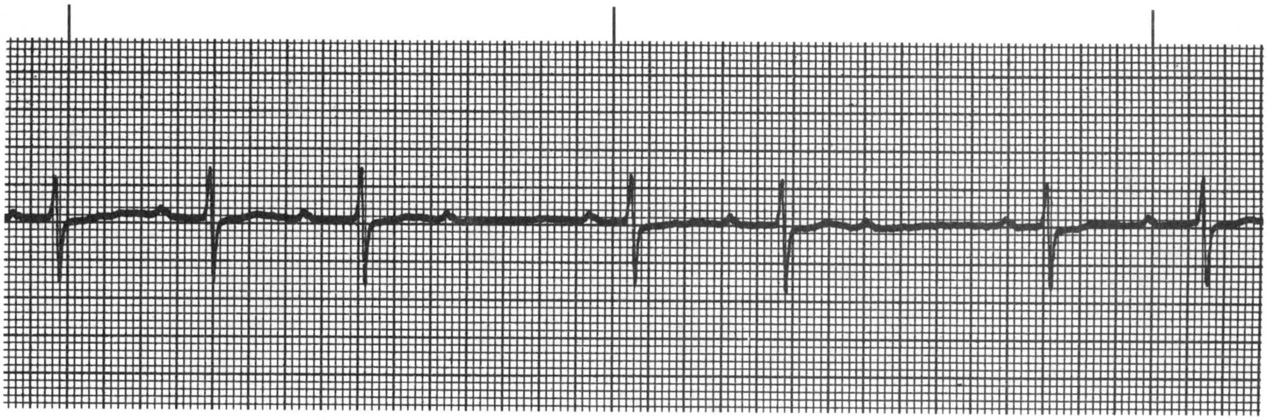

Strip 8-63. Rhythm:_____ Rate:_____ P wave:_____

PR interval:_____ QRS:_____

Rhythm interpretation:_____

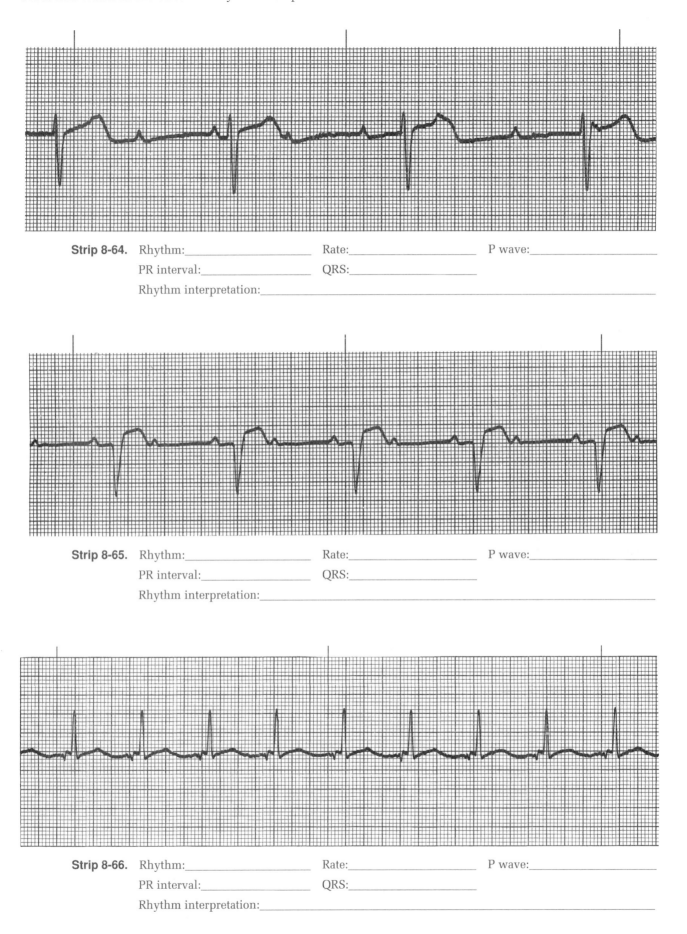

Strip 8-64. Rhythm:_____ Rate:_____ P wave:_____

PR interval:_____ QRS:_____

Rhythm interpretation:_____

Strip 8-65. Rhythm:_____ Rate:_____ P wave:_____

PR interval:_____ QRS:_____

Rhythm interpretation:_____

Strip 8-66. Rhythm:_____ Rate:_____ P wave:_____

PR interval:_____ QRS:_____

Rhythm interpretation:_____

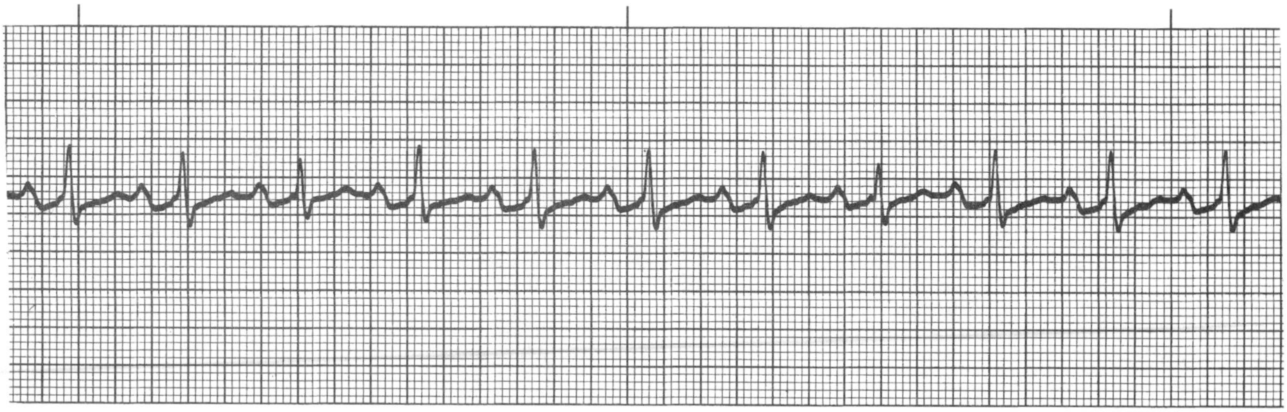

Strip 8-67. Rhythm:_____ Rate:_____ P wave:_____

PR interval:_____ QRS:_____

Rhythm interpretation:_____

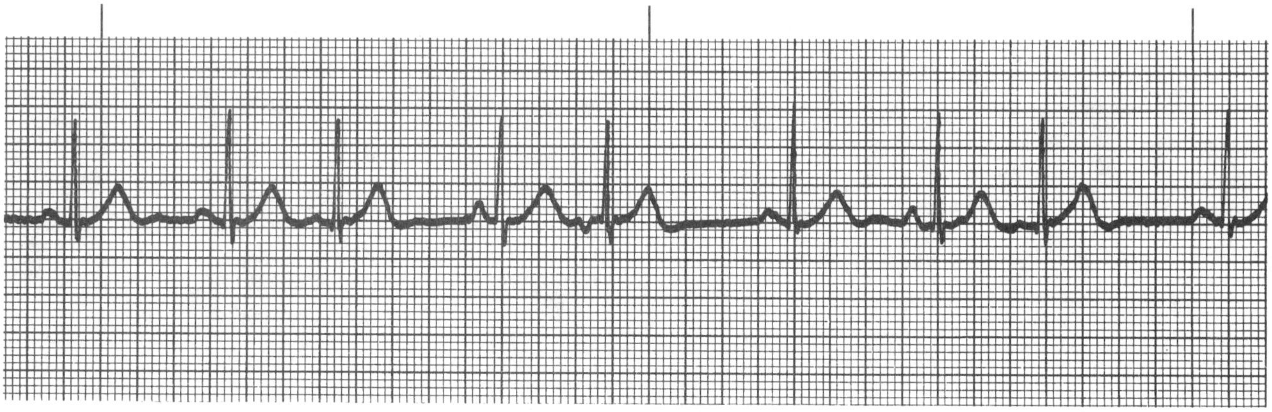

Strip 8-68. Rhythm:_____ Rate:_____ P wave:_____

PR interval:_____ QRS:_____

Rhythm interpretation:_____

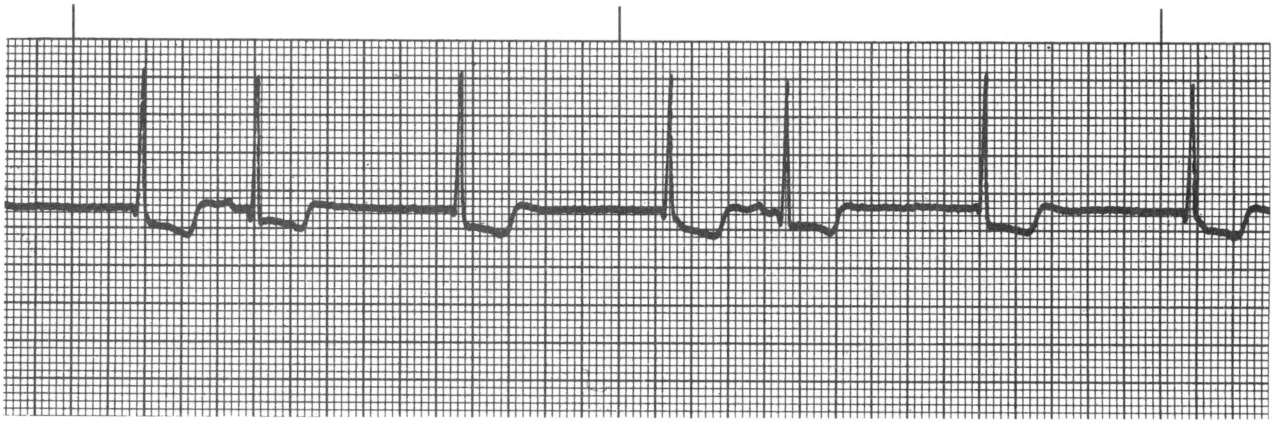

Strip 8-69. Rhythm:_____ Rate:_____ P wave:_____

PR interval:_____ QRS:_____

Rhythm interpretation:_____

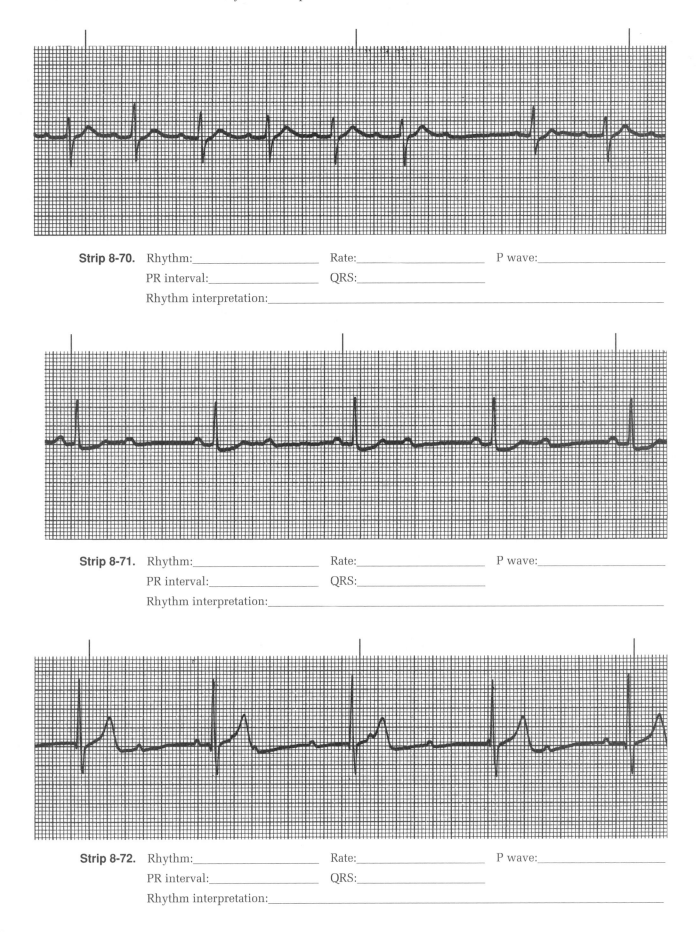

Strip 8-70. Rhythm:_____ Rate:_____ P wave:_____

PR interval:_____ QRS:_____

Rhythm interpretation:_____

Strip 8-71. Rhythm:_____ Rate:_____ P wave:_____

PR interval:_____ QRS:_____

Rhythm interpretation:_____

Strip 8-72. Rhythm:_____ Rate:_____ P wave:_____

PR interval:_____ QRS:_____

Rhythm interpretation:_____

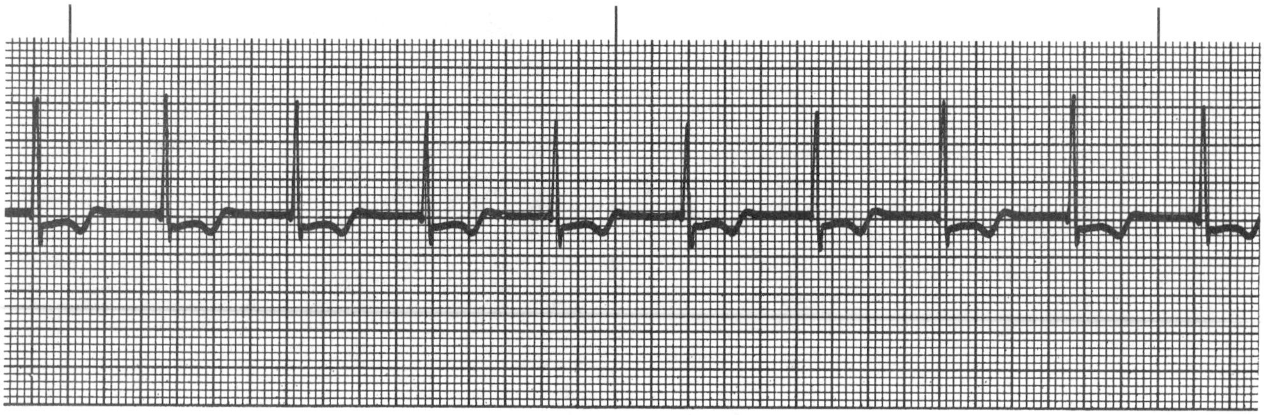

Strip 8-73. Rhythm:_____ Rate:_____ P wave:_____

PR interval:_____ QRS:_____

Rhythm interpretation:_____

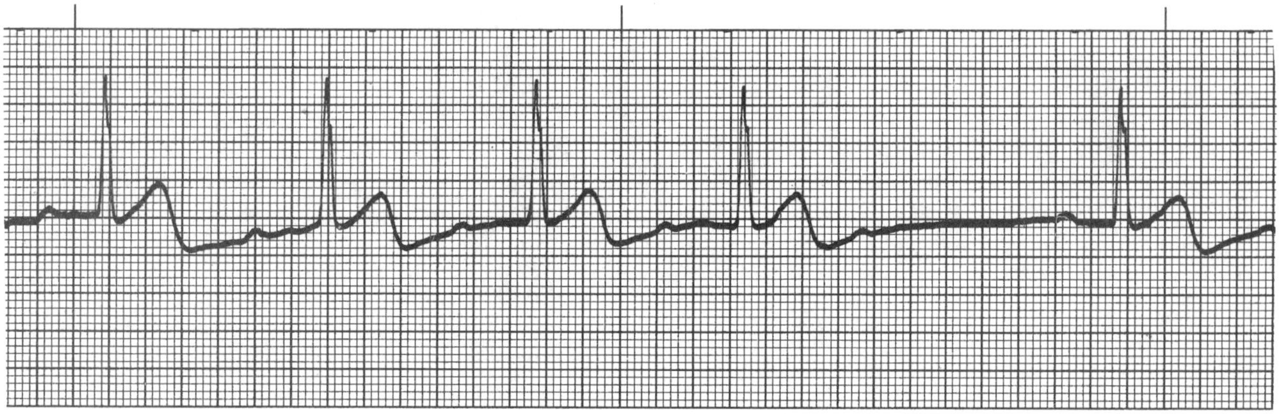

Strip 8-74. Rhythm:_____ Rate:_____ P wave:_____

PR interval:_____ QRS:_____

Rhythm interpretation:_____

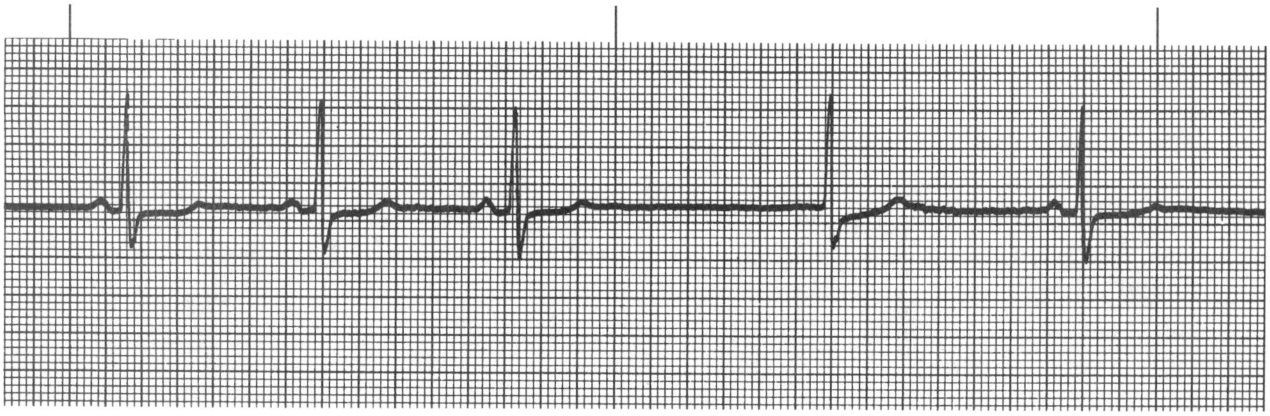

Strip 8-75. Rhythm:_____ Rate:_____ P wave:_____

PR interval:_____ QRS:_____

Rhythm interpretation:_____

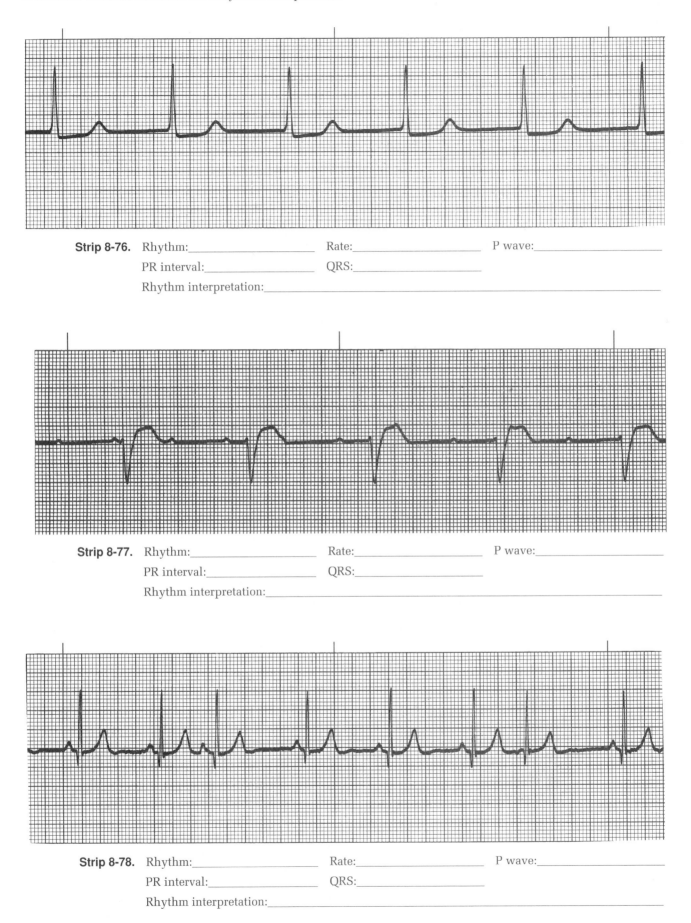

Strip 8-76. Rhythm:_____ Rate:_____ P wave:_____

PR interval:_____ QRS:_____

Rhythm interpretation:_____

Strip 8-77. Rhythm:_____ Rate:_____ P wave:_____

PR interval:_____ QRS:_____

Rhythm interpretation:_____

Strip 8-78. Rhythm:_____ Rate:_____ P wave:_____

PR interval:_____ QRS:_____

Rhythm interpretation:_____

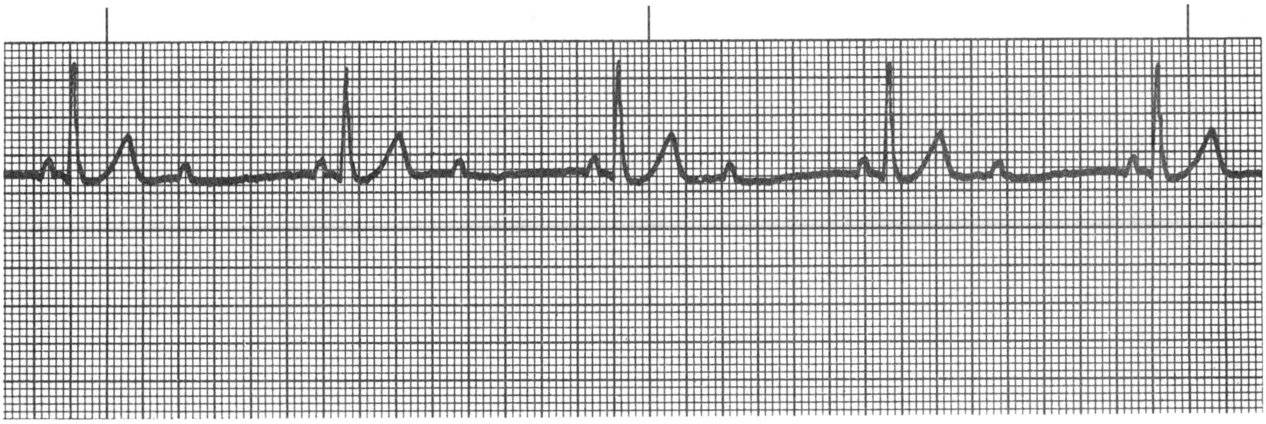

Strip 8-79. Rhythm:_____ Rate:_____ P wave:_____

PR interval:_____ QRS:_____

Rhythm interpretation:_____

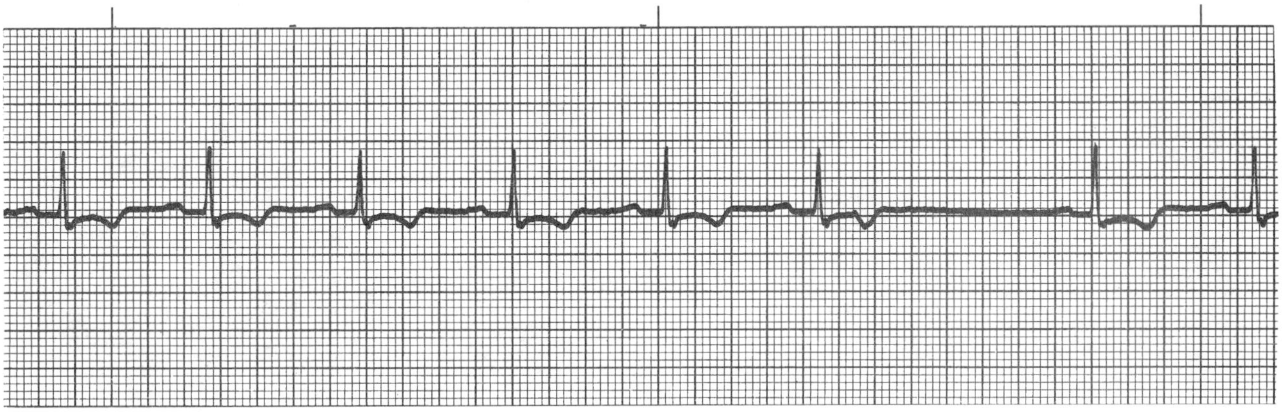

Strip 8-80. Rhythm:_____ Rate:_____ P wave:_____

PR interval:_____ QRS:_____

Rhythm interpretation:_____

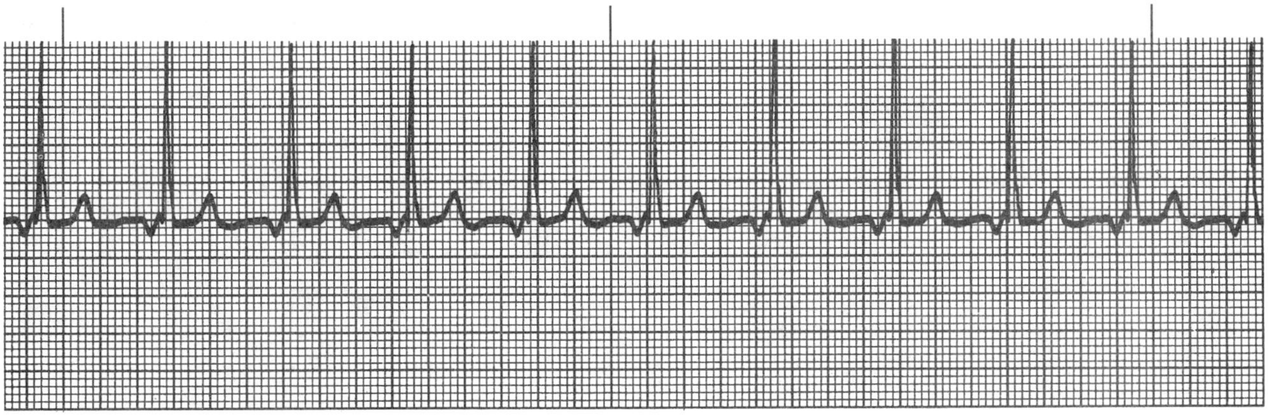

Strip 8-81. Rhythm:_____ Rate:_____ P wave:_____

PR interval:_____ QRS:_____

Rhythm interpretation:_____

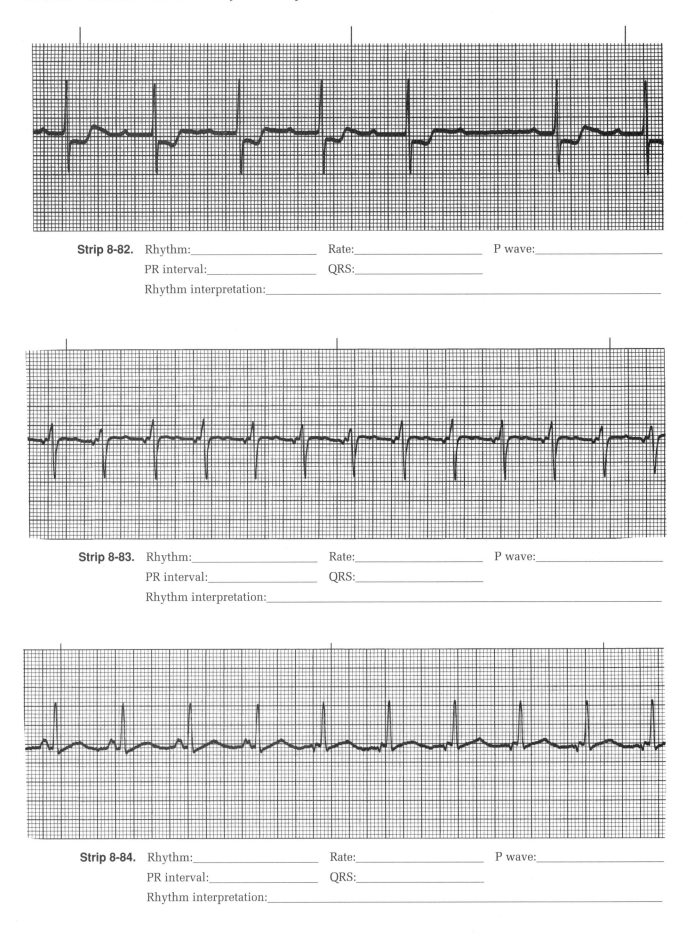

Strip 8-82. Rhythm:_____ Rate:_____ P wave:_____

PR interval:_____ QRS:_____

Rhythm interpretation:_____

Strip 8-83. Rhythm:_____ Rate:_____ P wave:_____

PR interval:_____ QRS:_____

Rhythm interpretation:_____

Strip 8-84. Rhythm:_____ Rate:_____ P wave:_____

PR interval:_____ QRS:_____

Rhythm interpretation:_____

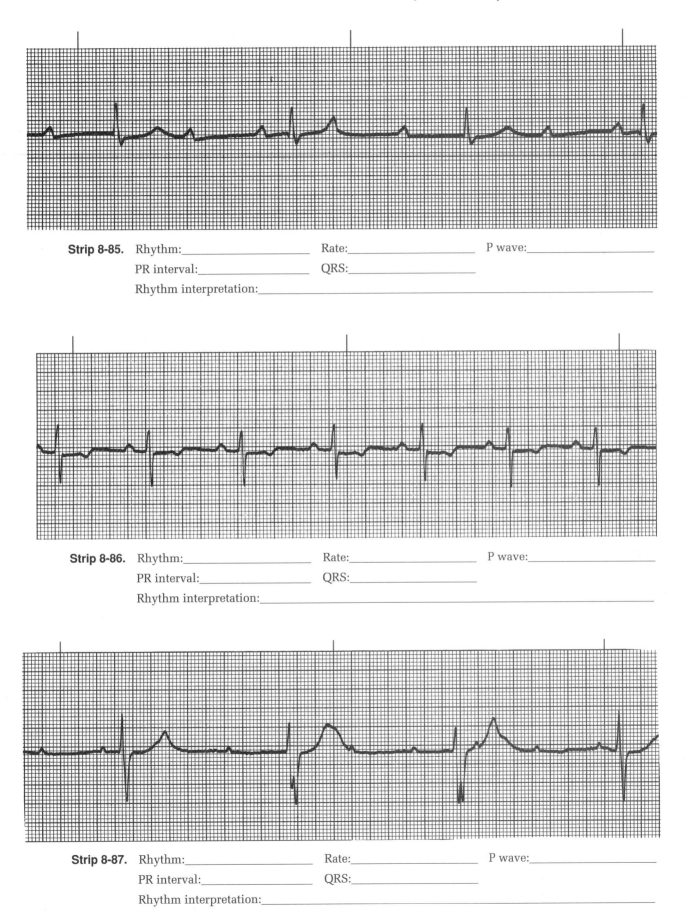

Strip 8-85. Rhythm:_____ Rate:_____ P wave:_____

PR interval:_____ QRS:_____

Rhythm interpretation:_____

Strip 8-86. Rhythm:_____ Rate:_____ P wave:_____

PR interval:_____ QRS:_____

Rhythm interpretation:_____

Strip 8-87. Rhythm:_____ Rate:_____ P wave:_____

PR interval:_____ QRS:_____

Rhythm interpretation:_____

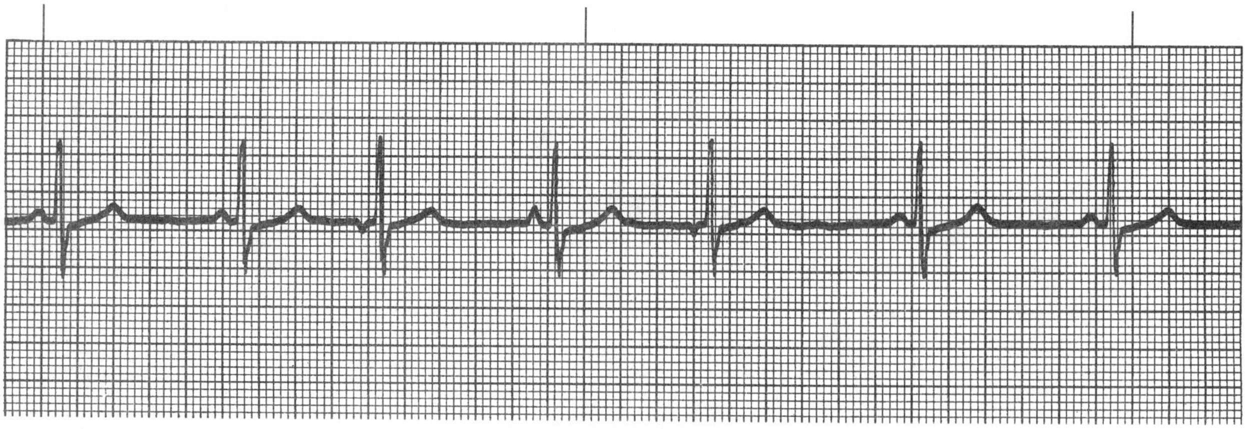

Strip 8-88. Rhythm:_____ Rate:_____ P wave:_____

PR interval:_____ QRS:_____

Rhythm interpretation:_____

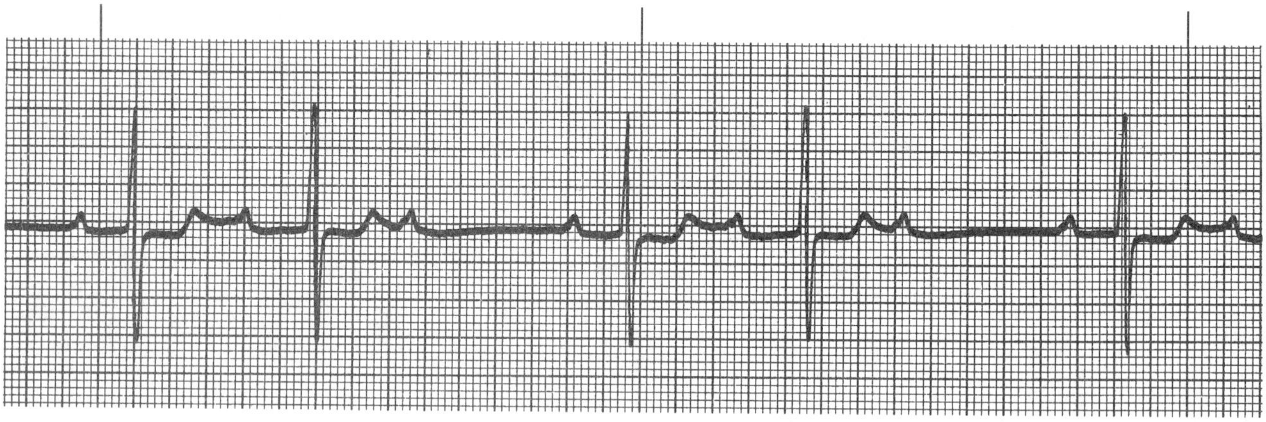

Strip 8-89. Rhythm:_____ Rate:_____ P wave:_____

PR interval:_____ QRS:_____

Rhythm interpretation:_____

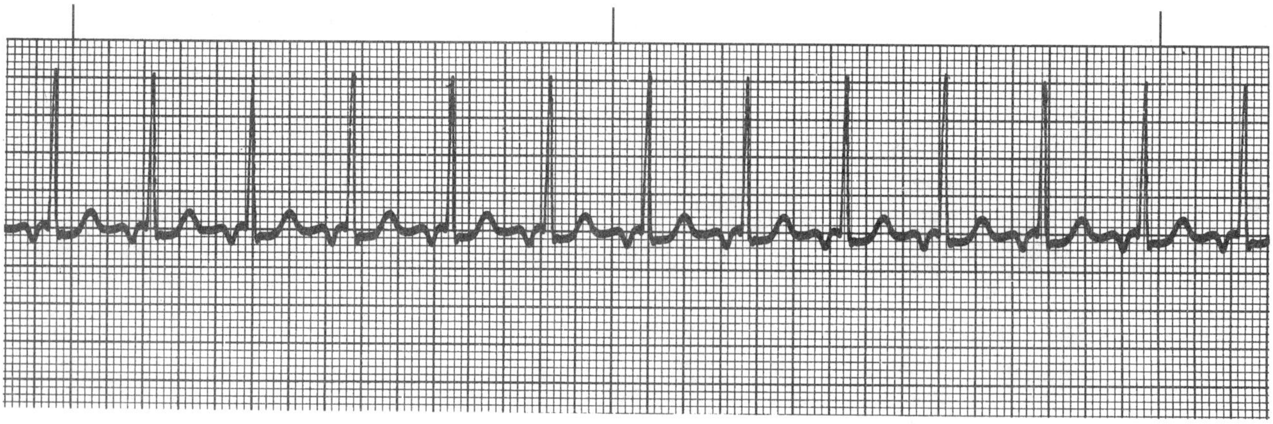

Strip 8-90. Rhythm:_____ Rate:_____ P wave:_____

PR interval:_____ QRS:_____

Rhythm interpretation:_____

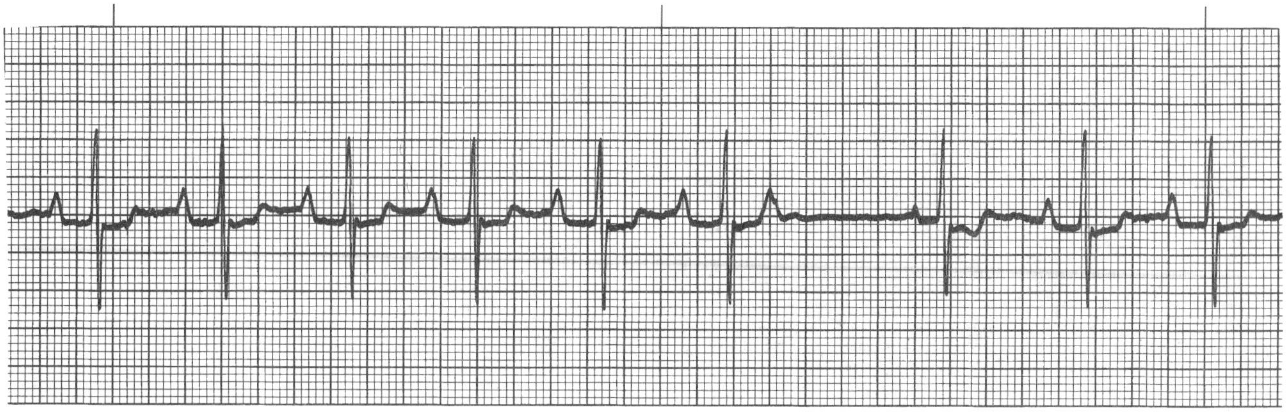

Strip 8-91. Rhythm:_____ Rate:_____ P wave:_____

PR interval:_____ QRS:_____

Rhythm interpretation:_____

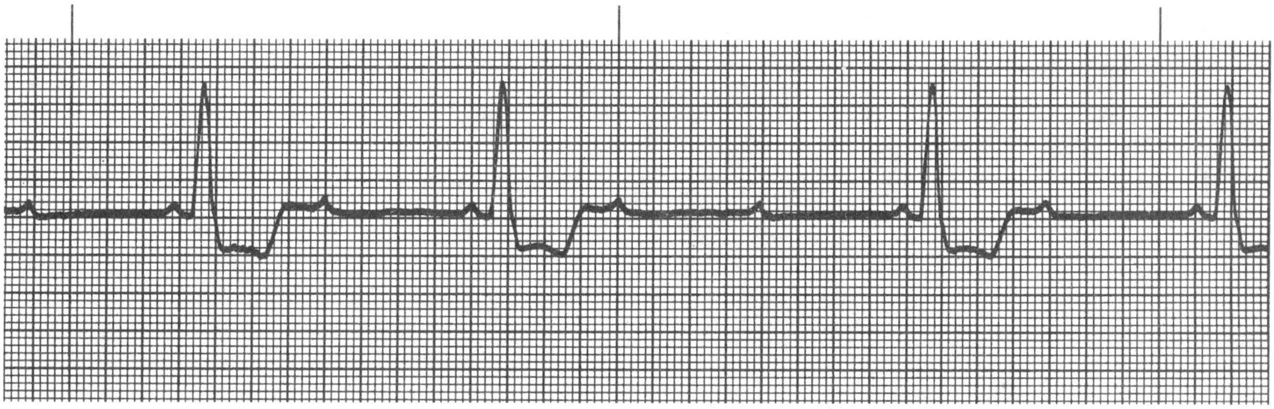

Strip 8-92. Rhythm:_____ Rate:_____ P wave:_____

PR interval:_____ QRS:_____

Rhythm interpretation:_____

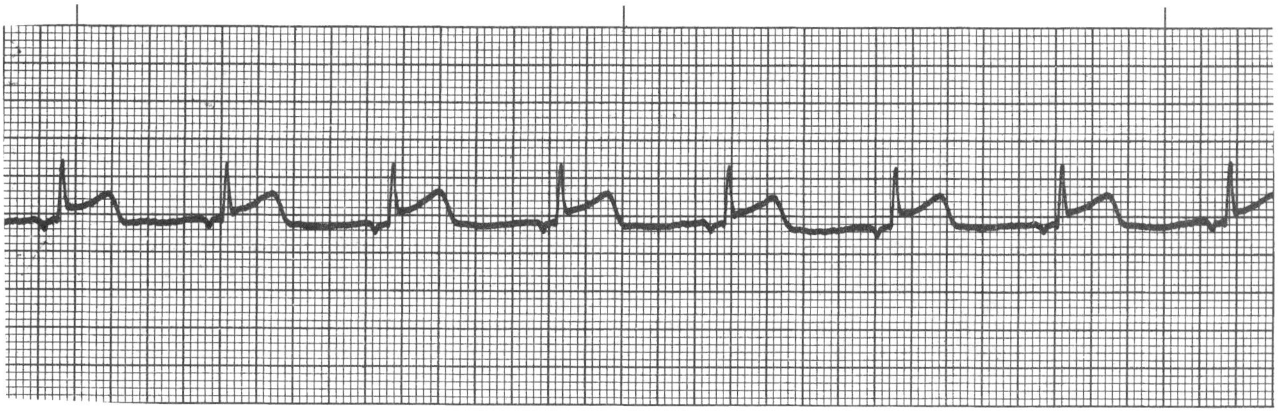

Strip 8-93. Rhythm:_____ Rate:_____ P wave:_____

PR interval:_____ QRS:_____

Rhythm interpretation:_____

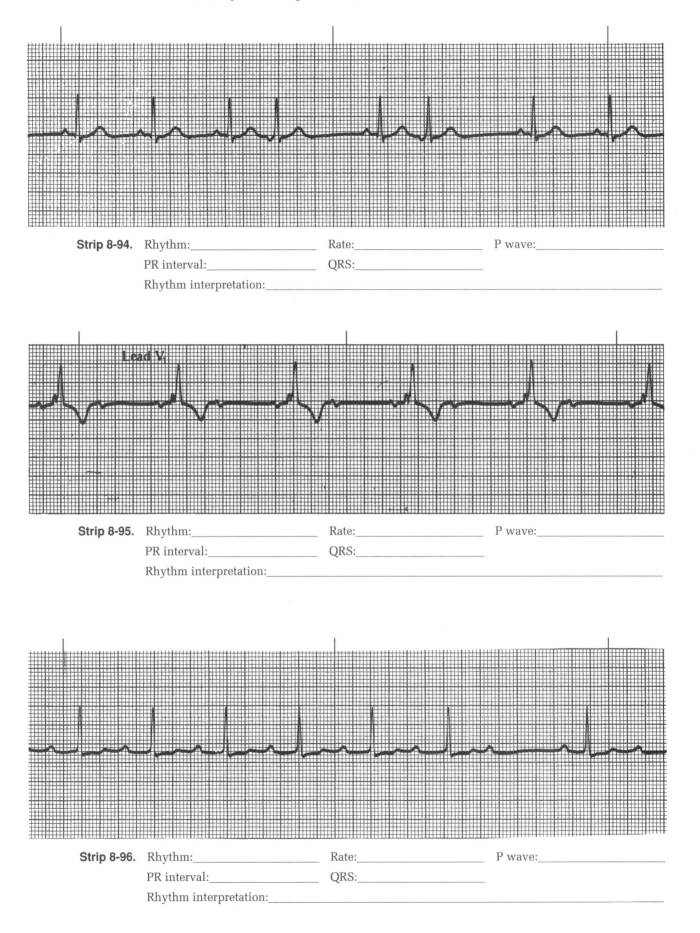

Strip 8-94. Rhythm:_____ Rate:_____ P wave:_____

PR interval:_____ QRS:_____

Rhythm interpretation:_____

Lead V₁

Strip 8-95. Rhythm:_____ Rate:_____ P wave:_____

PR interval:_____ QRS:_____

Rhythm interpretation:_____

Strip 8-96. Rhythm:_____ Rate:_____ P wave:_____

PR interval:_____ QRS:_____

Rhythm interpretation:_____

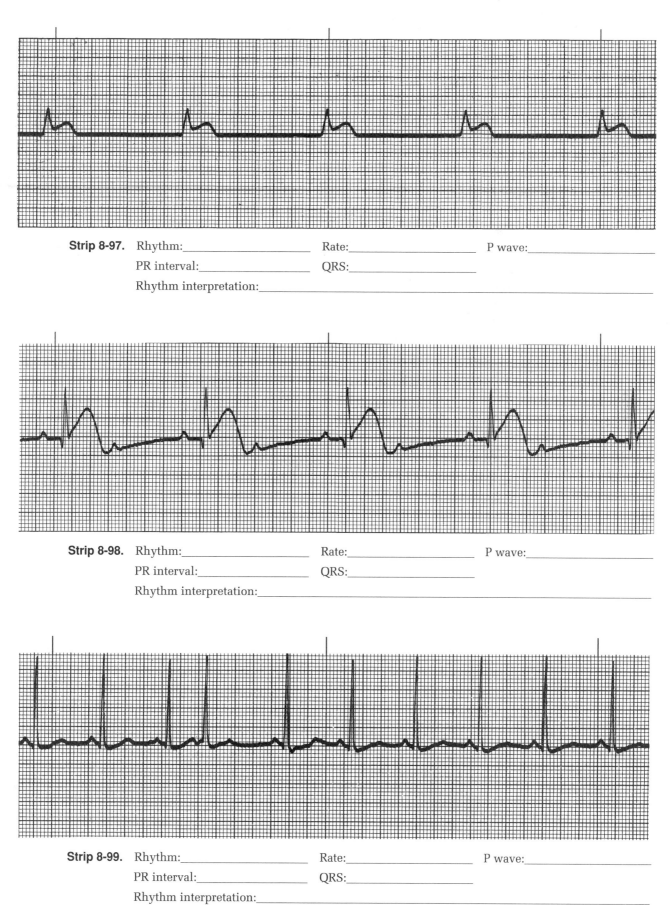

Strip 8-97. Rhythm:_____ Rate:_____ P wave:_____

PR interval:_____ QRS:_____

Rhythm interpretation:_____

Strip 8-98. Rhythm:_____ Rate:_____ P wave:_____

PR interval:_____ QRS:_____

Rhythm interpretation:_____

Strip 8-99. Rhythm:_____ Rate:_____ P wave:_____

PR interval:_____ QRS:_____

Rhythm interpretation:_____

9

Ventricular Arrhythmias and Bundle Branch Block

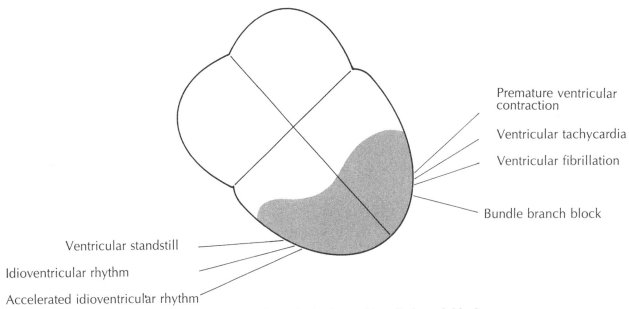

Premature ventricular contraction

Ventricular tachycardia

Ventricular fibrillation

Bundle branch block

Ventricular standstill

Idioventricular rhythm

Accelerated idioventricular rhythm

Figure 9-1. Ventricular arrhythmias and bundle branch block.

Ventricular arrhythmias (Fig. 9-1) originate in the ventricles below the branching portion of the bundle of His and include premature ventricular contractions (PVCs), ventricular tachycardia, ventricular fibrillation, idioventricular rhythm, accelerated idioventricular rhythm, and ventricular standstill. All of these rhythms are associated with a wide QRS complex (except ventricular fibrillation and ventricular standstill). The impulse focus in bundle branch block does not originate in ventricular tissue, but it is included in this rhythm group because of the location of the block within the intraventricular system and the resulting wide QRS. Most of these rhythms are, or have the potential to be, life-threatening and demand prompt recognition and treatment

BUNDLE BRANCH BLOCK

A bundle branch block (Fig. 9-2) (Box 9-1) refers to an obstruction in the transmission of the electrical impulse through one of the branches (either right or

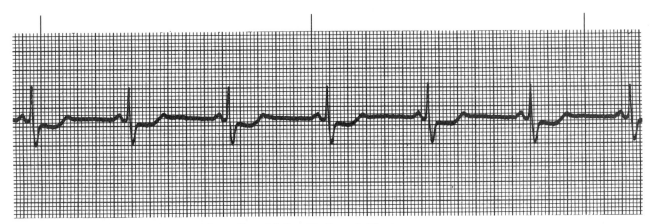

Figure 9-2. **Sinus Bradycardia with Bundle Branch Block**

Rhythm: Regular

Rate: 54

P waves: Sinus P waves are present

PR: 0.14 to 0.16 seconds

QRS: 0.12 seconds

Comment: ST segment depression is present.

left) of the bundle of His. Normally the electrical impulses travel through the right bundle branch and the left bundle branch and their fascicles simultaneously, causing synchronous depolarization of the right and left ventricles. Normal ventricular depolarization is completed within 0.10 seconds or less. A block in one bundle branch causes the ventricle on that side to be depolarized later than the ventricle on the intact side. This delay results in an abnormal QRS complex—one that is wide (0.12 seconds or greater in duration) and bizarre in size and shape. The presence of a bundle branch block can be recognized by a single monitoring lead by the appearance of the wide, bizarre QRS complex. However, differentiating between right and left bundle branch block requires a 12-lead ECG.

Right bundle branch block (RBBB) may be present in healthy individuals with apparently normal hearts. RBBB may be permanent or transient. Sometimes it appears only when the heart rate exceeds a certain critical value (rate-related BBB). Unlike RBBB, left bundle branch block (LBBB) nearly always indicates a diseased heart. LBBB may also be permanent or transient and may be rate-related.

Common causes of bundle branch block include: acute myocardial infarction; coronary and hypertensive heart disease; cardiac tumors; cardiomyopathy; pericarditis; myocarditis; congestive heart failure; syphilitic, rheumatic, and congenital heart disease; and degenerative disease of the electrical conduction system (particularly in older individuals).

A bundle branch block by itself is not significant and requires no treatment. However, a temporary transvenous pacemaker is indicated for the treatment of a right or left bundle branch block under the following conditions:

1. If a new right or left bundle branch block develops as a result of acute myocardial infarction

2. If a bundle branch block is complicated by first-degree, second-degree, or third-degree AV block or by a fascicular block, especially in the setting of an acute MI

PREMATURE VENTRICULAR CONTRACTION (PVC)

A premature ventricular contraction (PVC) (Figs. 9-3 through 9-11) (Box 9-2) is a premature, ectopic impulse that originates somewhere in one of the ventricles and is usually caused by enhanced automaticity. The stimulus will depolarize the ventricle abnormally, resulting in an abnormal QRS complex with the following characteristics:

1. The QRS is premature.

2. A P-wave is not associated with the PVC. Occasionally P-waves are seen preceding the PVC or in the ST or T-wave following the PVC, but these are associated with the underlying rhythm.

3. The QRS is wide (0.12 seconds or greater), distorted and bizarre, often notched, and appears different from the QRS complexes of the underlying rhythm.

4. The ST and T-wave are usually opposite the main QRS deflection. Because depolarization is abnormal, repolarization is also abnormal.

5. The pause associated with the PVC is usually compensatory—that is, the measurement between the R-wave preceding the PVC to the R-wave following the PVC is equal to two R-R intervals of the underlying regular rhythm (Figure 9-3). The compensatory pause occurs because the SA node is not depolarized by the ectopic ventricular beat, the discharge timing remains unchanged, and the basic underlying rhythm will resume on time following the PVC. Rarely, the SA node will be depolarized by the PVC, resulting in a noncompensatory pause (the measurement between the R-wave preceding the PVC to the R-wave following the PVC will be less than two R-R intervals of the underlying regular rhythm).

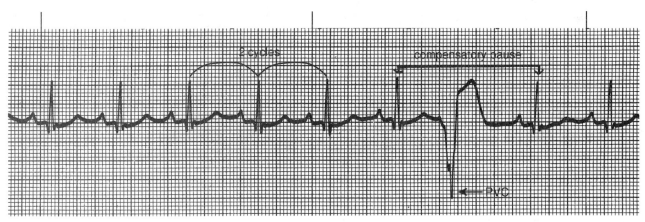

Figure 9-3. **Normal Sinus Rhythm with One PVC**

Rhythm: Basic rhythm regular; irregular with PVC

Rate: Basic rhythm rate 79

P waves: Sinus P waves with basic rhythm

PR: 0.16 to 0.20 seconds (basic rhythm)

QRS: 0.08 to 0.10 seconds (basic rhythm) 0.14 to 0.16 seconds (PVC)

Comment: The interval between the beat preceding the PVC and the beat following the PVC is equal to the time of two normal beats and represents a full compensatory pause.

PVCs occur in addition to the patient's underlying rhythm and appear in various combinations. They may appear as a single beat, every other beat (bigeminal pattern, Figure 9-4), every third beat (trigeminal pattern, Figure 9-5), every fourth beat (quadrigeminal pattern), in pairs, also called couplets (Figure 9-6), or in runs (Figure 9-7). A run of three or more consecutive PVCs is termed ventricular tachycardia. PVCs which are identical in size, shape, and direction arise from the same focus in the ventricles and are called uniform or unifocal PVCs. PVCs from different ectopic sites will differ in size, shape, and direction and are called multiform or multifocal PVCs (Figure 9-8). A PVC sandwiched between two normally conducted sinus beats, without greatly disturbing the regularity of the underlying rhythm, is called an interpolated PVC (Figure 9-9)—a full compensatory pause, usually associated with the PVC, is absent.

The "R-on-T" phenomenon (Figure 9-10) is a term used to indicate a PVC that has occurred during the vulnerable period of ventricular repolarization (on or near the peak of the T-wave). During this period some myocardial muscle fibers are completely repolarized, others are partially repolarized, while still others may be completely refractory. Stimulation of the ventricle at this time may precipitate repetitive ventricular contractions, resulting in ventricular tachycardia or fibrillation.

Like premature atrial contractions, PVCs are very common, becoming more frequent with age. They may occur in healthy hearts as well as in individuals with underlying heart disease. Some of the causes of PVCs include: anxiety; excessive caffeine and alcohol intake; certain drugs (digitalis, epinephrine, isoproterenol, aminophylline); hypoxia; acidosis; electrolyte imbalance (hypokalemia, hypomagnesemia); congestive heart failure; myocardial infarction;

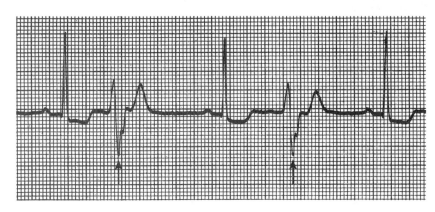

Figure 9-4. Bigeminal PVCs.

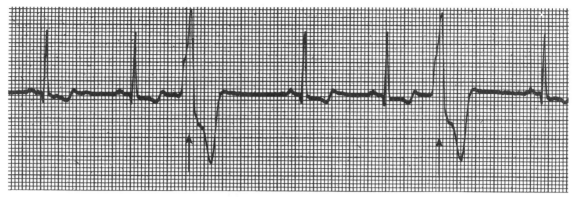

Figure 9-5. Trigeminal PVCs.

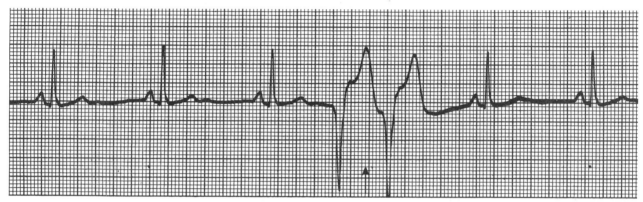

Figure 9-6. Paired PVCs.

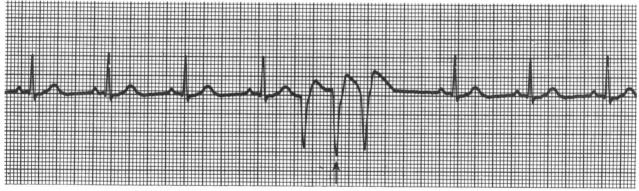

Figure 9-7. Run of PVCs (a paroxysm of ventricular tachycardia).

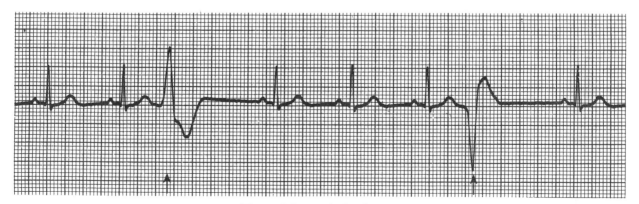

Figure 9-8. Multifocal PVCs.

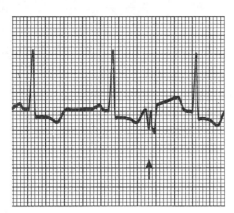

Figure 9-9. Interpolated PVC.

valvular, hypertensive or ischemic heart disease; cardiomyopathy; reperfusion following thrombolytic therapy or angioplasty; heart surgery or contact of the endocardium with catheters (pacing leads, pulmonary artery catheters).

Treatment of PVCs should be guided by the clinical setting. Because occasional PVCs are a normal finding in healthy individuals, no treatment may be indicated. Initially a search should be made for possible reversible causes. Elimination of certain drugs, oxygen therapy for hypoxemia, treatment of hypokalemia and hypomagnesemia may be effective in some patients. Frequent PVCs (greater than 5 per

minute), paired PVCs, runs of 3 or more consecutive PVCs, or R-on-T PVCs are usually treated, especially in patients with acute myocardial infarction or ischemic heart disease, because of the increased risk of ventricular tachycardia or ventricular fibrillation in this setting. In the acute setting, IV lidocaine or procainamide may be used. In the nonacute setting, oral antiarrhythmics may be given. PVCs resistant to conventional drug therapy may require electrophysiologic study.

On some occasions a ventricular beat may occur late instead of early. These beats are called ventricular escape beats (Figure 9-11). Escape beats are more likely to occur due to an increased vagal effect on the SA node rather than to enhanced automaticity, as is associated with the premature ventricular beat. Escape beats occur commonly following a pause in the underlying rhythm. The morphologic characteristics of the late beat will be the same as for the PVC. No treatment is required.

VENTRICULAR TACHYCARDIA

Ventricular tachycardia (Figures 9-12 and 9-13) (Box 9-3) is an arrhythmia originating in an ectopic focus in the ventricles, discharging impulses at a rate of 140–250 per minute. The rhythm is usually asso-

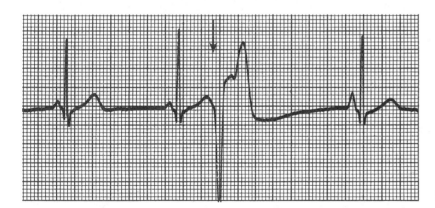

Figure 9-10. R-on-T PVC.

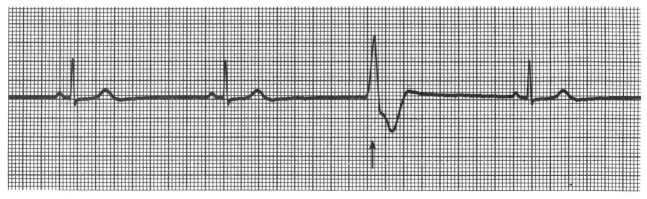

Figure 9-11. Ventricular escape beat.

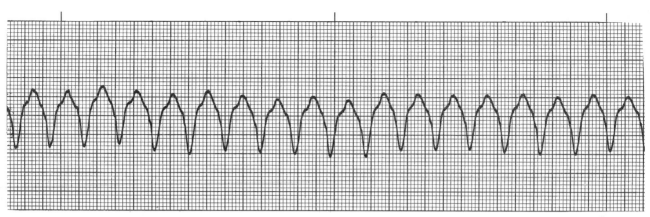

Figure 9-12. **Ventricular Tachycardia**

Rhythm:	Regular
Rate:	150
P waves:	None identified
PR:	Not measurable
QRS:	0.14–0.16 seconds

ciated with enhanced automaticity or reentry. On the ECG the rhythm appears as a series of wide QRS complexes at a rapid rate. There are no associated P-waves. The QRS complexes are distorted and bizarre, often notched, with a duration of 0.12 seconds or greater. As a rule the QRS complexes are identical (monomorphic). When the QRS complexes differ, the ventricular tachycardia is considered to be polymorphic. The QRS complexes are followed by large T-waves, opposite in direction to the main QRS deflection. The rhythm is usually regular, but may be slightly irregular.

Ventricular tachycardia usually occurs in patients with underlying heart disease. It commonly occurs in myocardial ischemia or infarction, cardiomyopathy, mitral valve prolapse, or congestive

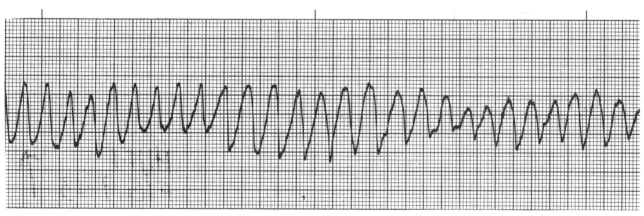

Figure 9-13. **Ventricular Tachycardia (Torsades de pointes)**

Rhythm:	Regular
Rate:	250
P waves:	None identified
PR:	Not measurable
QRS:	0.12–0.22 seconds (some much wider than others)
Comment:	This type of ventricular tachycardia is called torsades de pointes (twists of points). The QRS changes from negative to positive polarity and appears to twist around the isoelectric line. It is associated with a prolonged QT interval and is refractory to lidocaine and procainamide. Intravenous magnesium or overdrive pacing has been successful in the treatment of this rhythm.

Box 9-3. Ventricular Tachycardia: Identifying ECG Features

Rhythm: Regular

Rate: 140–250

P waves: No P-waves are associated with ventricular tachycardia. However, the SA node continues to beat independently and sinus P-waves may occasionally be seen before or after the PVC— usually the P waves are hidden in the QRS complexes.

PR: Not measurable

QRS: Wide (0.12 seconds or greater)

heart failure. Digitalis toxicity is also a common cause of ventricular tachycardia. Certain medications (quinidine, procainamide, tricyclic antidepressants) may prolong the QT interval, causing the ventricles to be particularly vulnerable to ventricular tachycardia. Other causes include electrolyte disturbances (especially hypokalemia and hypomagnesemia), mechanical stimulation of the endocardium by a pacing catheter or pulmonary artery catheter, and reperfusion following thrombolytic therapy or angioplasty.

Ventricular tachycardia may develop without any warning signs but is most often preceded by frequent or dangerous forms of PVCs (occurring in pairs, runs, or R-on-T type). Ventricular tachycardia may appear as a sustained rhythm (lasting longer than 30 seconds) or as a nonsustained rhythm (lasting less than 30 seconds) occurring in short bursts or paroxysms. A series of three or more consecutive PVCs is technically considered a burst of ventricular tachycardia.

The seriousness of ventricular tachycardia depends primarily on its duration. Nonsustained ventricular tachycardia, unless frequent, usually does not cause hemodynamic compromise, but can progress into sustained VT. Sustained ventricular tachycardia is a life-threatening arrhythmia for two major reasons. First, the rapid ventricular rate and loss of atrial kick reduce cardiac output, leading to hypotension and decreased perfusion to vital organs. Second, the condition may degenerate into ventricular fibrillation.

Treatment of ventricular tachycardia depends on the clinical setting and the ability of the patient to tolerate the arrhythmia. First check the pulse. If there is no pulse (pulseless VT), the rhythm must be treated as ventricular fibrillation. *If there is a pulse and the patient is stable* (conscious, acceptable vital signs, no complaints of anginal pain, and so forth), the following protocols should be followed:

1. Give lidocaine IV in a bolus dose of 1–1.5 mg/kg, followed thereafter by one-half the initial dose every 5 minutes until the rhythm is suppressed or resolved or a total dose of 3 mg/kg has been given. If rhythm is suppressed or resolved, start lidocaine maintenance infusion (1 gm lidocaine in 250 cc D_5W at 2 mg/minute [30 cc/hr]).

2. If rhythm is unresolved, give procainamide IV slowly at 20 mg/minute until the rhythm is suppressed, significant hypotension ensues, the QRS doubles its pretreatment width, or a total dose of 17 mg/kg (usually 1000 mg) has been given. If rhythm is suppressed or resolved, start procainamide maintenance infusion (1 gm procainamide in 250 cc D_5W at 2 mg/minute [30 cc/hr]).

3. If rhythm is unresolved, give bretylium 5 mg/kg (usually 500 mg) diluted in 50 cc D_5W over 8–10 minutes. If rhythm is unresolved, repeat bretylium at a dose of 10 mg/kg diluted in 50 cc D,W over 8–10 minutes. Bretylium may be repeated every 10–30 minutes until a total of 30 mg/kg is given. If rhythm is suppressed or resolved, start bretylium maintenance infusion (1 gm in 250 cc D_5W at 2 mg/minute [30 cc/hr]).

4. If the rhythm is unresponsive to drug therapy, sedate the patient and perform cardioversion beginning at 100 joules, increasing joules (200, 300, 360) with subsequent attempts.

If there is a pulse and the patient is unstable (unconscious, hypotensive, or complaining of anginal pain), the following protocols should be followed:

1. Sedate the patient (if not unconscious).

2. Cardiovert the rhythm at 100 joules initially, increasing the joules (200, 300, 360) with subsequent attempts.

3. Begin drug therapy as under stable VT protocols, alternating with cardioversion attempts (drug/shock/drug/shock).

Treatment of chronic, recurrent ventricular tachycardia includes therapy with oral antidysrhythmic drugs. Further evaluation may include specialized electrophysiologic testing and endocardial mapping, with long-term options including use of the implantable cardioverter defibrillator (ICD) or reentry circuit ablation. The ICD is a special, surgically implanted device developed to deliver an electric shock directly to the heart during a life-threatening tachycardia. Destruction (ablation) of the reentry circuit involves delivering short pulses of radiofrequency current through an intracardiac catheter. It produces a small burn that effectively blocks the part of the circuit supporting the reentrant-type wave.

A unique variant form of ventricular tachycardia called *torsade de pointes* (Figure 9-13) in which the

QRS complexes seem to twist around the baseline, changing back and forth from negative to positive polarity, is commonly an immediate forerunner to ventricular fibrillation. This polymorphic type of ventricular tachycardia is associated with a prolonged QT interval and is often caused by drugs conventionally recommended in treating ventricular tachycardia (e.g., quinidine or procainamide). Other causes include phenothiazine or tricyclic antidepressant overdose, and electrolyte disturbances (especially hypokalemia and hypomagnesemia). Drugs used to treat "ordinary" ventricular tachycardia are usually ineffective and some may paradoxically exacerbate the arrhythmia. Treatment protocols include:

1. Elimination of predisposing factors—rhythm has tendency to recur unless precipitating factors are eliminated.

2. Administration of magnesium sulfate bolus (1–2 gm of a 50% solution diluted in 10 cc D_5W) over 1–2 minutes followed by maintenance infusion of 1–2 gm/hr.

3. Overdrive pacing, especially if rhythm is precipitated by bradycardia.

4. Cardioversion beginning at 100 joules, increasing joules (200, 300, 360) with subsequent attempts.

VENTRICULAR FIBRILLATION

In ventricular fibrillation (Figures 9-14 and 9-15) (Box 9-4) a disorganized, chaotic, electrical focus in the ventricles takes over control of the heart. The ventricles do not beat in any coordinated fashion but instead quiver asynchronously and ineffectively, just as the atria respond in atrial fibrillation. The ECG tracing shows an irregular, chaotic baseline with wave deflections of varying size, shape, and height with no QRS complexes present. If the fibrillatory waves are large the arrhythmia is considered to be "coarse" ventricular fibrillation. If the fibrillatory waves are small the arrhythmia is considered to be "fine" ventricular fibrillation. The distinction between the two may be significant since coarse ventricular fibrillation usually indicates a more recent onset and is more likely to be reversed by defibrillation. Fine ventricular fibrillation usually indicates that the arrhythmia has been present longer and may require drug therapy first, then defibrillation, before arrhythmia can be reversed. In addition, fine ventricular fibrillation must be differentiated from asystole.

Ventricular fibrillation is the most common cause of sudden cardiac death. It usually occurs in the presence of significant heart disease, most commonly coronary artery disease, myocardial ischemia, and acute myocardial infarction. Other causes include: cardiomyopathy, mitral valve prolapse, cardiac trauma, drug toxicity (digitalis, quinidine, procainamide), hypoxia, electrolyte imbalance (hypokalemia, hyperkalemia), and accidental electrical shock.

Ventricular fibrillation may occur spontaneously, but it is most often preceded by ventricular tachycardia or frequent or dangerous forms of PVCs (occurring in pairs, runs, multifocal, or R-on-T type). Once ventricular fibrillation occurs there is no cardiac output, peripheral pulses and blood pressure are absent, and the patient becomes unconscious im-

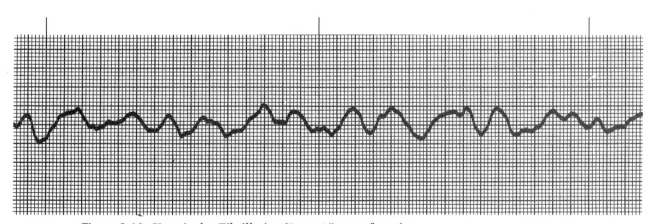

Figure 9-14. Ventricular Fibrillation ("coarse" wave forms)

Rhythm:	Chaotic
Rate:	0 (no QRS complexes are present)
P waves:	None; wave deflections are chaotic and vary in size, shape, and height
PR:	Not measurable
QRS:	Absent

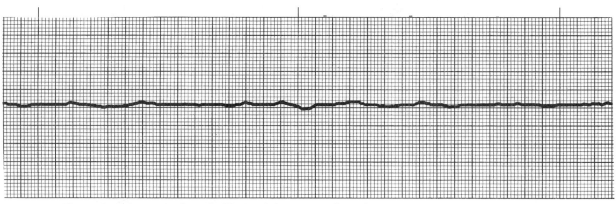

Figure 9-15. Ventricular Fibrillation ("fine" wave forms)

Rhythm:	Chaotic
Rate:	0 (no QRS complexes are present)
P waves:	Absent; wave deflections are chaotic and vary in size, shape, and height
PR:	Not measurable
QRS:	Absent

mediately. Cyanosis and seizures may also be present. Death is imminent unless the arrhythmia is treated immediately. Treatment protocols include:

1. Check the pulse and rapidly assess the patient—if there is a pulse and/or the patient is conscious, ventricular fibrillation is not the problem. ECG artifacts produced by loose or dry electrodes, patient movement, or muscle tremors, may resemble ventricular fibrillation.

2. If there is no pulse and the patient is unconscious, administer a precordial thump (witnessed arrest in monitored patient only).

3. Defibrillate starting at 200 joules; if unsuccessful, defibrillate at 300 and 360 in rapid succession.

4. Start CPR; establish an IV line; intubate patient.

5. Give epinephrine 1 mg IV; continue CPR for 1 minute to circulate drug; defibrillate at 360 joules.

Repeat epinephrine every 3–5 minutes. Note: if IV access is not available, give 2–2½ times the IV dose via the endotracheal tube.

6. Give lidocaine 1–1.5 mg/kg IV; continue CPR to circulate drug; defibrillate at 360 joules. IV lidocaine may be repeated at half-dose increments every 5 minutes until a total dose of 3 mg/kg has been given. Note: if IV access is not available, give 2–2½ times the IV dose via an endotracheal tube. If rhythm resolves, start lidocaine drip (1 gm in 250 cc D_5W) at 2 mg/minute [30 cc/hr]).

7. Give bretylium 5 mg/kg (usually 500 mg) IV undiluted; continue CPR for 1 minute to circulate drug; defibrillate at 360 joules. Bretylium may be increased to 10 mg/kg until total dose of 30 mg/kg has been given. If rhythm resolves, start bretylium drip (1 gm in 250 cc D_5W at 2 mg/minute [30 cc/hr]).

8. Continue drugs, circulation, defibrillation attempts until rhythm resolves or a decision is made to stop resuscitative efforts.

Box 9-4. Ventricular Fibrillation: Identifying ECG Features

Rhythm:	Chaotic
Rate:	0 (no QRS complexes are present)
P waves:	Absent; wave deflections seen are chaotic and vary in size, shape, and height; wave deflections may be small (described as "fine") or large (described as "coarse")
PR:	Not measurable
QRS:	Absent

IDIOVENTRICULAR RHYTHM (VENTRICULAR ESCAPE RHYTHM)

Idioventricular rhythm (IVR) (Figure 9-16) (Box 9-5) is an arrhythmia originating in an escape pacemaker site in the ventricles, with a heart rate between 30–40 per minute (sometimes less). Since the impulse focus is in the ventricles, there is no associated atrial activity and P-waves will not be present. The ECG tracing is characterized by an absence of P-

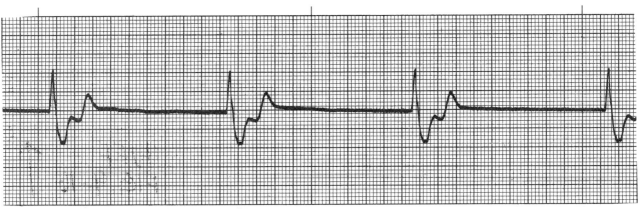

Figure 9-16. **Idioventricular Rhythm**

Rhythm:	Irregular
Rate:	30
P waves:	Absent
PR:	Not measurable
QRS:	0.22–0.24 seconds

waves, with wide QRS complexes occurring regularly at a rate of 40 or less.

Idioventricular rhythm occurs when 1) the rate of impulse formation of the higher pacemaker centers (SA node and AV node) become less than that of the escape pacemaker in the ventricles, or 2) the impulses from the higher pacing centers are blocked and fail to reach the ventricles. The ventricular escape rhythm may be transient or continuous. Transient idioventricular rhythm is seen as three or more ventricular beats lasting only a few seconds or minutes, is usually related to increased vagal effect on the higher pacing centers, and is not significant. Continuous idioventricular rhythm is seen in advanced heart disease or heart failure and is usually a terminal event, occurring just before ventricular standstill. Continuous idioventricular rhythm is generally symptomatic, associated with hypotension and a marked decrease in cardiac output. Treatment of the rhythm includes:

1. Administer atropine 0.5–1 mg IV—may repeat every 3–5 minutes until heart rate increases or a total dose of 0.04 mg/kg (usually 2–3 mg) is given.

Box 9-5. Idioventricular Rhythm: Identifying ECG Features

Rhythm:	Usually regular
Rate:	30–40 (sometimes slower)
P waves:	Absent
PR:	Not measurable
QRS:	Wide (0.12 seconds or greater)

2. Initiate transcutaneous pacing.

3. If hypotensive, start dopamine infusion (400 mg dopamine in 500 cc D₅W) at 2.5–5 micrograms/kg/minute.

4. Consider insertion of temporary transvenous pacemaker.

ACCELERATED IDIOVENTRICULAR RHYTHM

Accelerated idioventricular rhythm (AIVR) (Figure 9-17) (Box 9-6) is an arrhythmia originating in an ectopic pacemaker site in the ventricles with a rate between 50–100 per minute. The term "accelerated" denotes a rhythm that exceeds the inherent ventricular escape rate of 30–40 but is not fast enough to be ventricular tachycardia. This rhythm is usually related to enhanced automaticity of the ventricular tissue. Accelerated idioventricular rhythm has the same ECG characteristics as idioventricular rhythm and is differentiated by the heart rate.

Accelerated idioventricular rhythm is common following acute myocardial infarction and is frequently a reperfusion rhythm (either spontaneous reperfusion or following thrombolytic therapy or angioplasty). It is also seen in patients with cardiomyopathy. Accelerated idioventricular rhythm is a transient arrhythmia that is usually well tolerated and produces no hemodynamic effects. Brief episodes of AIVR frequently alternate with periods of normal sinus rhythm. Treatment is usually not required.

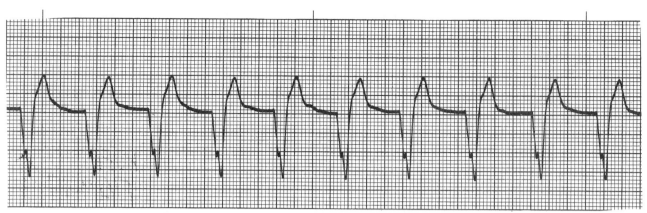

Figure 9-17. **Accelerated Idioventricular Rhythm**

Rhythm: Regular

Rate: 84

P waves: None identified

PR: Not measurable

QRS: 0.16 seconds

Box 9-6. **Accelerated Idioventricular Rhythm: Identifying ECG Features**

Rhythm: Usually regular

Rate: 50–100

P waves: Absent

PR: Not measurable

QRS: Wide (0.12 seconds or greater)

VENTRICULAR STANDSTILL (VENTRICULAR ASYSTOLE)

Ventricular standstill or asystole (Figures 9-18 and 9-19) (Box 9-7) is the absence of all electrical activity within the ventricles. The ECG tracing will show either P-waves without QRS complexes or a straight line. If P-waves are present the arrhythmia

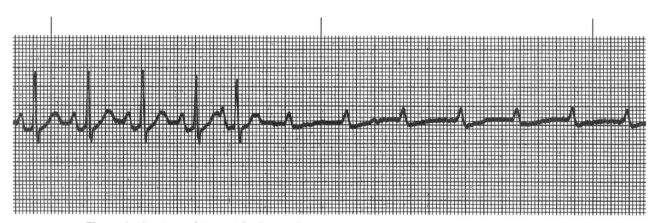

Figure 9-18. **Normal Sinus Rhythm with One PAC Changing to Ventricular Standstill**

Rhythm: Basic rhythm regular

Rate: Basic rhythm 100

P waves: Sinus P waves are present

PR: 0.16 to 0.18 seconds (basic rhythm)

QRS: 0.06 seconds (basic rhythm)

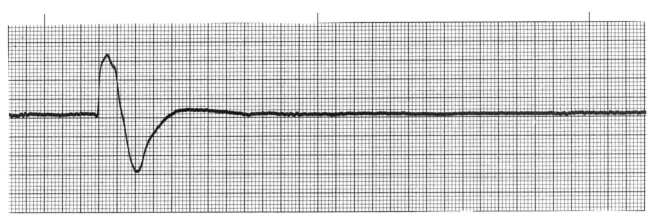

Figure 9-19. One Wide Ventricular Complex Changing to Ventricular Standstill

Rhythm:	0
Rate:	0
P waves:	None identified
PR:	Not measurable
QRS:	0.28 seconds or wider

Box 9-7. Ventricular Standstill: Identifying ECG Features

Rhythm:	0 (no QRS complexes are present)
Rate:	0 (no QRS complexes are present)
P waves:	ECG tracing will show either P-waves without QRS complexes or a straight line
PR:	Not measurable
QRS:	Absent

was most likely preceded by some type of advanced AV block (second-degree Mobitz II or third-degree). Ventricular standstill with a straight line is usually the terminal arrhythmia following ventricular tachycardia, ventricular fibrillation, or idioventricular rhythm. Prognosis is extremely poor despite resuscitative efforts.

Once ventricular standstill occurs there is no cardiac output, peripheral pulses and blood pressure are absent, and the patient becomes unconscious immediately. Cyanosis and seizure activity may also be present. Death is imminent unless the arrhythmia is treated immediately. Treatment protocols include:

1. Check pulse and rapidly assess the patient—if there is a pulse and/or the patient is conscious, ventricular standstill is not the problem.

2. Check monitor lead system—a loose electrode pad or lead wire will show a straight line. Check monitor rhythm in 2 leads if possible—fine waveform ventricular fibrillation may mimic ventricular standstill.

3. Start CPR; establish IV line; intubate patient.

4. Give epinephrine 1 mg IV—continue CPR to circulate drug; drug may be repeated every 3–5 minutes. Note: if IV access is not available, give 2–2½ times the IV dose via endotracheal tube.

5. Give atropine 1 mg IV—continue CPR to circulate drug; drug may be repeated every 3–5 minutes until total dose of 0.04 mg/kg (usually 2–3 mg) is given. Note: if IV access is not available, give 2–2½ times the IV dose VIA endotracheal tube.

6. Apply transcutaneous pacemaker. Consider insertion of temporary transvenous pacemaker

7. Continue administration of epinephrine, atropine, and CPR until rhythm is resolved or a decision is made to discontinue resuscitative efforts.

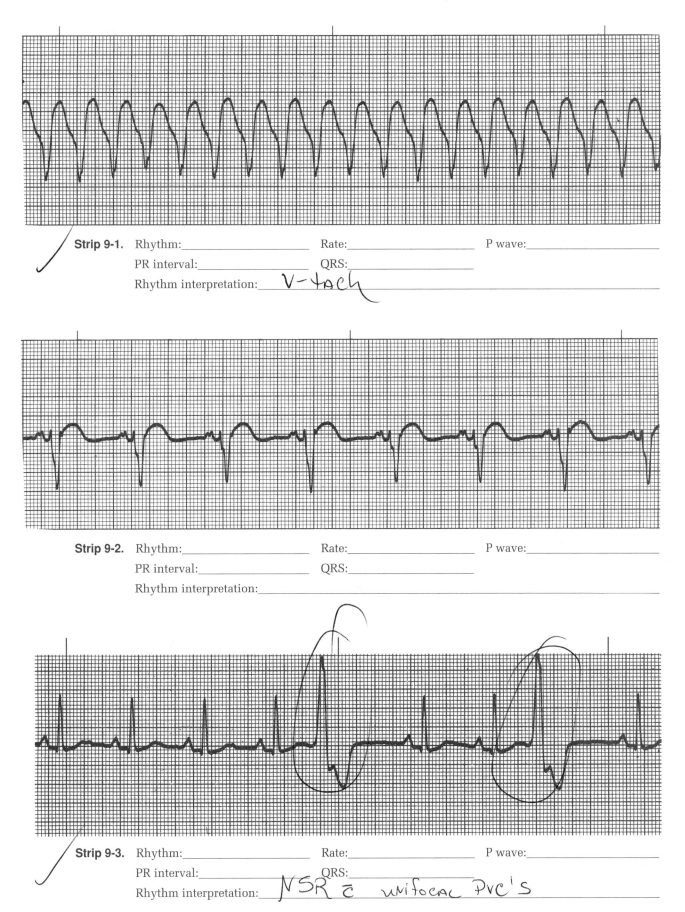

Strip 9-1. Rhythm:_____ Rate:_____ P wave:_____

PR interval:_____ QRS:_____

Rhythm interpretation:___V-tach_____

Strip 9-2. Rhythm:_____ Rate:_____ P wave:_____

PR interval:_____ QRS:_____

Rhythm interpretation:_____

Strip 9-3. Rhythm:_____ Rate:_____ P wave:_____

PR interval:_____ QRS:_____

Rhythm interpretation:___NSR c̄ uNifocal PVC's_____

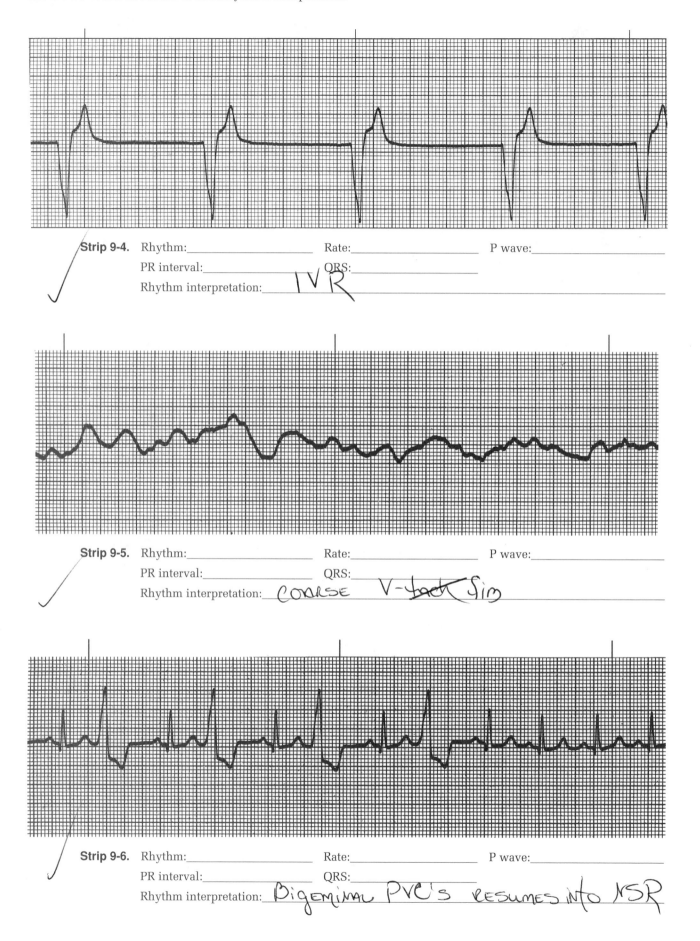

Strip 9-4. Rhythm:_____ Rate:_____ P wave:_____

PR interval:_____ QRS:_____

Rhythm interpretation:____IVR_____

Strip 9-5. Rhythm:_____ Rate:_____ P wave:_____

PR interval:_____ QRS:_____

Rhythm interpretation:____COARSE   V-tach fim_____

Strip 9-6. Rhythm:_____ Rate:_____ P wave:_____

PR interval:_____ QRS:_____

Rhythm interpretation:____Bigeminal PVC's resumes into NSR

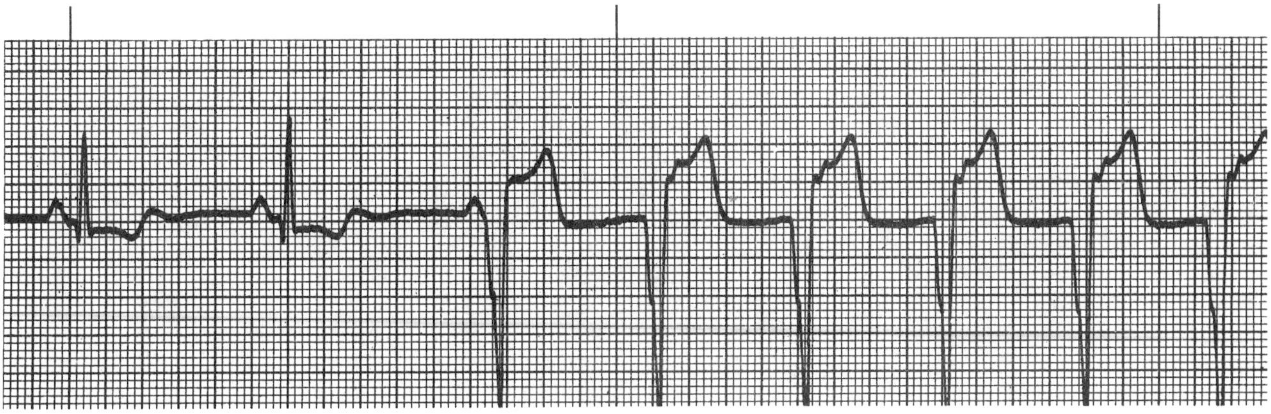

Strip 9-7. Rhythm:_____ Rate:_____ P wave:_____

PR interval:_____ QRS:_____

Rhythm interpretation:_____

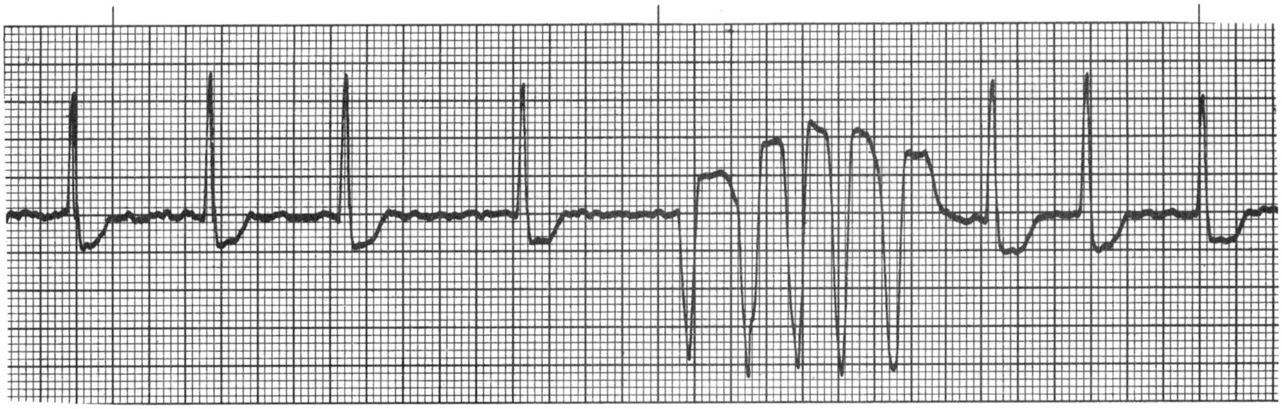

Strip 9-8. Rhythm:_____ Rate:_____ P wave:_____

PR interval:_____ QRS:_____

Rhythm interpretation: 5 beat run of V tach

A fib c̄

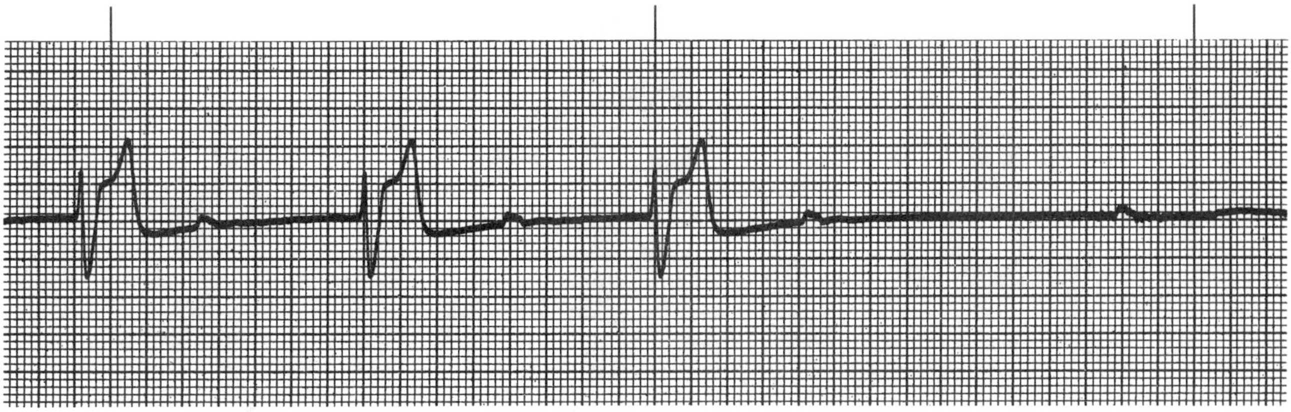

Strip 9-9. Rhythm:_____ Rate:_____ P wave:_____

PR interval:_____ QRS:_____

Rhythm interpretation:_____

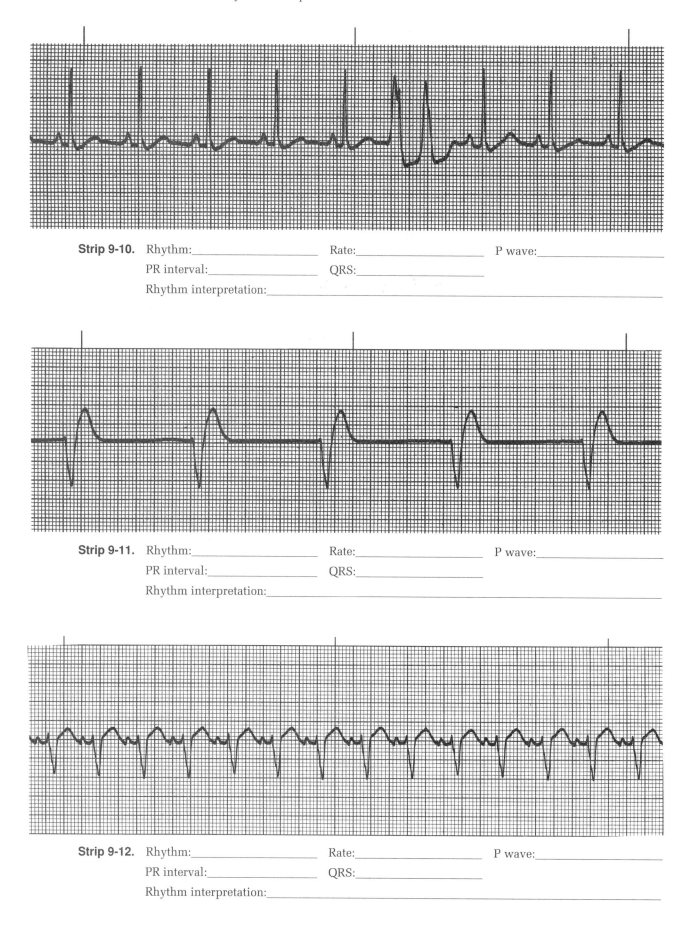

Strip 9-10. Rhythm:_____ Rate:_____ P wave:_____

PR interval:_____ QRS:_____

Rhythm interpretation:_____

Strip 9-11. Rhythm:_____ Rate:_____ P wave:_____

PR interval:_____ QRS:_____

Rhythm interpretation:_____

Strip 9-12. Rhythm:_____ Rate:_____ P wave:_____

PR interval:_____ QRS:_____

Rhythm interpretation:_____

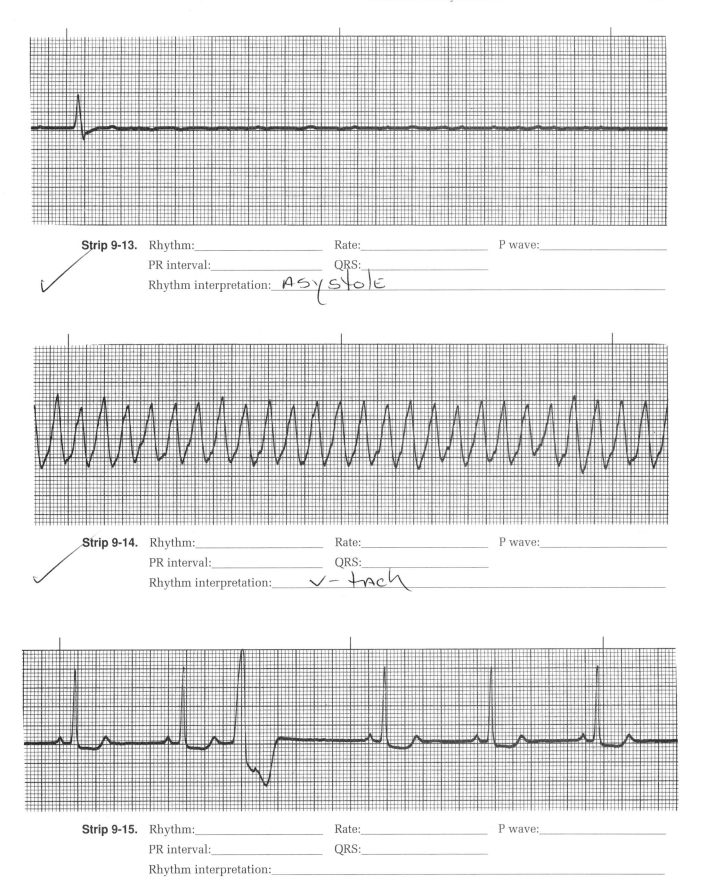

Strip 9-13. Rhythm:_____ Rate:_____ P wave:_____

PR interval:_____ QRS:_____

Rhythm interpretation:_ASYSTOLE_____

Strip 9-14. Rhythm:_____ Rate:_____ P wave:_____

PR interval:_____ QRS:_____

Rhythm interpretation:_____V-trach_____

Strip 9-15. Rhythm:_____ Rate:_____ P wave:_____

PR interval:_____ QRS:_____

Rhythm interpretation:_____

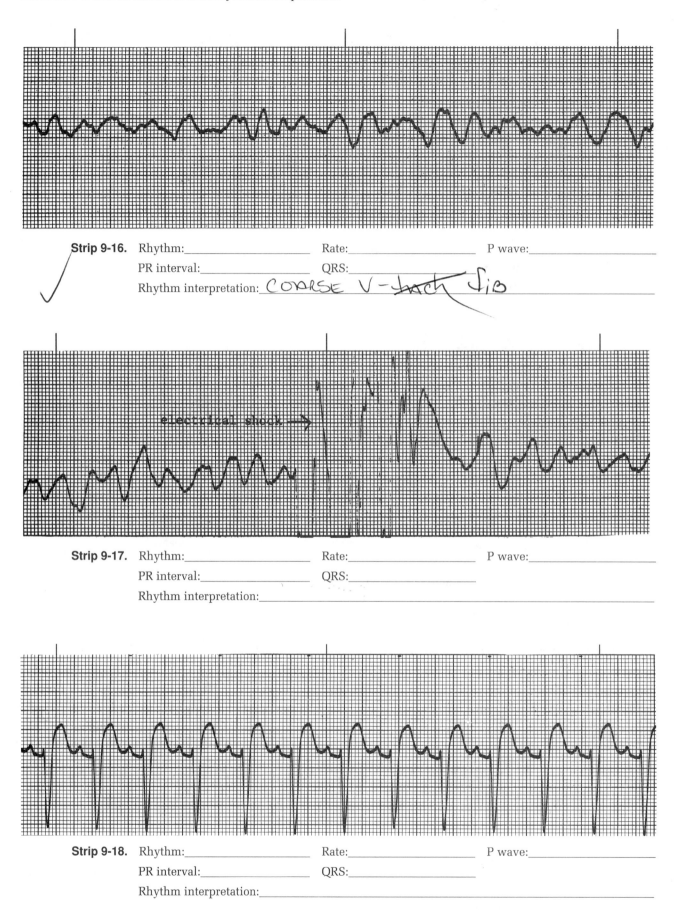

Strip 9-16. Rhythm:_____ Rate:_____ P wave:_____

PR interval:_____ QRS:_____

Rhythm interpretation: *COARSE V-tach fib*

✓

Strip 9-17. Rhythm:_____ Rate:_____ P wave:_____

PR interval:_____ QRS:_____

Rhythm interpretation:_____

electrical shock →

Strip 9-18. Rhythm:_____ Rate:_____ P wave:_____

PR interval:_____ QRS:_____

Rhythm interpretation:_____

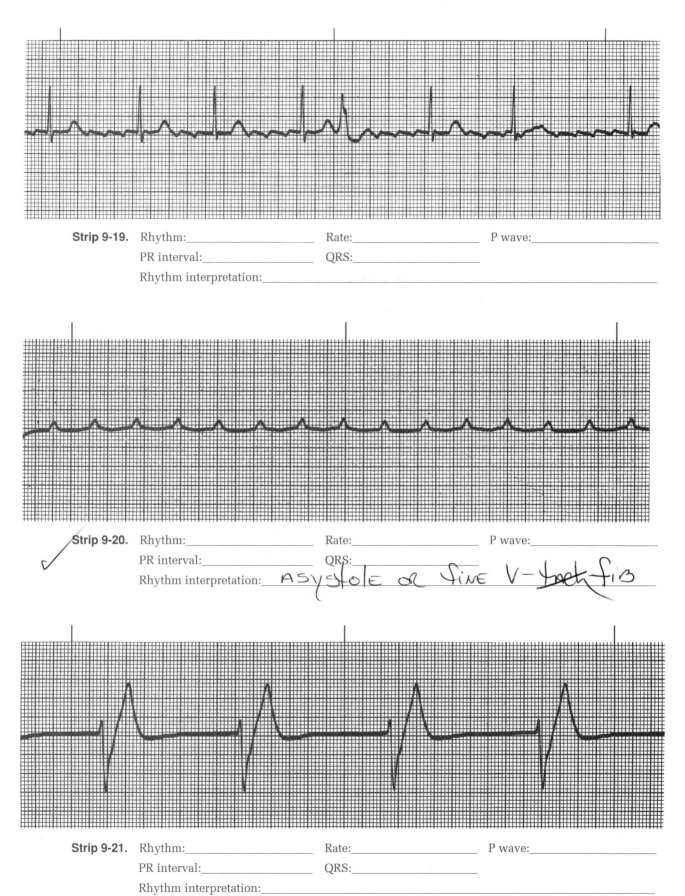

Strip 9-19. Rhythm:_____ Rate:_____ P wave:_____

PR interval:_____ QRS:_____

Rhythm interpretation:_____

Strip 9-20. Rhythm:_____ Rate:_____ P wave:_____

PR interval:_____ QRS:_____

Rhythm interpretation: ASYSTOLE OR fine V-tach-fib

Strip 9-21. Rhythm:_____ Rate:_____ P wave:_____

PR interval:_____ QRS:_____

Rhythm interpretation:_____

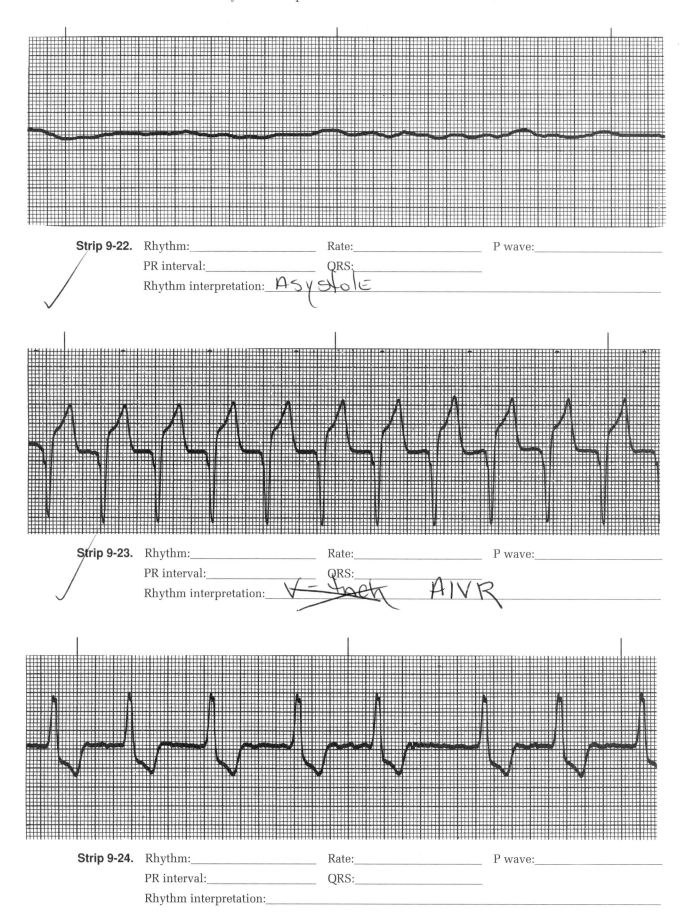

Strip 9-22. Rhythm:_____ Rate:_____ P wave:_____

PR interval:_____ QRS:_____

Rhythm interpretation: ASystole _____

Strip 9-23. Rhythm:_____ Rate:_____ P wave:_____

PR interval:_____ QRS:_____

Rhythm interpretation: ~~V-tach~~ AIVR _____

Strip 9-24. Rhythm:_____ Rate:_____ P wave:_____

PR interval:_____ QRS:_____

Rhythm interpretation:_____

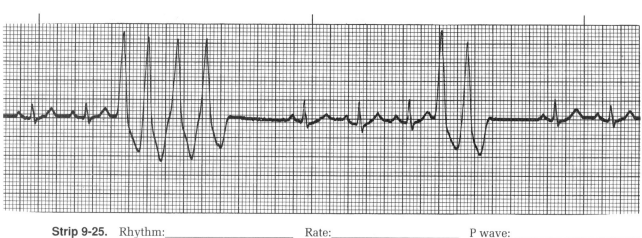

Strip 9-25. Rhythm:_____ Rate:_____ P wave:_____

PR interval:_____ QRS:_____

Rhythm interpretation:_____

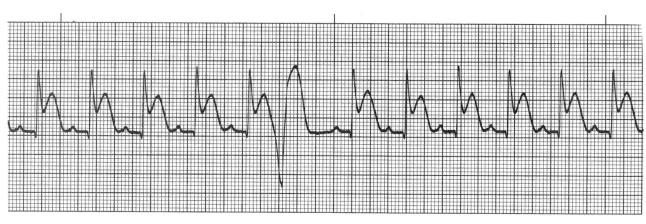

Strip 9-26. Rhythm:_____ Rate:_____ P wave:_____

PR interval:_____ QRS:_____

Rhythm interpretation:_____

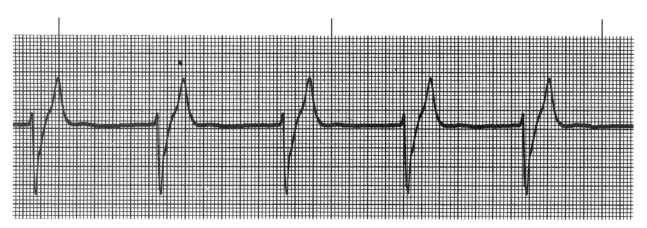

Strip 9-27. Rhythm:_____ Rate:_____ P wave:_____

PR interval:_____ QRS:_____

Rhythm interpretation:_____

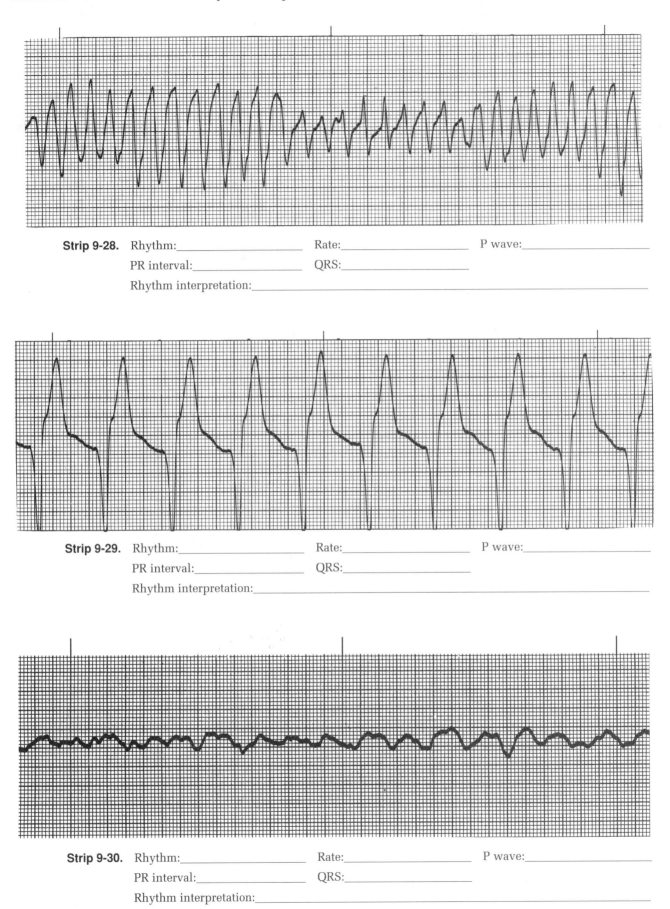

Strip 9-28. Rhythm:_____ Rate:_____ P wave:_____

PR interval:_____ QRS:_____

Rhythm interpretation:_____

Strip 9-29. Rhythm:_____ Rate:_____ P wave:_____

PR interval:_____ QRS:_____

Rhythm interpretation:_____

Strip 9-30. Rhythm:_____ Rate:_____ P wave:_____

PR interval:_____ QRS:_____

Rhythm interpretation:_____

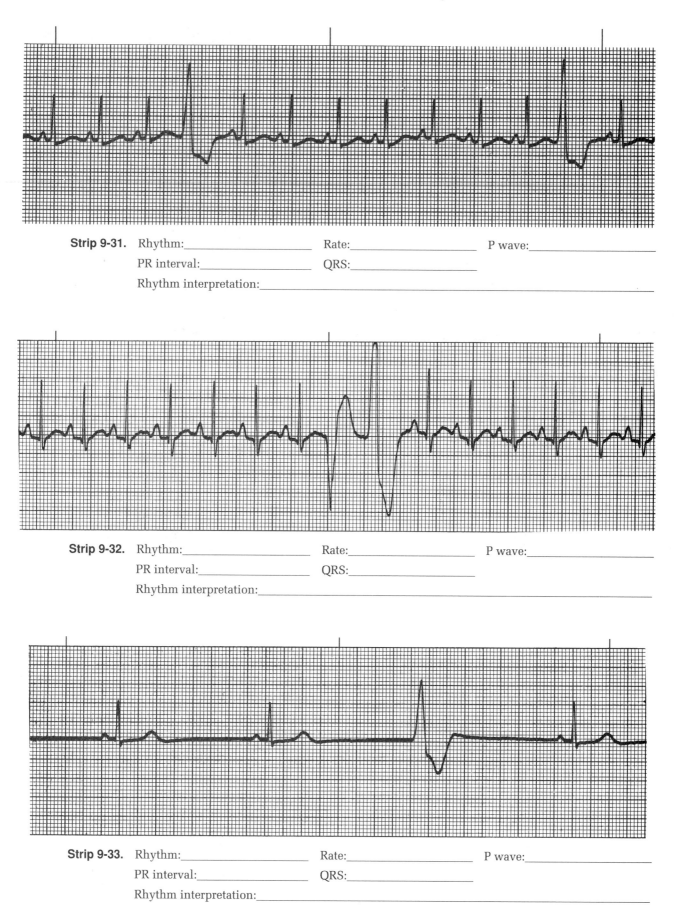

Strip 9-31. Rhythm:_____ Rate:_____ P wave:_____

PR interval:_____ QRS:_____

Rhythm interpretation:_____

Strip 9-32. Rhythm:_____ Rate:_____ P wave:_____

PR interval:_____ QRS:_____

Rhythm interpretation:_____

Strip 9-33. Rhythm:_____ Rate:_____ P wave:_____

PR interval:_____ QRS:_____

Rhythm interpretation:_____

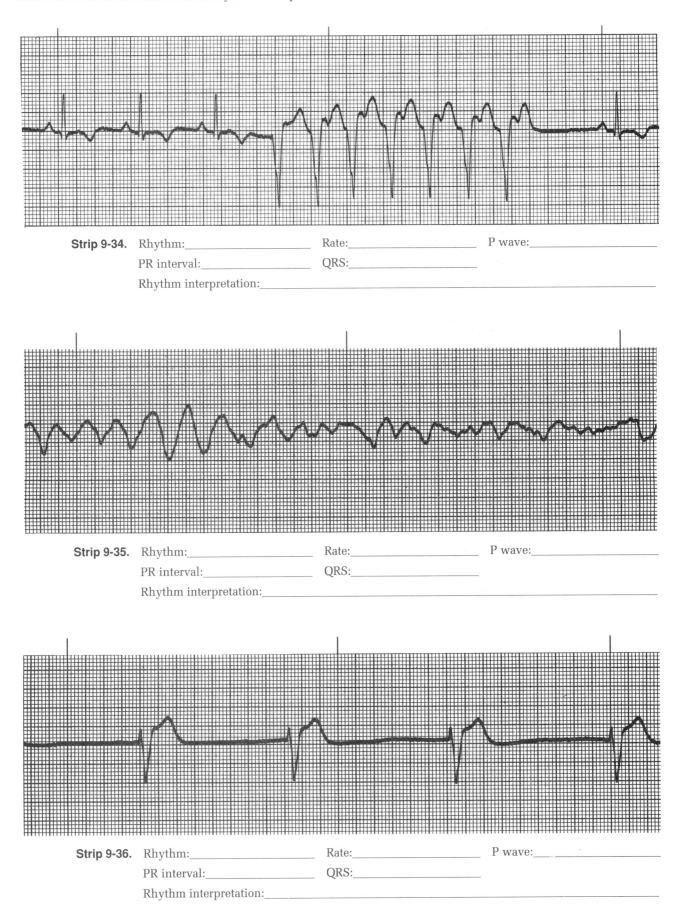

Strip 9-34. Rhythm:_____ Rate:_____ P wave:_____

PR interval:_____ QRS:_____

Rhythm interpretation:_____

Strip 9-35. Rhythm:_____ Rate:_____ P wave:_____

PR interval:_____ QRS:_____

Rhythm interpretation:_____

Strip 9-36. Rhythm:_____ Rate:_____ P wave:___ _____

PR interval:_____ QRS:_____

Rhythm interpretation:_____

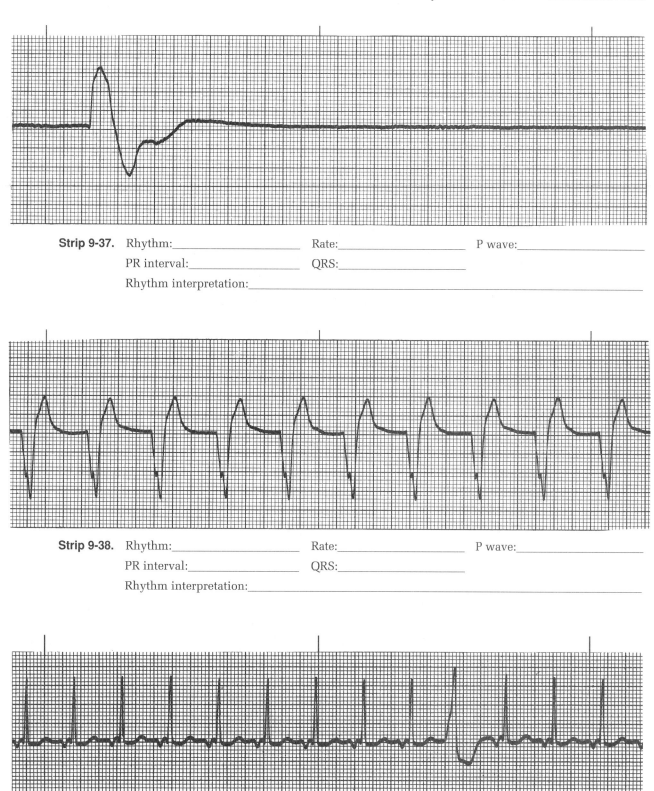

Strip 9-37. Rhythm:_____ Rate:_____ P wave:_____

PR interval:_____ QRS:_____

Rhythm interpretation:_____

Strip 9-38. Rhythm:_____ Rate:_____ P wave:_____

PR interval:_____ QRS:_____

Rhythm interpretation:_____

Strip 9-39. Rhythm:_____ Rate:_____ P wave:_____

PR interval:_____ QRS:_____

Rhythm interpretation:_____

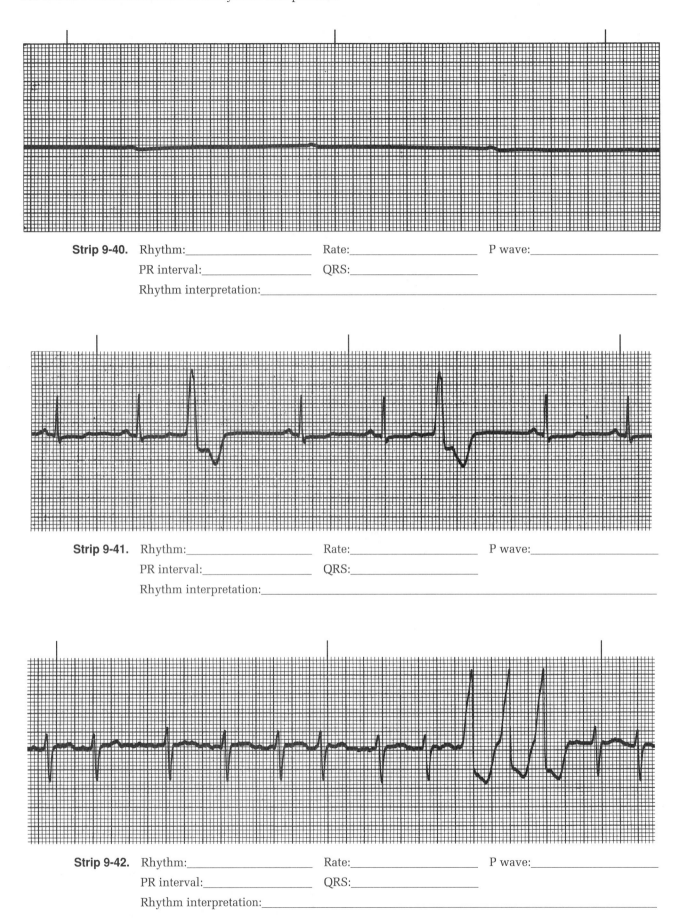

Strip 9-40. Rhythm:_____ Rate:_____ P wave:_____

PR interval:_____ QRS:_____

Rhythm interpretation:_____

Strip 9-41. Rhythm:_____ Rate:_____ P wave:_____

PR interval:_____ QRS:_____

Rhythm interpretation:_____

Strip 9-42. Rhythm:_____ Rate:_____ P wave:_____

PR interval:_____ QRS:_____

Rhythm interpretation:_____

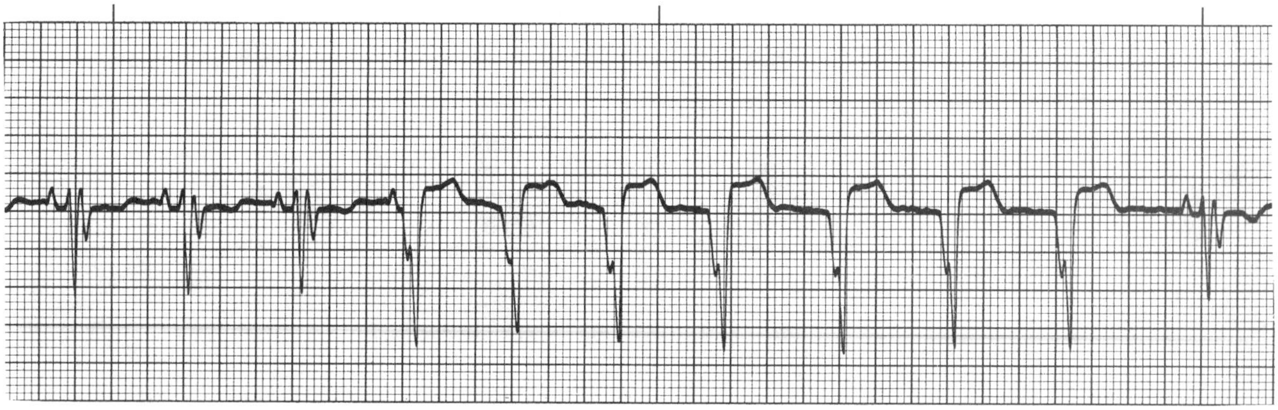

Strip 9-43. Rhythm:_____ Rate:_____ P wave:_____

PR interval:_____ QRS:_____

Rhythm interpretation:_____

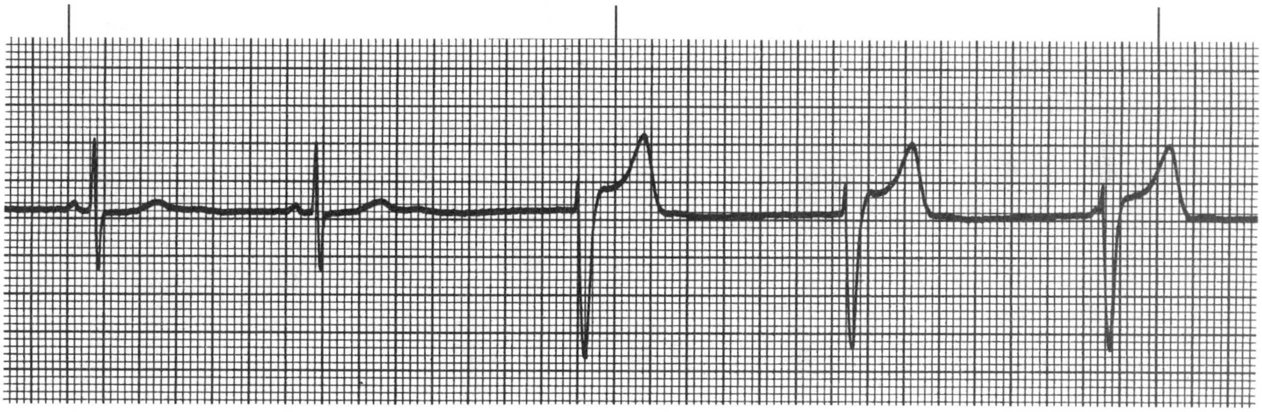

Strip 9-44. Rhythm:_____ Rate:_____ P wave:_____

PR interval:_____ QRS:_____

Rhythm interpretation:_____

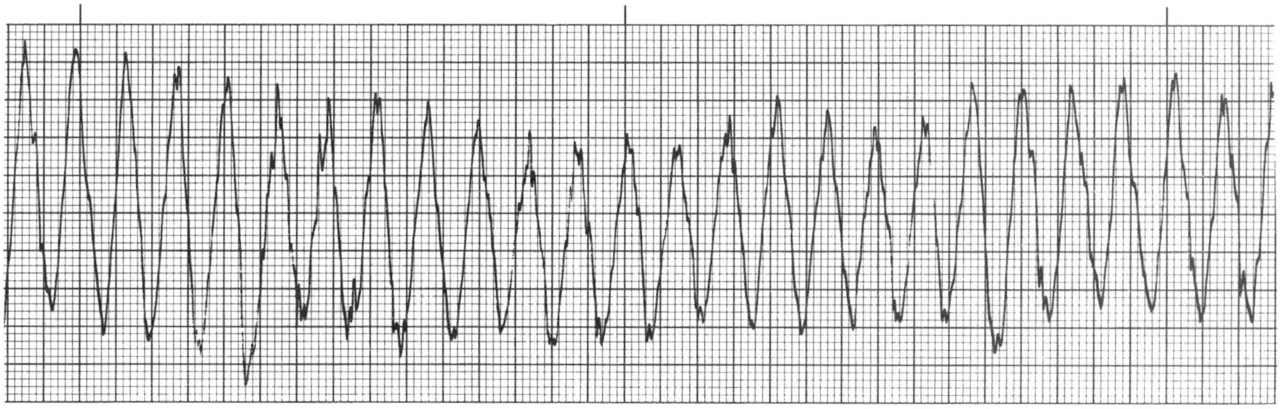

Strip 9-45. Rhythm:_____ Rate:_____ P wave:_____

PR interval:_____ QRS:_____

Rhythm interpretation:_____

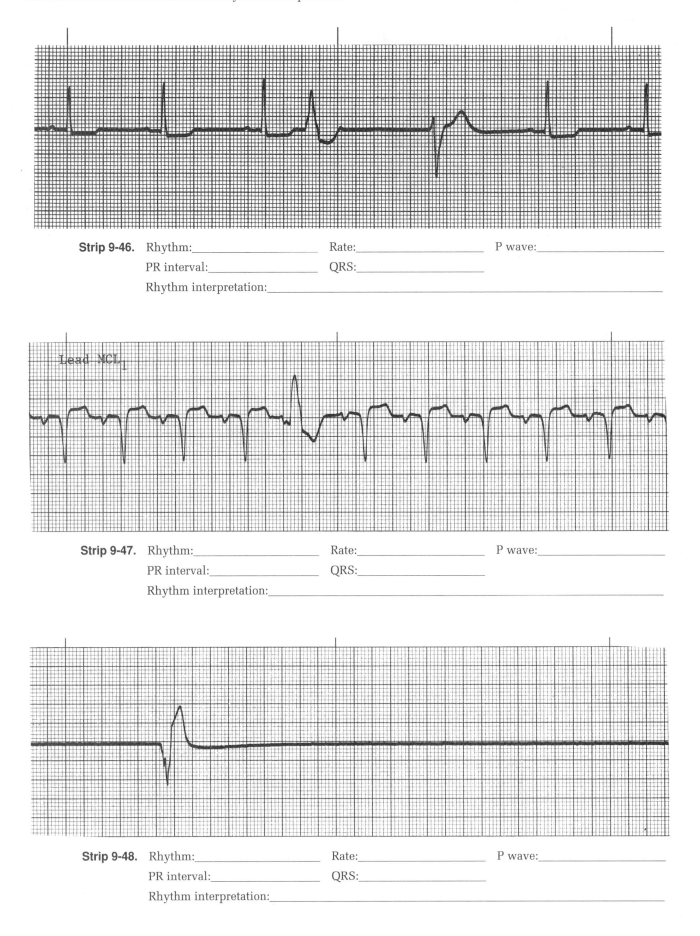

Strip 9-46. Rhythm:_____ Rate:_____ P wave:_____

PR interval:_____ QRS:_____

Rhythm interpretation:_____

Strip 9-47. Rhythm:_____ Rate:_____ P wave:_____

PR interval:_____ QRS:_____

Rhythm interpretation:_____

Strip 9-48. Rhythm:_____ Rate:_____ P wave:_____

PR interval:_____ QRS:_____

Rhythm interpretation:_____

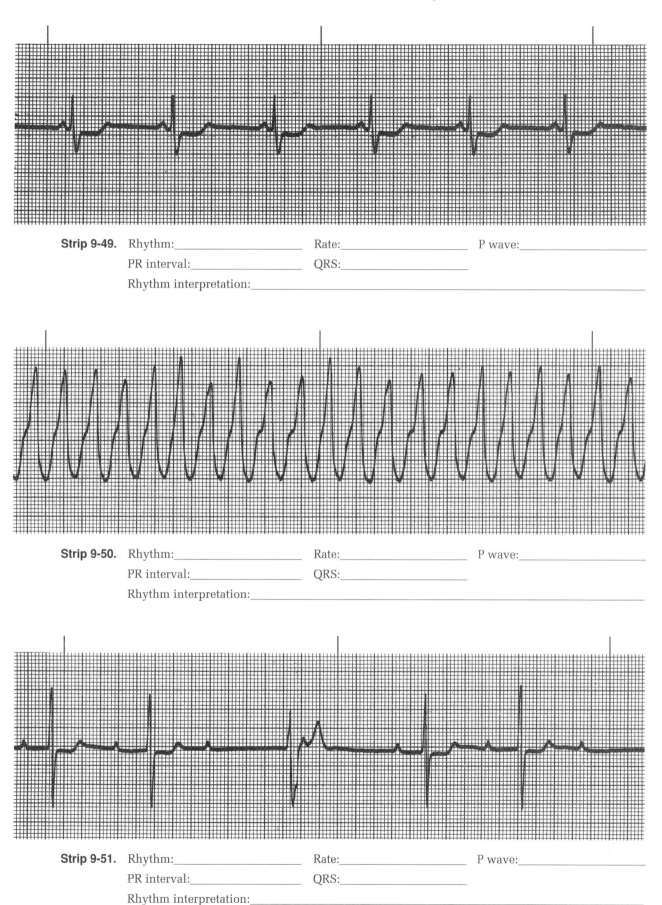

Strip 9-49. Rhythm:_____ Rate:_____ P wave:_____

PR interval:_____ QRS:_____

Rhythm interpretation:_____

Strip 9-50. Rhythm:_____ Rate:_____ P wave:_____

PR interval:_____ QRS:_____

Rhythm interpretation:_____

Strip 9-51. Rhythm:_____ Rate:_____ P wave:_____

PR interval:_____ QRS:_____

Rhythm interpretation:_____

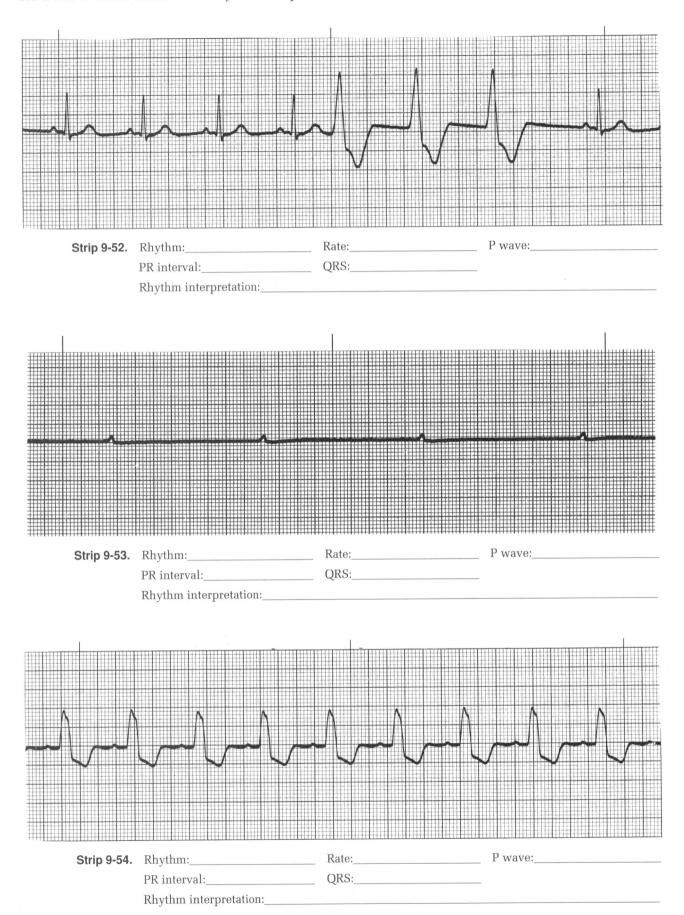

Strip 9-52. Rhythm:_____ Rate:_____ P wave:_____

PR interval:_____ QRS:_____

Rhythm interpretation:_____

Strip 9-53. Rhythm:_____ Rate:_____ P wave:_____

PR interval:_____ QRS:_____

Rhythm interpretation:_____

Strip 9-54. Rhythm:_____ Rate:_____ P wave:_____

PR interval:_____ QRS:_____

Rhythm interpretation:_____

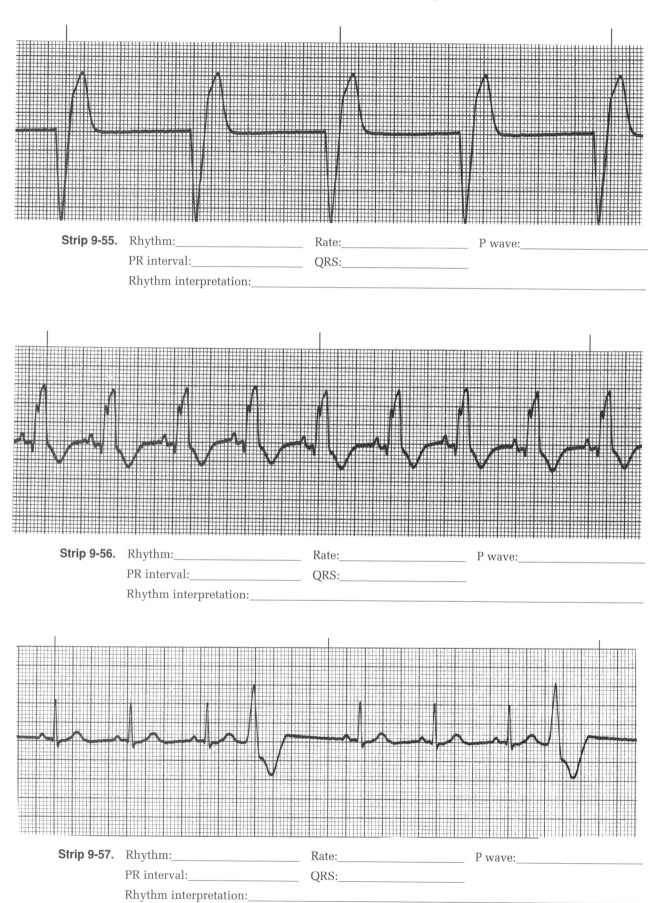

Strip 9-55. Rhythm:_____ Rate:_____ P wave:_____

PR interval:_____ QRS:_____

Rhythm interpretation:_____

Strip 9-56. Rhythm:_____ Rate:_____ P wave:_____

PR interval:_____ QRS:_____

Rhythm interpretation:_____

Strip 9-57. Rhythm:_____ Rate:_____ P wave:_____

PR interval:_____ QRS:_____

Rhythm interpretation:_____

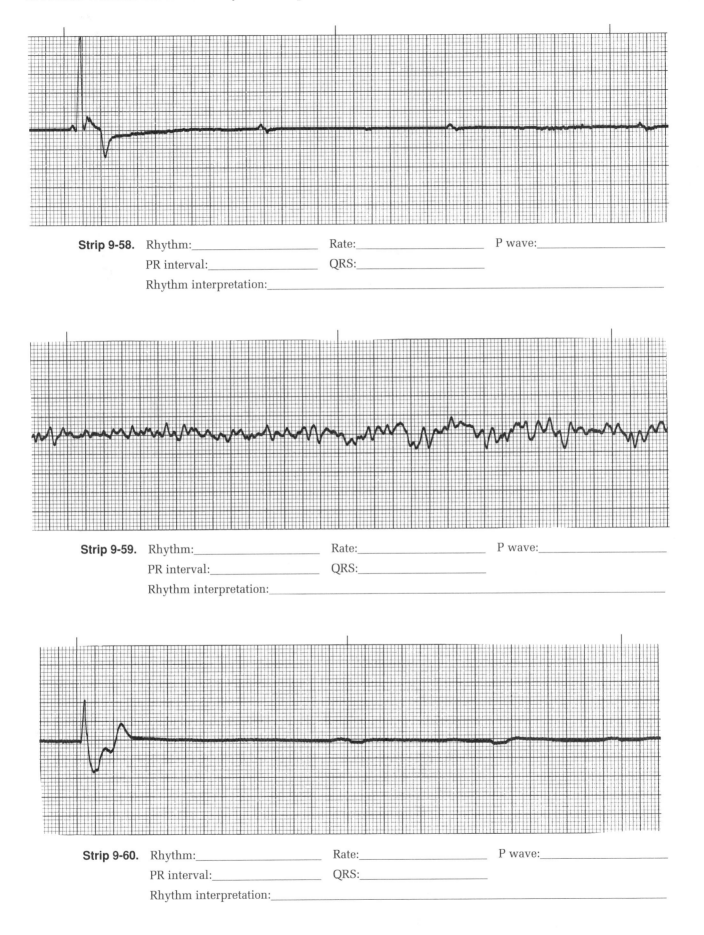

Strip 9-58. Rhythm:_____ Rate:_____ P wave:_____

PR interval:_____ QRS:_____

Rhythm interpretation:_____

Strip 9-59. Rhythm:_____ Rate:_____ P wave:_____

PR interval:_____ QRS:_____

Rhythm interpretation:_____

Strip 9-60. Rhythm:_____ Rate:_____ P wave:_____

PR interval:_____ QRS:_____

Rhythm interpretation:_____

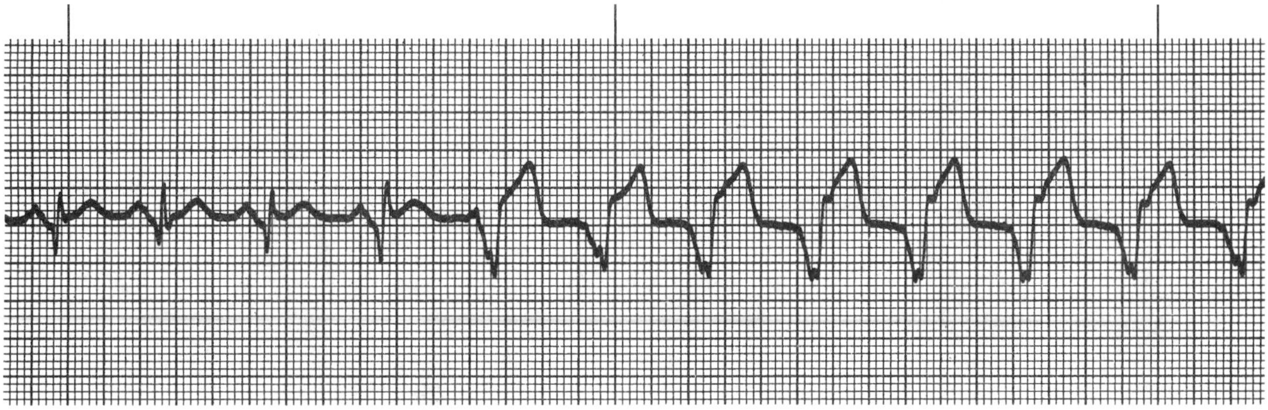

Strip 9-61. Rhythm:_____ Rate:_____ P wave:_____

PR interval:_____ QRS:_____

Rhythm interpretation:_____

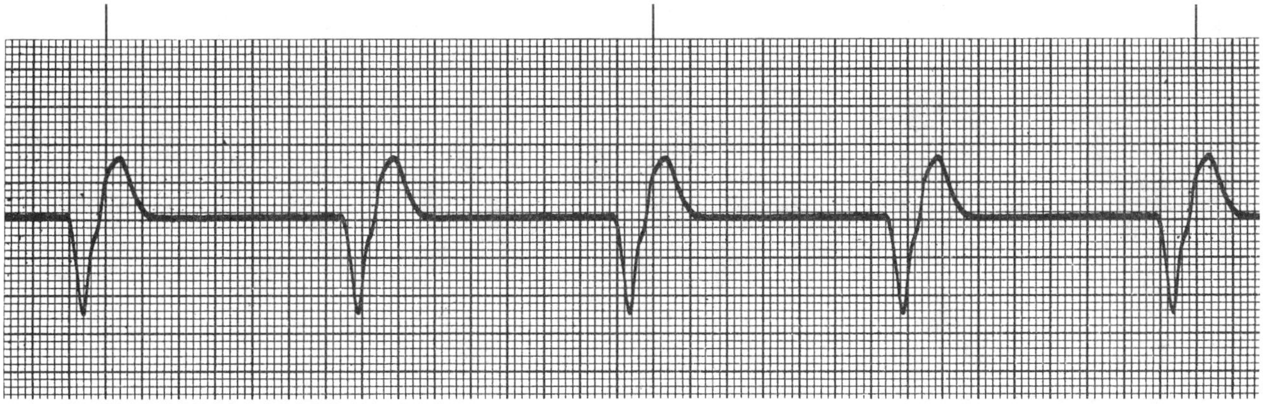

Strip 9-62. Rhythm:_____ Rate:_____ P wave:_____

PR interval:_____ QRS:_____

Rhythm interpretation:_____

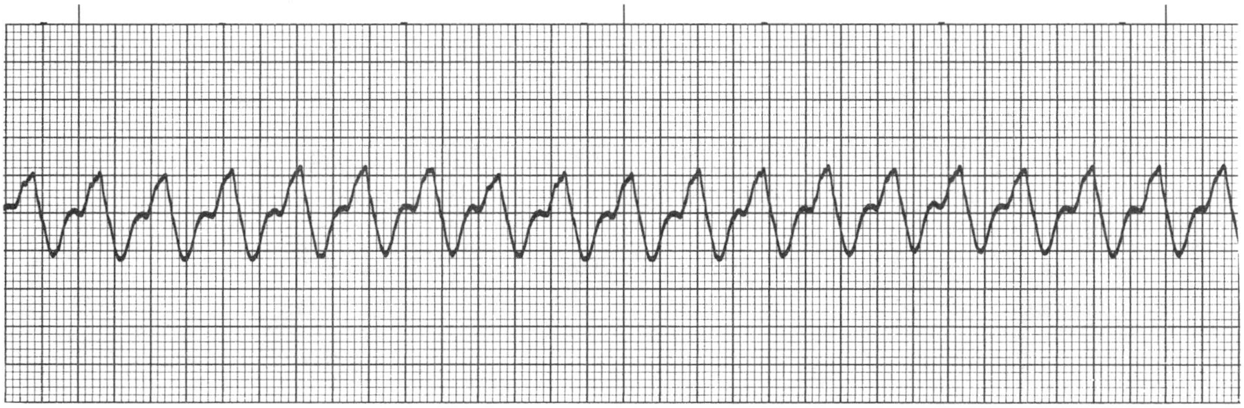

Strip 9-63. Rhythm:_____ Rate:_____ P wave:_____

PR interval:_____ QRS:_____

Rhythm interpretation:_____

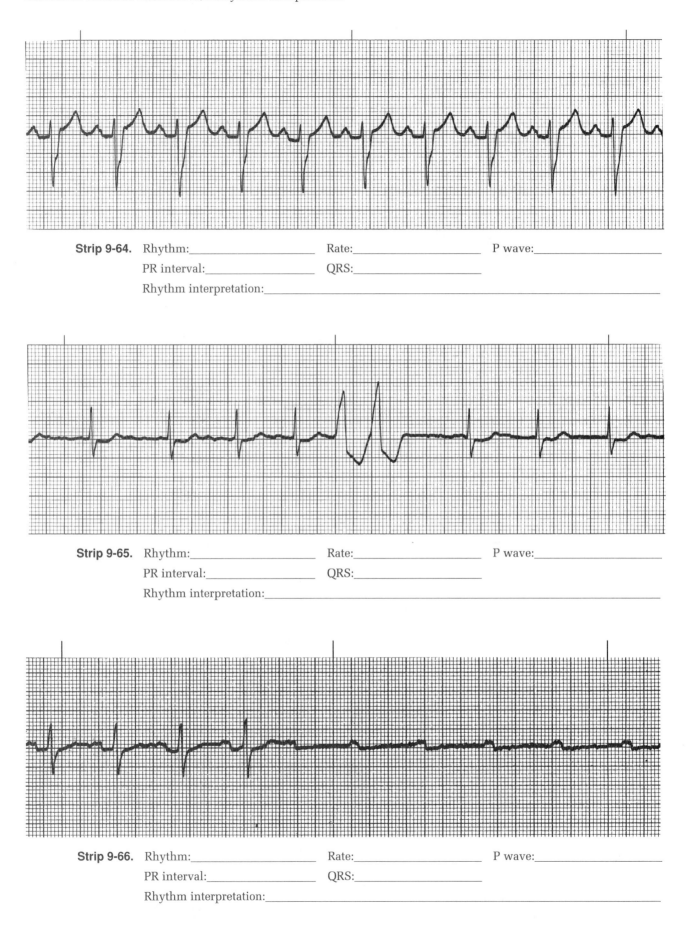

Strip 9-64. Rhythm:_____ Rate:_____ P wave:_____

PR interval:_____ QRS:_____

Rhythm interpretation:_____

Strip 9-65. Rhythm:_____ Rate:_____ P wave:_____

PR interval:_____ QRS:_____

Rhythm interpretation:_____

Strip 9-66. Rhythm:_____ Rate:_____ P wave:_____

PR interval:_____ QRS:_____

Rhythm interpretation:_____

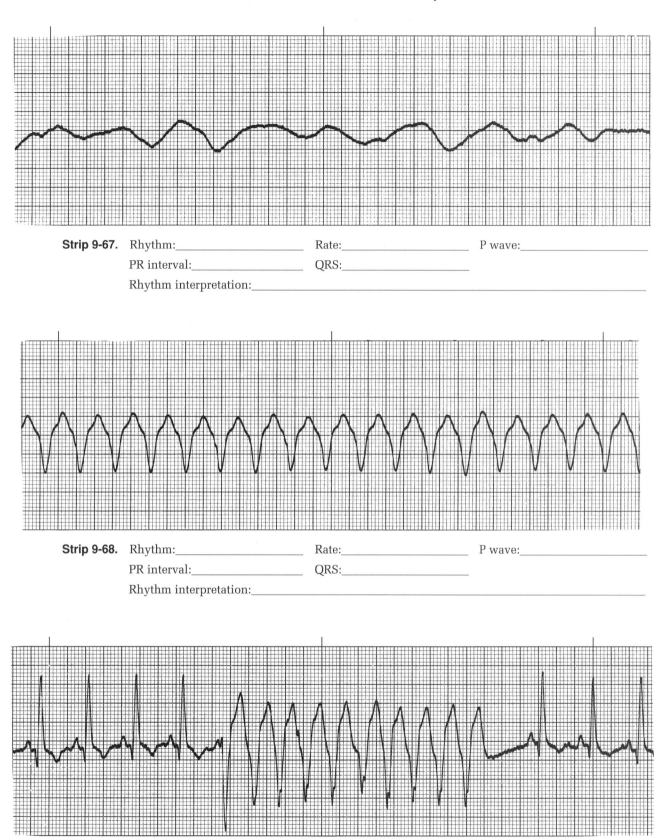

Strip 9-67. Rhythm:_____ Rate:_____ P wave:_____

PR interval:_____ QRS:_____

Rhythm interpretation:_____

Strip 9-68. Rhythm:_____ Rate:_____ P wave:_____

PR interval:_____ QRS:_____

Rhythm interpretation:_____

Strip 9-69. Rhythm:_____ Rate:_____ P wave:_____

PR interval:_____ QRS:_____

Rhythm interpretation:_____

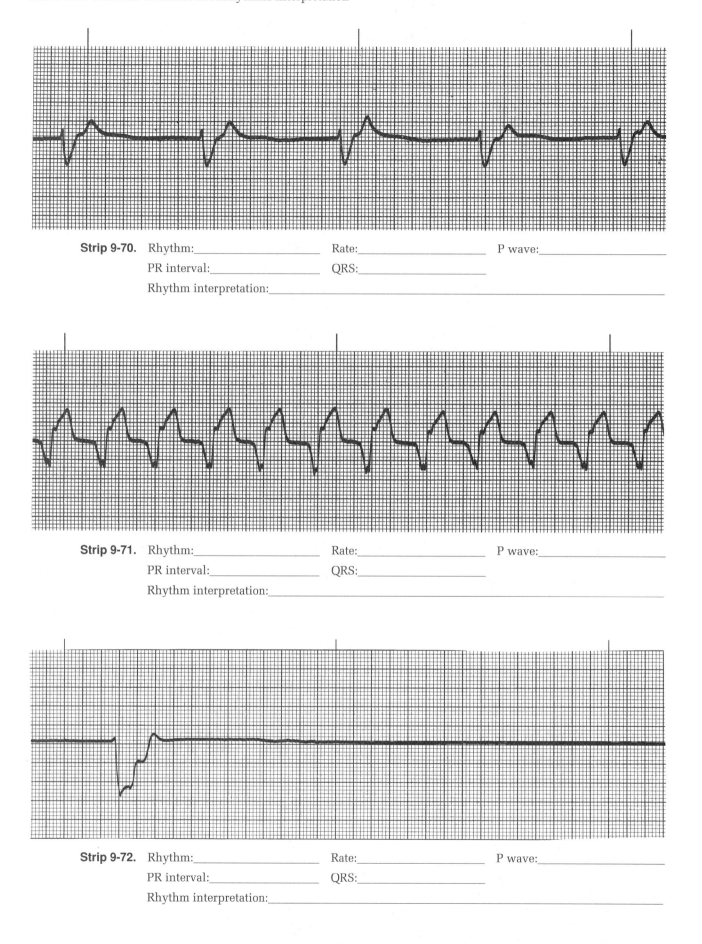

Strip 9-70. Rhythm:_____ Rate:_____ P wave:_____

PR interval:_____ QRS:_____

Rhythm interpretation:_____

Strip 9-71. Rhythm:_____ Rate:_____ P wave:_____

PR interval:_____ QRS:_____

Rhythm interpretation:_____

Strip 9-72. Rhythm:_____ Rate:_____ P wave:_____

PR interval:_____ QRS:_____

Rhythm interpretation:_____

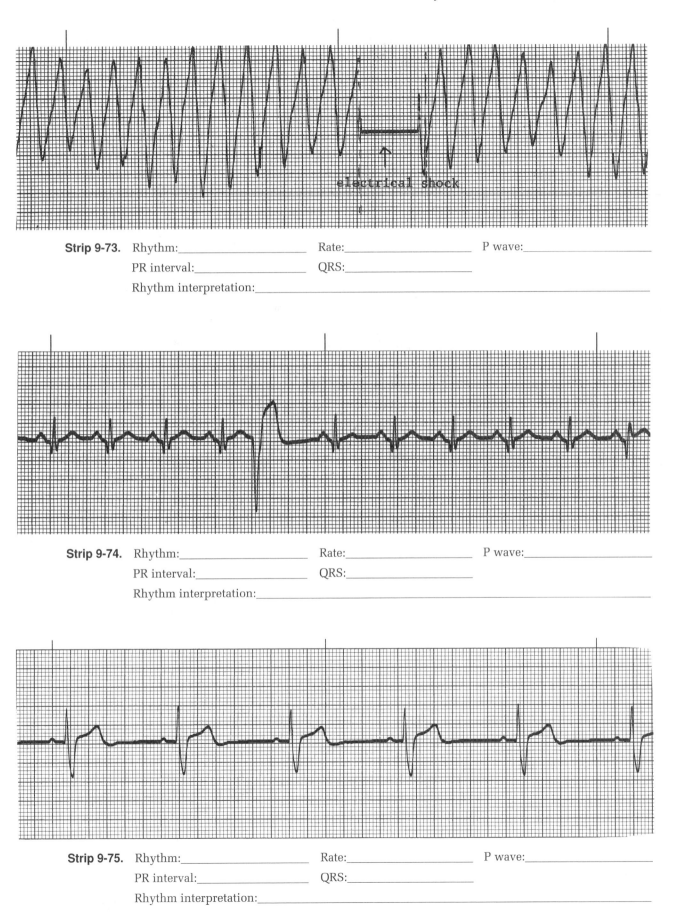

electrical shock

Strip 9-73. Rhythm:_____ Rate:_____ P wave:_____

PR interval:_____ QRS:_____

Rhythm interpretation:_____

Strip 9-74. Rhythm:_____ Rate:_____ P wave:_____

PR interval:_____ QRS:_____

Rhythm interpretation:_____

Strip 9-75. Rhythm:_____ Rate:_____ P wave:_____

PR interval:_____ QRS:_____

Rhythm interpretation:_____

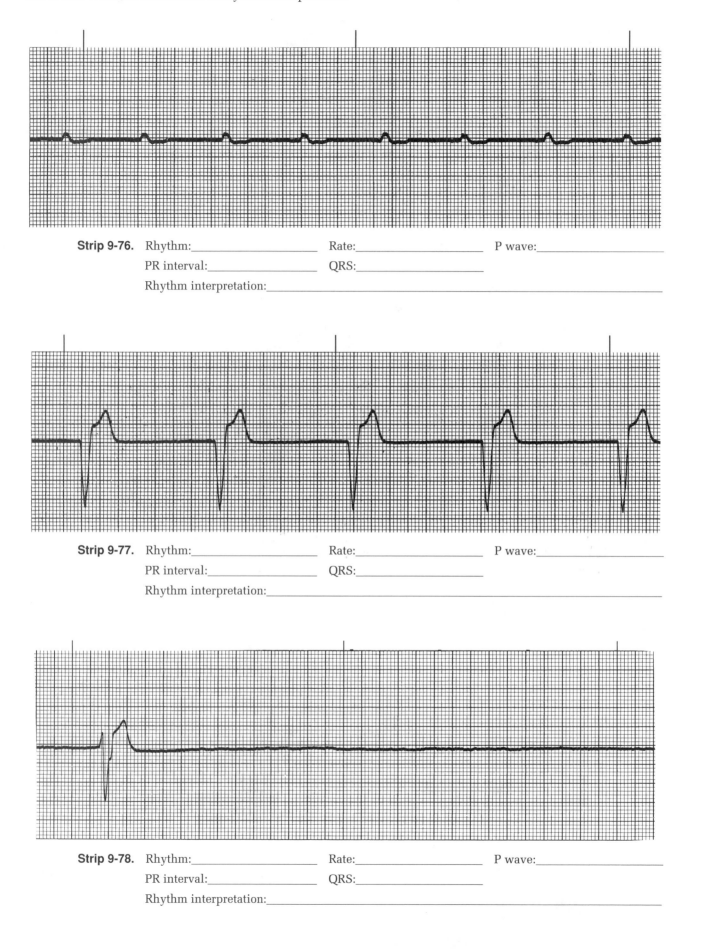

Strip 9-76. Rhythm:_____ Rate:_____ P wave:_____

PR interval:_____ QRS:_____

Rhythm interpretation:_____

Strip 9-77. Rhythm:_____ Rate:_____ P wave:_____

PR interval:_____ QRS:_____

Rhythm interpretation:_____

Strip 9-78. Rhythm:_____ Rate:_____ P wave:_____

PR interval:_____ QRS:_____

Rhythm interpretation:_____

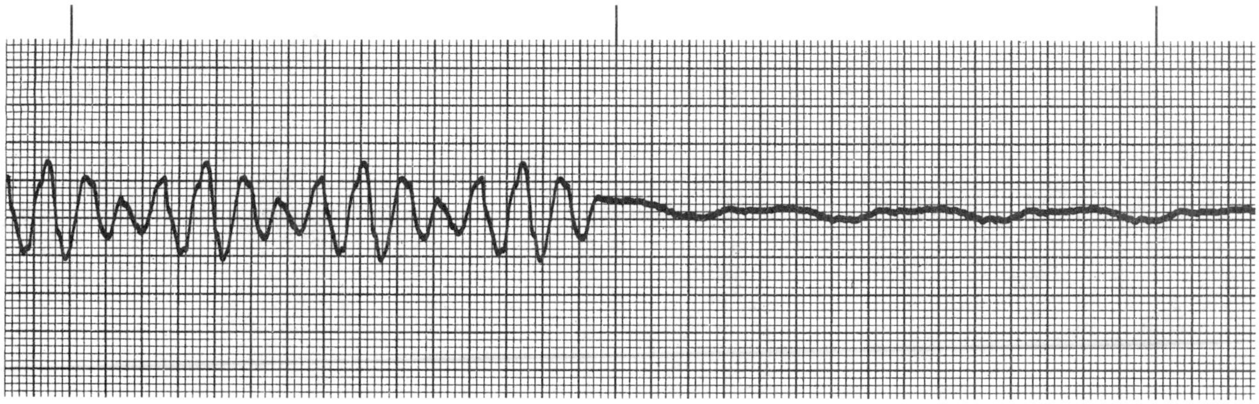

Strip 9-79. Rhythm:_____ Rate:_____ P wave:_____

PR interval:_____ QRS:_____

Rhythm interpretation:_____

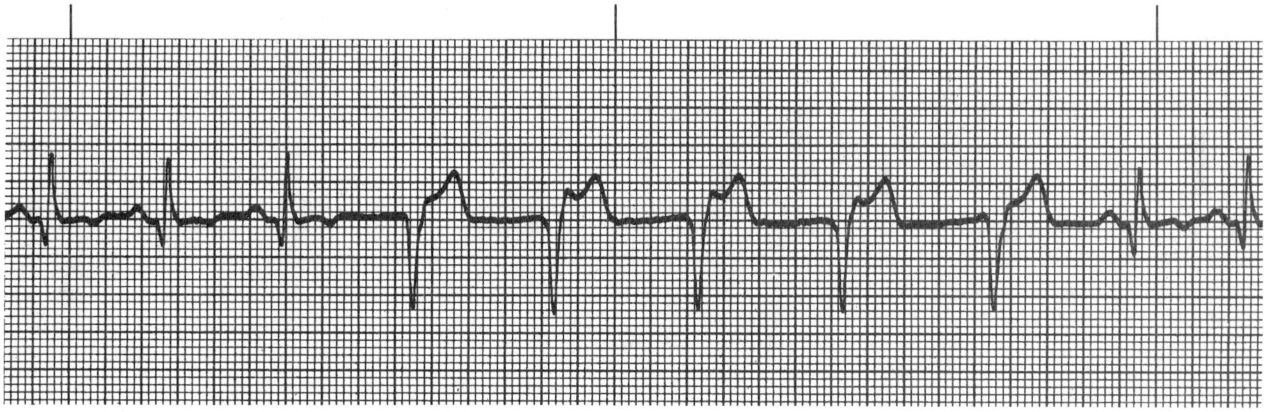

Strip 9-80. Rhythm:_____ Rate:_____ P wave:_____

PR interval:_____ QRS:_____

Rhythm interpretation:_____

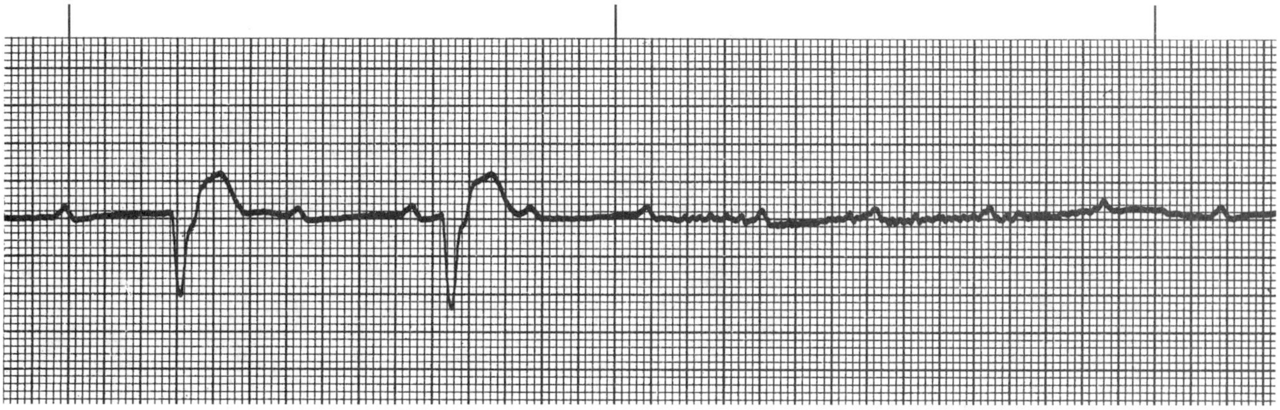

Strip 9-81. Rhythm:_____ Rate:_____ P wave:_____

PR interval:_____ QRS:_____

Rhythm interpretation:_____

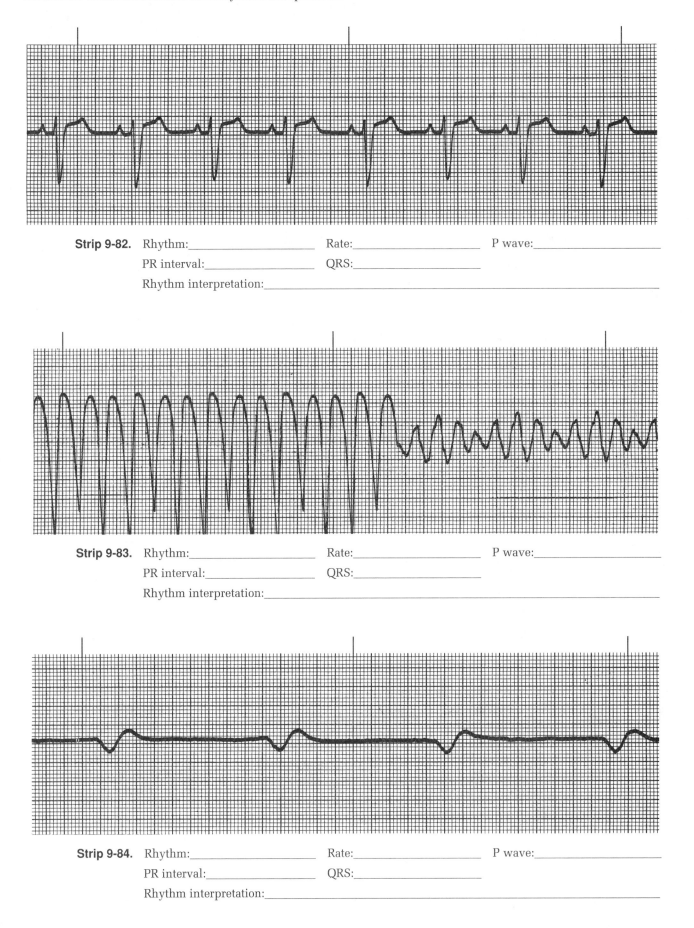

Strip 9-82. Rhythm:_____ Rate:_____ P wave:_____

PR interval:_____ QRS:_____

Rhythm interpretation:_____

Strip 9-83. Rhythm:_____ Rate:_____ P wave:_____

PR interval:_____ QRS:_____

Rhythm interpretation:_____

Strip 9-84. Rhythm:_____ Rate:_____ P wave:_____

PR interval:_____ QRS:_____

Rhythm interpretation:_____

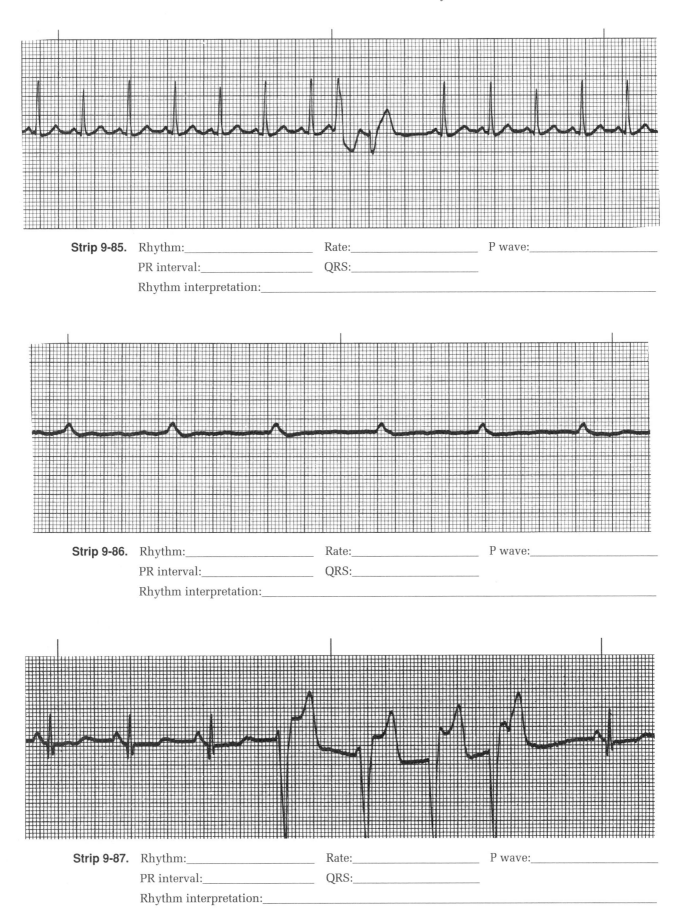

Strip 9-85. Rhythm:_____ Rate:_____ P wave:_____

PR interval:_____ QRS:_____

Rhythm interpretation:_____

Strip 9-86. Rhythm:_____ Rate:_____ P wave:_____

PR interval:_____ QRS:_____

Rhythm interpretation:_____

Strip 9-87. Rhythm:_____ Rate:_____ P wave:_____

PR interval:_____ QRS:_____

Rhythm interpretation:_____

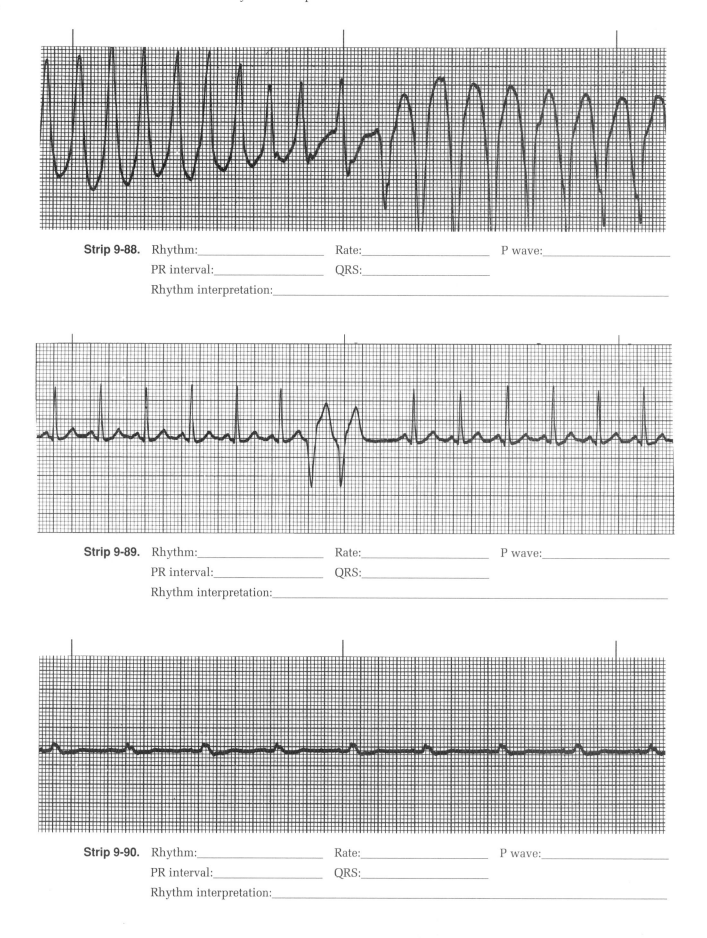

Strip 9-88. Rhythm:_____ Rate:_____ P wave:_____

PR interval:_____ QRS:_____

Rhythm interpretation:_____

Strip 9-89. Rhythm:_____ Rate:_____ P wave:_____

PR interval:_____ QRS:_____

Rhythm interpretation:_____

Strip 9-90. Rhythm:_____ Rate:_____ P wave:_____

PR interval:_____ QRS:_____

Rhythm interpretation:_____

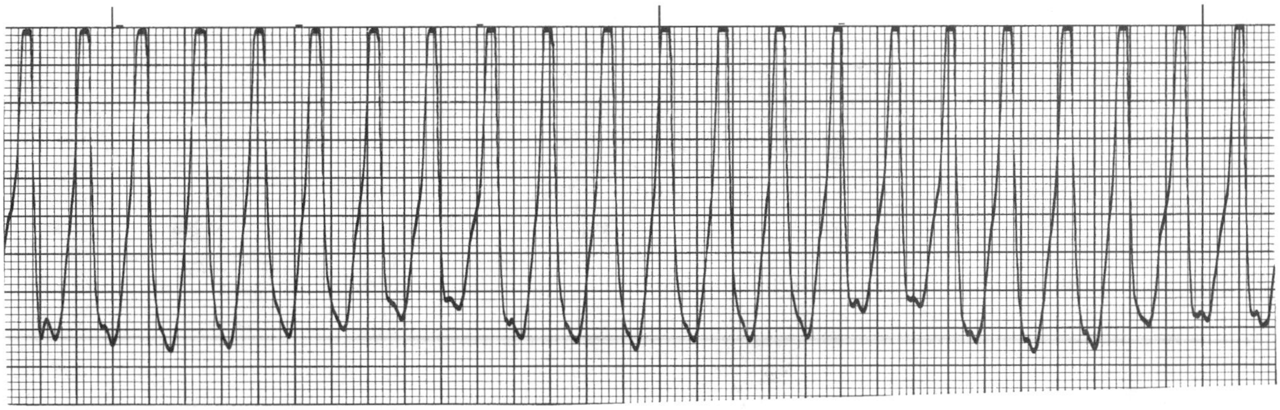

Strip 9-91. Rhythm:_____ Rate:_____ P wave:_____

PR interval:_____ QRS:_____

Rhythm interpretation:_____

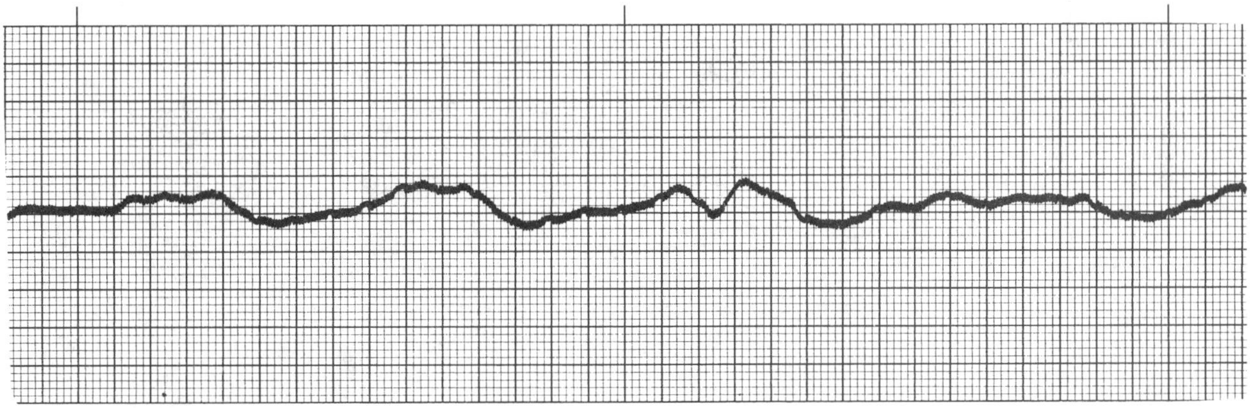

Strip 9-92. Rhythm:_____ Rate:_____ P wave:_____

PR interval:_____ QRS:_____

Rhythm interpretation:_____

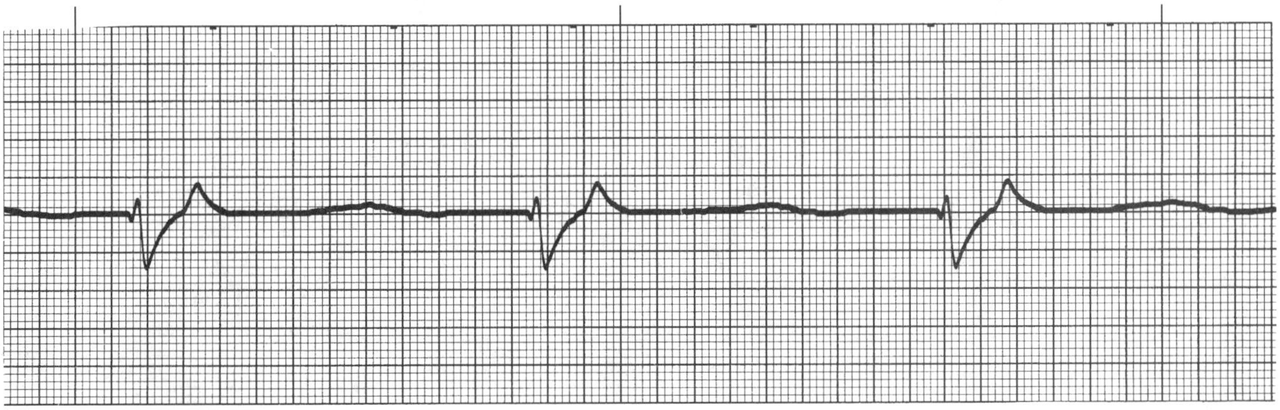

Strip 9-93. Rhythm:_____ Rate:_____ P wave:_____

PR interval:_____ QRS:_____

Rhythm interpretation:_____

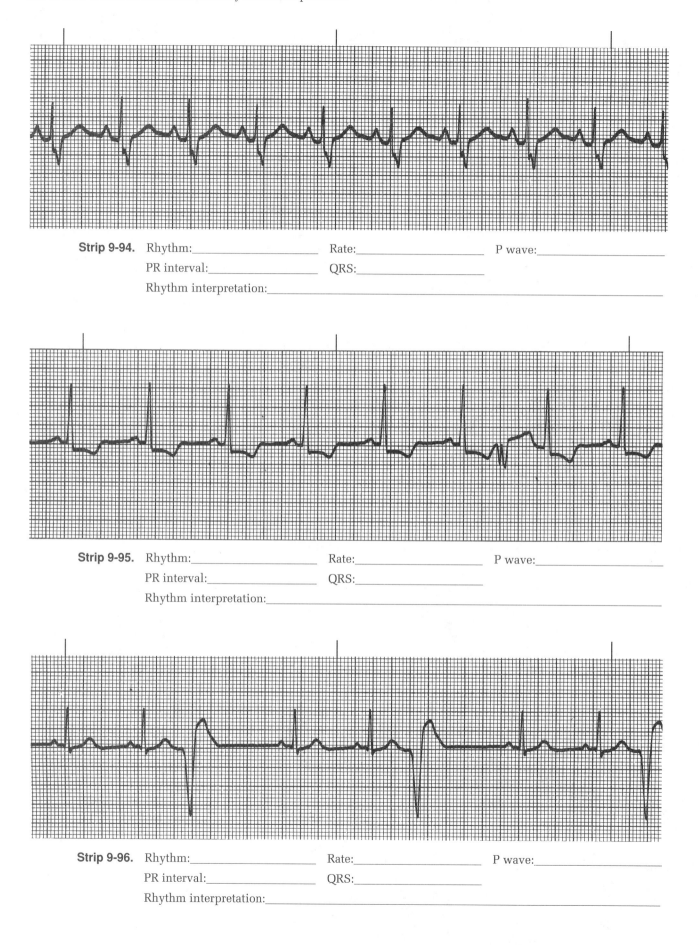

Strip 9-94. Rhythm:_____ Rate:_____ P wave:_____

PR interval:_____ QRS:_____

Rhythm interpretation:_____

Strip 9-95. Rhythm:_____ Rate:_____ P wave:_____

PR interval:_____ QRS:_____

Rhythm interpretation:_____

Strip 9-96. Rhythm:_____ Rate:_____ P wave:_____

PR interval:_____ QRS:_____

Rhythm interpretation:_____

10

Pacemakers

A pacemaker is a battery-powered device that delivers an electrical stimulus to the myocardium, resulting in contraction. Pacemakers are used primarily when the patient's own heart rate is excessively slow: symptomatic sinus bradycardia, sinus arrest, sick sinus syndrome (a degenerative process of the sinus node that produces alternating periods of bradycardia and tachycardia), slow atrial fibrillation; or when there is a potential for ventricular standstill to occur, as in second-degree AV block Mobitz II or third-degree AV block. Pacemakers can also be used for PVCs and ventricular tachycardia refractory to drug therapy. In this situation the pacing rate is set higher than the ectopic focus rate (overdrive pacing) in an attempt to suppress an ectopic focus.

A pacemaker functions in one of two ways: as a fixed-rate pacemaker or as a demand pacemaker. Fixed-rate pacemakers initiate impulses at a set rate regardless of the patient's intrinsic rate. The fixed-rate pacemaker competes with the patient's own heart rhythm and is potentially dangerous because the pacing stimulus may fall during the vulnerable period of the cardiac cycle and induce serious ventricular arrhythmias. This type of pacemaker is used primarily when the patient has no intrinsic heart rate, such as during cardiac arrest. Demand pacemakers are designed with a sensing mechanism that inhibits discharge when the patient's heart rate is adequate and a pacing mechanism that triggers the pacemaker to fire when no intrinsic activity occurs within a pre-determined period. Many different types of demand pacemakers are available:

1. Single chamber pacemakers which sense and pace either the atrium or the ventricle
2. Dual chamber pacemakers which sense and pace both the atrium and the ventricle

An advantage of the dual chamber pacemakers is their ability to restore the AV synchronous sequence of the heart (atrial kick) that contributes 20–30% of cardiac output. More advanced pacemakers are able to produce varying heart rates that are responsive to increased myocardial needs (e.g., exercise), and some are incorporated with antitachycardia and defibrillator features designed to abolish rapid dysrhythmias.

All pacemakers have some components in common—the pulse generator and the pacing catheter. The pulse generator houses the battery that creates the electrical signal, and contains the various controls or settings for pacemaker function (electrical output or mA, sensitivity or mV, heart rate setting, mode of pacing, specialized settings, and so forth). The pacing catheter (often called the lead or electrode) serves as a transmission line between the pulse generator and the endocardium. Electrical impulses are conducted from the pulse generator to the endocardium while information about intrinsic electrical activity is relayed from the catheter tip back to the generator for processing.

Pacemakers may be temporary or permanent. There are two types of temporary pacing systems: the external (transcutaneous) pacemaker and the temporary transvenous pacemaker. With the external pacemaker system, large pacing pads are placed on the anterior and posterior chest (Figure 10-1). Placement of the pacing pads will affect the current required to obtain ventricular capture. The placement that offers the most direct current pathway to the heart will usually produce the lowest threshold. The pacing pads are attached to a pacing cable which is then connected to a defibrillator/monitor. ECG leads are also attached to the patient. A pacing rate is set and the mA dial turned up until consistent capture is seen. The myocardium is stimulated indirectly by electric currents transmitted through the chest wall. There are also defibrillator/monitor/external pacing systems available which have the capability to monitor, externally pace, and defibrillate the patient through one set of chest pads. With this system, pacing pads are usually placed on the anterior chest, with one pacing pad below the right clavicle and one below the left breast.

External pacemakers are non-invasive, quick and easy to apply, and designed to function in the demand mode. Successful transcutaneous pacing requires a higher current output (mA) than conventional transvenous pacing. Delivery of this stronger current may cause chest wall pain and skin burns (although the larger pacing pad minimizes the risk of burns.) Transcutaneous pacing is effective as a treatment when meaningful contractile activity is present (e.g., in the hemodynamically significant bradycardias such as symptomatic sinus bradycardia, second-degree AV block Mobitz II and third-degree AV block). External pacing is usually not effective for treatment of ventricular standstill or

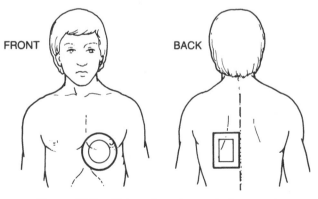

Figure 10-1. External pacing pad placement.

pulseless electrical activity (PEA) that occurs in the setting of cardiac arrest. This is because the primary problem in these situations is the inability of the myocardium to contract when appropriately stimulated. External pacemakers are used as a temporary measure in emergency situations where transvenous access is not readily available. Transvenous pacing is still the treatment of choice for patients requiring a temporary but longer period of pacemaker support.

With the temporary transvenous pacemaker (Figure 10-2), the pacing electrode is inserted by transvenous route into the right ventricle and connected via a bridging cable to an external pulse generator. The endocardium is stimulated directly by electric currents transmitted from the pulse generator. Controls on the face of the pulse generator allow operator manipulation of pacing parameters. Removable batteries are contained within the generator housing.

Like transcutaneous pacing, the temporary transvenous pacemaker is also used to treat the hemodynamically significant bradycardias and is usually not effective when meaningful contractile activity is absent (ventricular standstill and PEA). For significant unresolved rhythm or conduction disorders, permanent pacing is required.

Implantation of a permanent pacemaker (Figure 10-3) does not automatically follow temporary pacing. The procedure is performed only after careful analysis of each patient's clinical situation. Insertion of the permanent pacemaker is usually accomplished using the transvenous approach. The pacing catheter is inserted into a major (often subclavian) vein and advanced into the heart, where it is in contact with the endocardium of the right atrium or right ventricle or both. The pulse generator is implanted in the subcutaneous tissue below the right or left clavicle. The procedure is generally done using IV conscious sedation in combination with local anesthesia. In situations where endocardial pacing cannot be achieved, the permanent pacemaker is inserted by a transthoracic surgical approach using general anesthesia. The pacing catheter is attached to the epicardial surface of the left or right ventricle and the generator implanted in a subcutaneous pocket in the abdominal wall.

Basic functions of all pacemakers include the ability to sense, fire, and capture. Appropriate sensing implies that the pulse generator is able to "see" intrinsic patient beats. Firing means that the pulse generator has delivered a stimulus to the heart. Capturing means that the heart has responded to the stimulus. Most difficulties encountered with cardiac pacing result from abnormalities in sensing, firing, and/or capturing. Most of these difficulties can be traced to parameter settings, battery failure, problems at the interface of the catheter tip and endocardium, or problems with generator or lead integrity

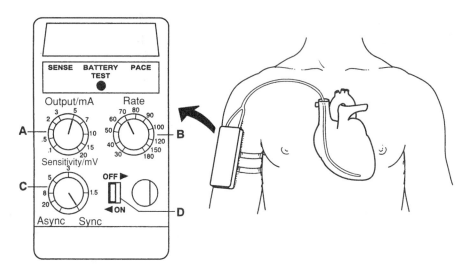

Figure 10-2. Temporary pacemaker.

A. Output or mA Dial
   Controls the amount of electrical energy delivered to the endocardium.
B. Rate Dial
   Determines the rate in beats per minute at which the stimulus is to be delivered.
C. Sensitivity or mV Dial
   Controls the ability of the generator to sense intrinsic activity.
   In maximum clockwise position, this provides demand (synchronous) pacing.
   In maximum counterclockwise position, this provides fixed rate (asynchronous) pacing.
D. On/Off Control
   Activates/inactivates the pulse generator.

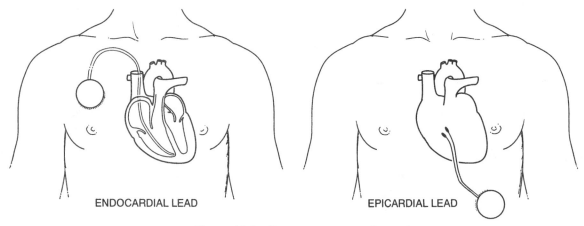

ENDOCARDIAL LEAD

EPICARDIAL LEAD

Figure 10-3. Permanent pacemaker.

(loose connections, break in pacing catheter, and so forth).

The temporary transvenous ventricular demand pacemaker is the simplest and most common type of pacing used in the acute clinical setting. This pacemaker is single chamber, paces and senses only in the ventricle, and is inhibited only by ventricular activity—in other words, when ventricular activity is sensed the pacemaker is inhibited (withholds a pacing stimulus), but when ventricular activity is not sensed the pacemaker will discharge impulses at a preset rate. Further discussion and ECG tracing focus on the temporary transvenous ventricular demand pacemaker.

PACEMAKER TERMS

Ventricular Capture

Capture indicates that the ventricle has responded to a pacing stimulus (Figure 10-4, Complex A). This is reflected on the ECG tracing by a stimulus artifact (a spike), followed by a wide QRS complex. Ventricular pacing causes sequential depolarization instead of synchronous depolarization. This means that one ventricle (usually the right) will be depolarized before the other. The prolonged depolarization time results in a wide QRS complex.

Native Beat

A native beat (also called intrinsic beat) is produced by the patient's own electrical conduction system. This beat is shown in Figure 10-4, complex B.

Fusion Beat

A fusion beat (Figure 10-4, Complex C) occurs when the pacemaker fires an electrical impulse at the same time that the patient's normal electrical impulse has activated the ventricles. The two forces simultaneously depolarize the ventricles, resulting in a fusion beat. The fusion beat has the characteristics of both pacemaker and patient forces, although one usually dominates the other. The resulting complex is

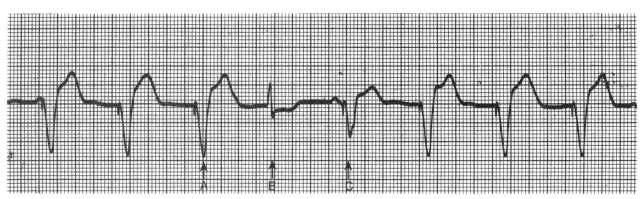

Figure 10-4. Ventricular capture (complex A), native beat (complex B), and fusion beat (complex C).

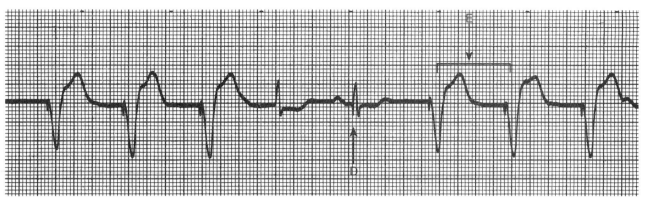

Figure 10-5. Pseudofusion beat (complex D) and automatic interval (complex E).

different in configuration and height from that caused by either of the forces alone. Fusion beats are normal.

Pseudofusion Beat

A pseudofusion beat (Figure 10-5, Complex D) occurs when a pacemaker spike falls within the QRS complex of a native beat but does not alter the height or configuration of the complex. The pacing stimulus had no effect on depolarization because the ventricle was already fully stimulated by the intrinsic beat. Pseudofusion beats are normal.

Automatic Interval

The automatic interval (Figure 10-5, Complex E) refers to the heart rate at which the pacemaker is set. This interval is measured from one pacing spike to the next consecutive pacing spike.

Pacemaker Rhythm

Pacemaker rhythm (Figure 10-6) occurs when the heart's rhythm is completely pacemaker induced.

This is reflected by an ECG tracing in which no patient beats are seen and all QRS complexes are induced by the pacemaker.

PACEMAKER MALFUNCTIONS

The most common malfunctions associated with the temporary transvenous ventricular demand pacemaker involve failure to capture and undersensing. These malfunctions are discussed below.

Failure to Capture

Failure to capture (Figure 10-7) means that the ventricles failed to respond to a pacing stimulus. This is reflected on the ECG by a pacing spike that occurs on time at the automatic interval rate, but is not followed by a QRS complex. Failure to capture is common with temporary pacemakers and often results from:

1. *Lead dislodgement.* An electrode tip must be in contact with the endocardium for the electrical stimulus to cause depolarization.

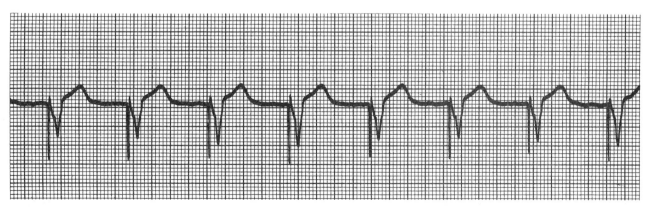

Figure 10-6. Pacemaker rhythm.

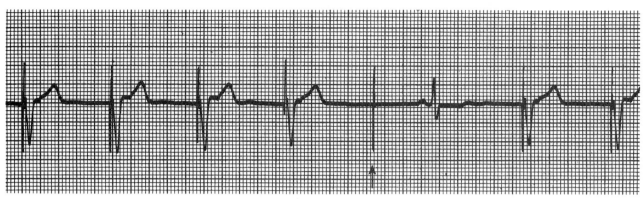

Figure 10-7. Loss of capture.

2. *Increase in stimulation threshold.* The minimum amount of current required to cause a ventricular response is called "threshold" and is determined during pacemaker insertion. The milliamperes (mA) dial is usually set at two times the insertion threshold. Over a period of days inflammation or fibrosis of tissue surrounding the catheter tip may raise the stimulation threshold, resulting in failure to capture. Effective capture is usually regained by simply increasing the milliamperes on the mA dial (see Figure 10-9). Table 10-1 summarizes the causes and appropriate interventions for failure to capture.

Undersensing

Undersensing (Figure 10-8) occurs when the pulse generator does not sense the patient's intrinsic beats. This problem is reflected on the ECG by a pacing spike that occurs earlier than it should following a native or paced beat. Ventricular capture may or may not occur. Under normal circumstances the generator senses the beat before it and does not fire a stimulus until the time indicated by the automatic interval setting. Undersensing often results from:

Table 10-1. Failure to Capture

Causes	Interventions
Electrical milliamps (mA) set too low	Increase the mA setting on pulse generator until consistent capture is achieved. Increasing the mA is achieved by turning the mA dial clockwise to a higher number.
Dislodgement of lead	Do overpenetrated chest x-ray to determine catheter position.
	If catheter is out of position, a temporary intervention is to place patient on left side (gravity may allow catheter to contact endocardium).
	Reposition the pacing catheter.

1. *Sensitivity setting set too low* (Figure 10-9). High sensitivity settings (low number on sensitivity dial) instruct the pulse generator to sense virtually all intrinsic activity (even low voltage signals), whereas low sensitivity settings (high number on sensitivity dial) instruct the generator to virtually ignore all intrinsic activity (even high voltage signals). The lowest number on the dial correlates with demand (synchronous) pacing, while the highest number correlates with fixed-rate (asynchronous) pacing.

2. *Lead dislodgement.* The electrode tip must be in contact with the endocardium before information about intrinsic activity can be received and relayed back to the generator for processing. Table 10-2 summarizes the causes and appropriate interventions for undersensing.

ANALYZING PACEMAKER RHYTHM STRIPS (VENTRICULAR DEMAND TYPE)

When analyzing pacemaker rhythm strips you will again need to use either calipers or an index card. I have found the following steps to be helpful.

Step 1. Place an index card (or caliper) above two consecutive paced beats. Mark on index card the interval from one pacing spike to the next. This is called the automatic interval and indicates the heart rate at which the pacemaker is set. The automatic interval measurement will assist you in determining if the pacemaker fired on time, too early, too late, or not at all.

Step 2. Start at left side of rhythm strip. Each pacing spike should be analyzed systematically to assess if the pacemaker is functioning appropriately.

Step 3. Identify pacing spike to be analyzed (only one spike should be analyzed at a time). Using

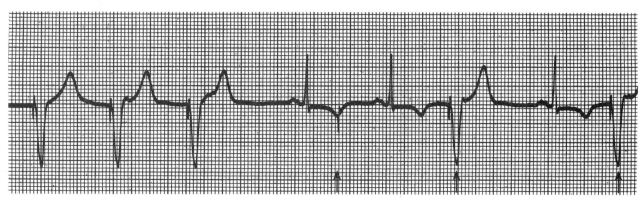

Figure 10-8. Undersensing.

Output (mA)

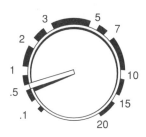

The output (mA) dial controls the amount of electrical energy delivered to the myocardium. Turning the dial to a higher number increases the mA.

Sensitivity (mV)

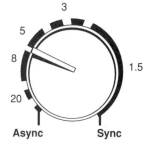

The sensitivity (mV) dial controls the ability of the generator to sense intrinsic activity. Turning the dial to a low number increases the sensitivity. Turning the dial to a high number decreases the sensitivity.

Figure 10-9. Output (mA) and sensitivity (mV) dials on a temporary pulse generator.

Table 10-2. Undersensing

Causes	Interventions
Sensitivity setting too low	Increase sensitivity on pulse generator by turning the sensitivity dial clockwise to a lower number.
Dislodgement of lead	Do overpenetrated chest x-ray to determine catheter position.
	If catheter is out of position, a temporary intervention is to place patient on left side (gravity may allow catheter to contact endocardium).
	The pacemaker may be turned off until physician can assess the problem if:
	Initial interventions had no effect.
	Patient's heart rate is adequate.
	The pacing spike is falling in the T-wave and there is a great potential for lethal arrhythmias to be induced.
	Reposition the pacing catheter.

marked index card (step 1), place left mark on spike of paced beat or R-wave of native beat immediately preceding pacing spike being analyzed. Observe the relationship of the spike being analyzed to the right mark on index card:

a. If spike being analyzed coincides with right mark, the possible answers include:

ventricular capture beat (normal)

fusion beat (normal)

pseudofusion beat (normal)

failure to capture (abnormal)

b. If spike being analyzed occurs earlier than right mark, the answer is:

undersensing malfunction (abnormal)

Study Figures 10-10 and 10-11—these strips have been analyzed for you.

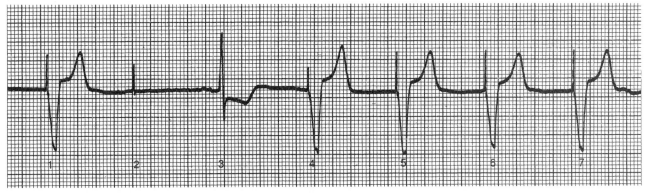

Figure 10-10. Pacemaker Analysis Strip #1.

1. The automatic interval can be measured from #4 to #5. The heart rate is 63.
2. #2 can be analyzed by placing left mark on index card on spike of beat just before it; #2 matches right mark on index card; #2 occurs on time but does not cause ventricular depolarization so it indicates failure to capture.
3. #3 is a native beat—it doesn't need analyzing.
4. #4 can be analyzed by placing left mark on R wave of native QRS just before it; #4 matches right mark on index card; #4 occurs on time and causes ventricular depolarization, indicating ventricular capture beat.
5. #5, #6, and #7 are all analyzed by placing left mark on spikes immediately preceding each beat to be analyzed—all occur on time and cause ventricular depolarization, indicating ventricular capture beats.

Interpretation: Failure to capture (one occurrence).

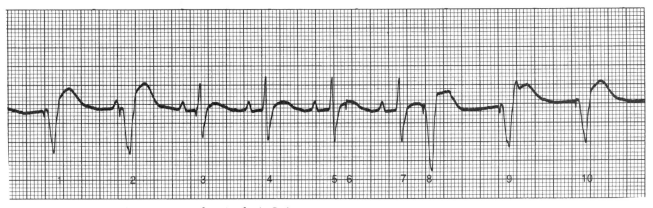

Figure 10-11. Pacemaker Analysis Strip #2.

1. The automatic interval can be measured from #1 to #2. The heart rate is 72.
2. #2 can be analyzed by placing left mark on index card on spike of beat immediately before it; #2 matches right mark on index card; #2 occurs on time and causes ventricular depolarization indicating ventricular capture beat.
3. #3 is a native beat (note spike at beginning of R wave); place left mark on spike of beat immediately before it; #3 matches right mark; #3 has a spike in it and is different from the other native beats (#4, #5, #7) in height so this represents a fusion beat.
4. #4 and #5 are native beats and do not need analyzing.
5. #6 can be analyzed by placing left mark on R wave of native beat just before it; #6 occurs much earlier than right mark; #6 indicates that generator did not sense preceding beat and represents undersensing problem.
6. #7 is a native beat.
7. #8 can be analyzed by placing left mark on R wave of native beat just before it; #8 occurs much earlier than right mark; #8 indicates the generator did not sense preceding beat and represents an undersensing problem. (Note: #6 represents an undersensing problem without capture while #8 represents an undersensing problem with capture.)
8. #9 can be analyzed by placing left mark on spike of beat just before it; #9 matches right mark; #9 occurs on time and causes ventricular depolarization indicating ventricular capture beat.
9. #10 can be analyzed by placing left mark on spike of beat just before it; #10 matches right mark; #10 occurs on time and causes ventricular depolarization indicating ventricular capture beat.

Interpretation: Undersensing malfunction (two occurrences).

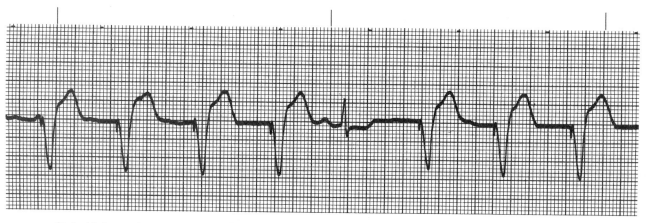

Strip 10-1. Automatic interval rate:_____

Analysis:_____

Interpretation:_____

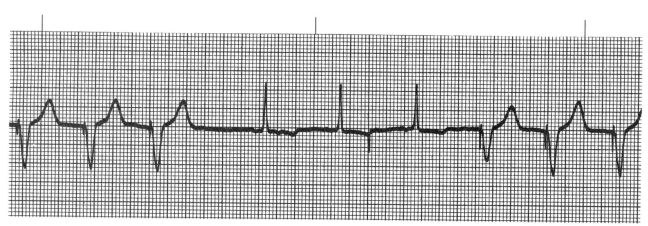

Strip 10-2. Automatic interval rate:_____

Analysis:_____

Interpretation:_____

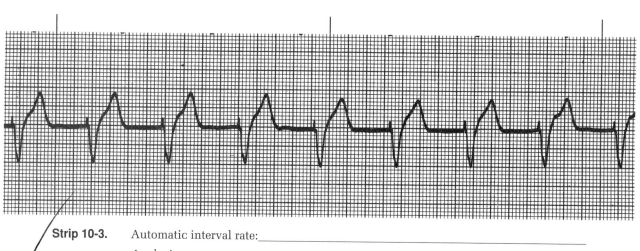

Strip 10-3. Automatic interval rate:_____

Analysis:_____

Interpretation:_____VENT. pacing_____

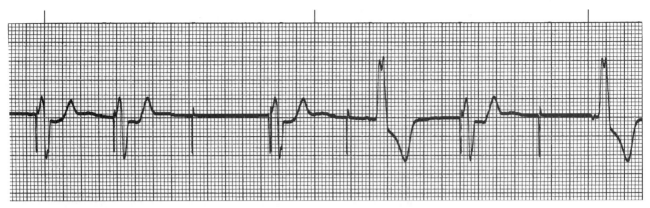

Strip 10-4. Automatic interval rate:_____

Analysis:_____

Interpretation:_____

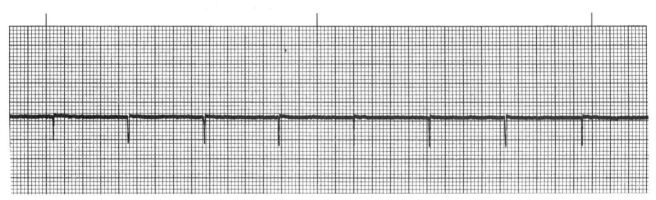

Strip 10-5. Automatic interval rate:_____

Analysis:_____

Interpretation:_____

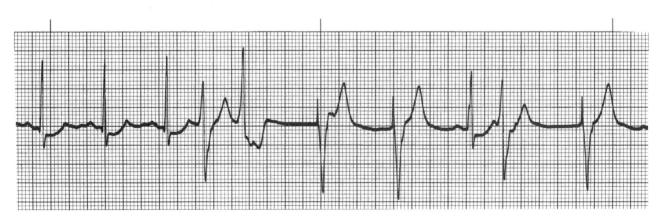

Strip 10-6. Automatic interval rate:_____

Analysis:_____

Interpretation:_____

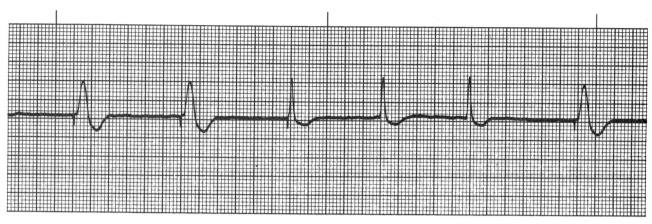

Strip 10-7.   Automatic interval rate:_____

Analysis:_____

Interpretation:_____

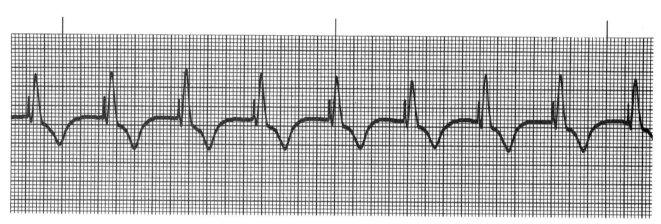

Strip 10-8.   Automatic interval rate:_____

Analysis:_____

Interpretation:_____

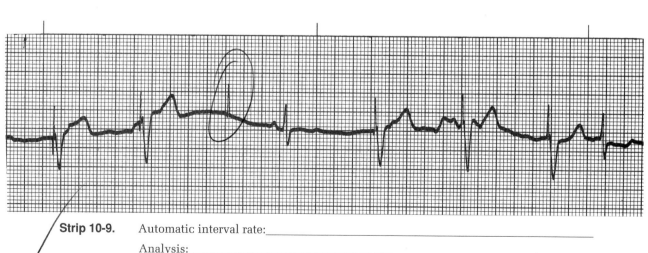

Strip 10-9.   Automatic interval rate:_____

Analysis:_____

Interpretation:_____V-pacing c̄ failure to capture_____

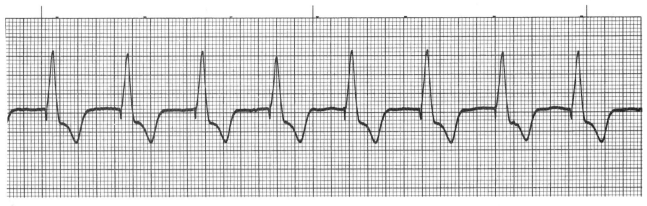

Strip 10-10. Automatic interval rate:_____

Analysis:_____

Interpretation:_____

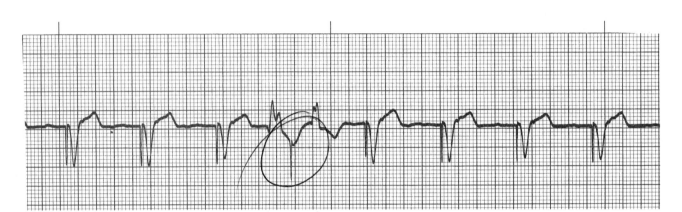

Strip 10-11. Automatic interval rate:_____

Analysis:_____

Interpretation:___V-pacing c̄ failure to sense_____

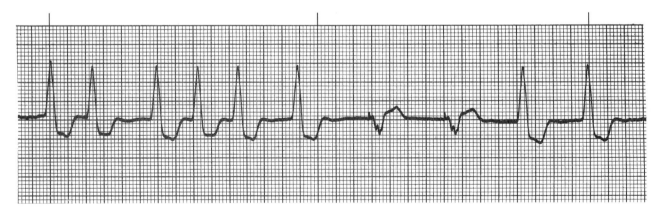

Strip 10-12. Automatic interval rate:_____

Analysis:_____

Interpretation:_____

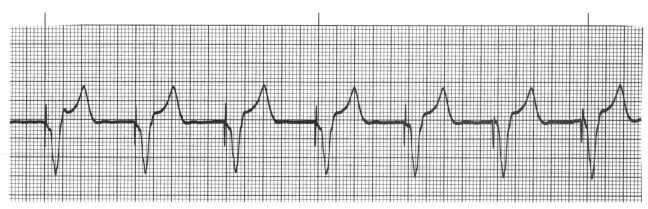

Strip 10-13.   Automatic interval rate:_____

Analysis:_____

Interpretation:_____

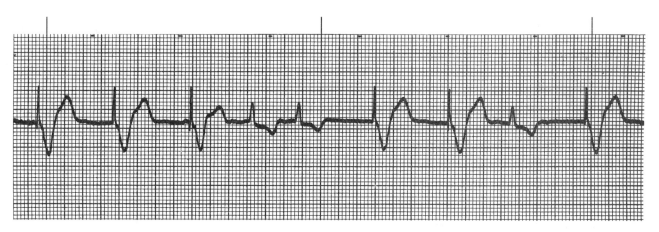

Strip 10-14.   Automatic interval rate:_____

Analysis:_____

Interpretation:_____

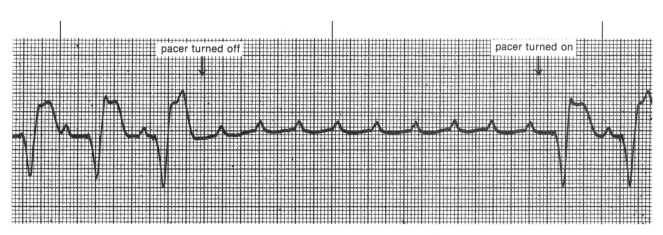

Strip 10-15.   Automatic interval rate:_____

Analysis:_____

Interpretation:_____

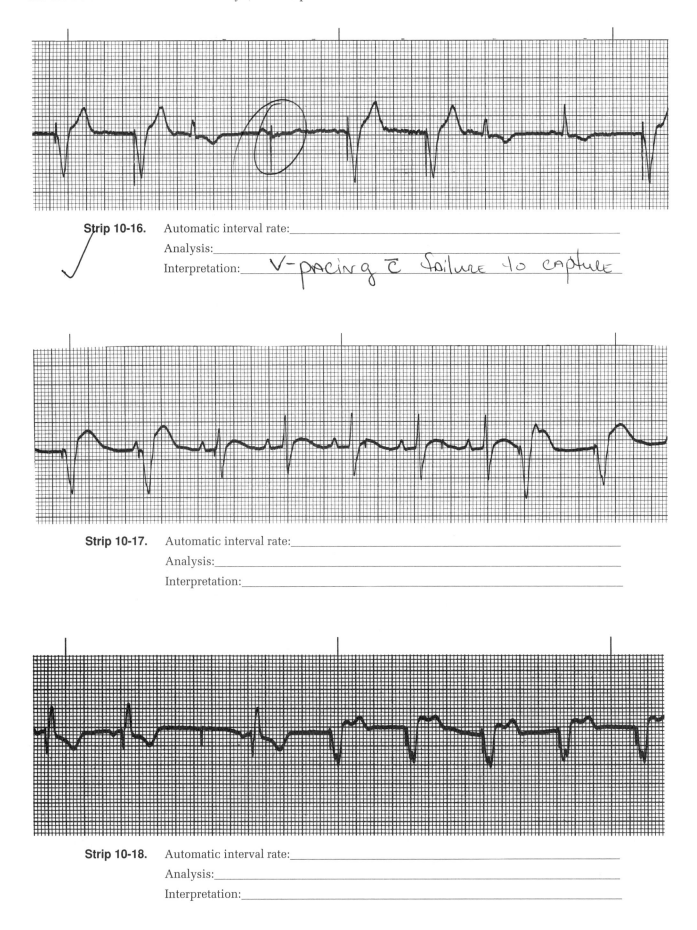

Strip 10-16. Automatic interval rate:_____

Analysis:_____

Interpretation:___ V-pacing c̄ failure to capture

Strip 10-17. Automatic interval rate:_____

Analysis:_____

Interpretation:_____

Strip 10-18. Automatic interval rate:_____

Analysis:_____

Interpretation:_____

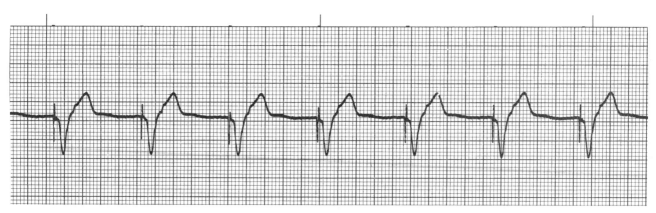

Strip 10-25. Automatic interval rate:_____

Analysis:_____

Interpretation:_____

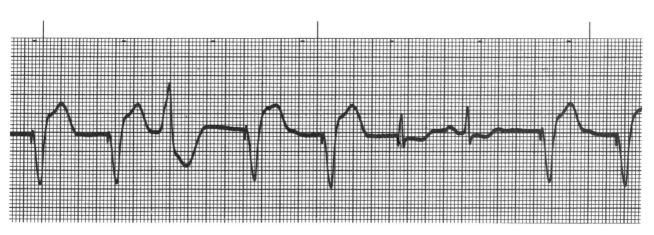

Strip 10-26. Automatic interval rate:_____

Analysis:_____

Interpretation:_____

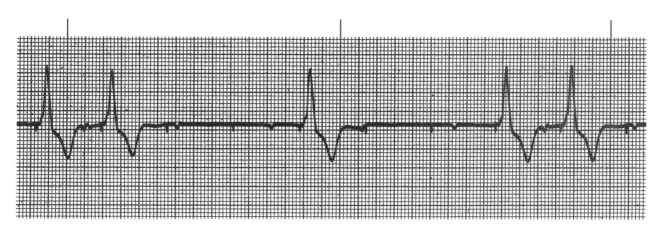

Strip 10-27. Automatic interval rate:_____

Analysis:_____

Interpretation:_____

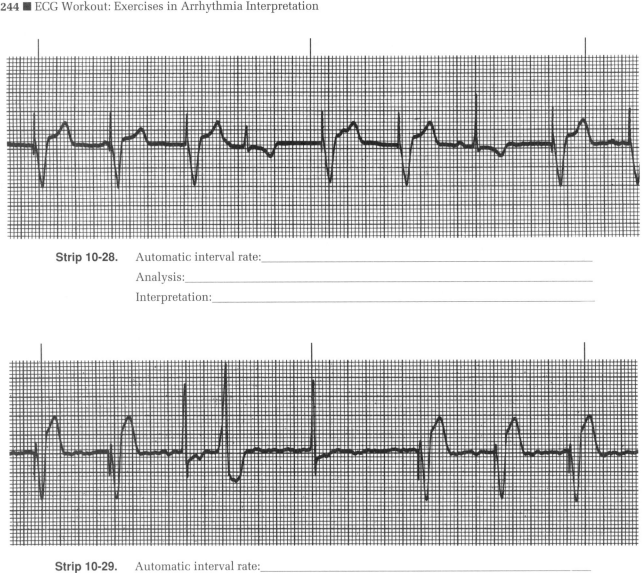

Strip 10-28. Automatic interval rate:_____

Analysis:_____

Interpretation:_____

Strip 10-29. Automatic interval rate:_____

Analysis:_____

Interpretation:_____

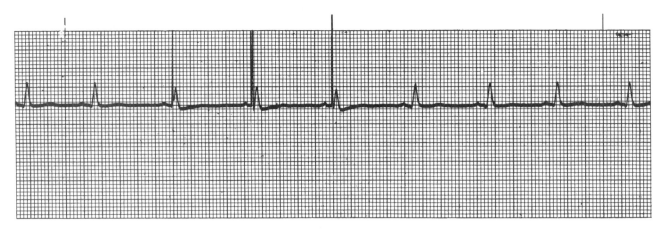

Strip 10-30. Automatic interval rate:_____

Analysis:_____

Interpretation:_____

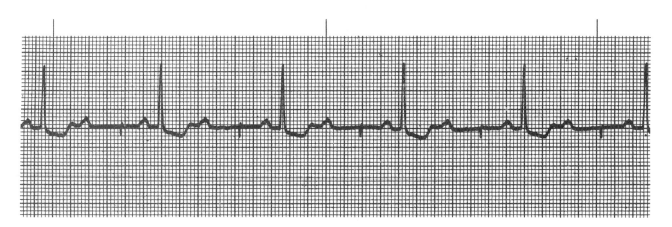

Strip 10-31. Automatic interval rate:_____

Analysis:_____

Interpretation:_____

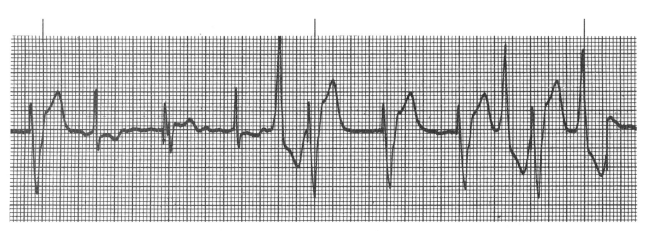

Strip 10-32. Automatic interval rate:_____

Analysis:_____

Interpretation:_____

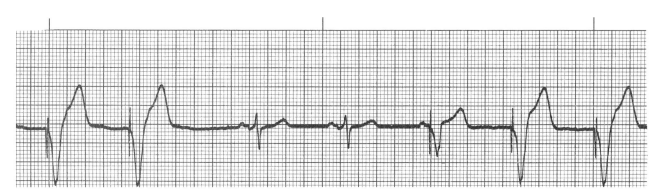

Strip 10-33. Automatic interval rate:_____

Analysis:_____

Interpretation:_____

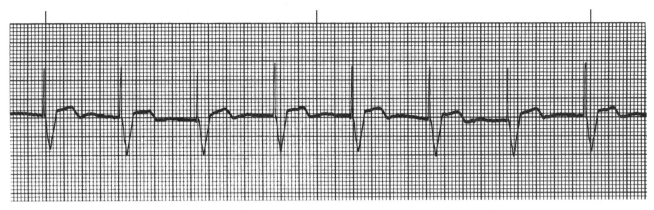

Strip 10-34.   Automatic interval rate:_____

Analysis:_____

Interpretation:_____

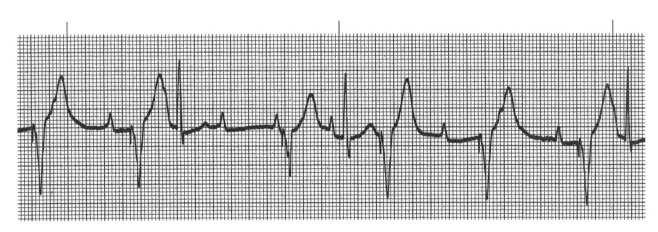

Strip 10-35.   Automatic interval rate:_____

Analysis:_____

Interpretation:_____

Post-Test

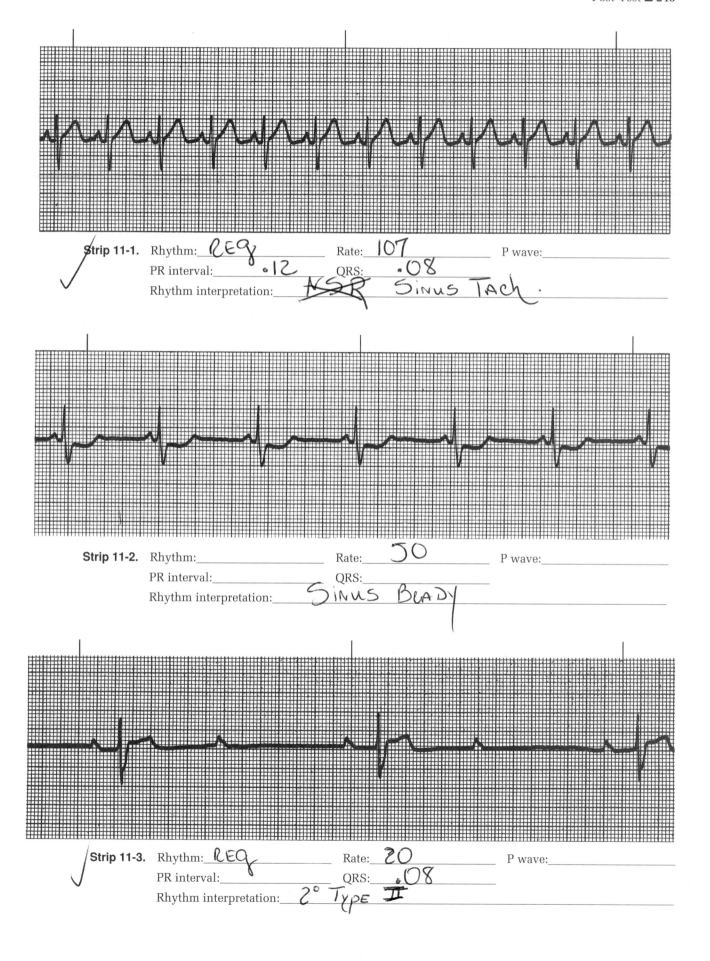

Strip 11-1. Rhythm: REg   Rate: 107   P wave: _____
PR interval: .12   QRS: .08
Rhythm interpretation: ~~NSR~~ Sinus Tach.

Strip 11-2. Rhythm: _____   Rate: 50   P wave: _____
PR interval: _____   QRS: _____
Rhythm interpretation: Sinus Brady

Strip 11-3. Rhythm: REg   Rate: 20   P wave: _____
PR interval: _____   QRS: .08
Rhythm interpretation: 2° Type II

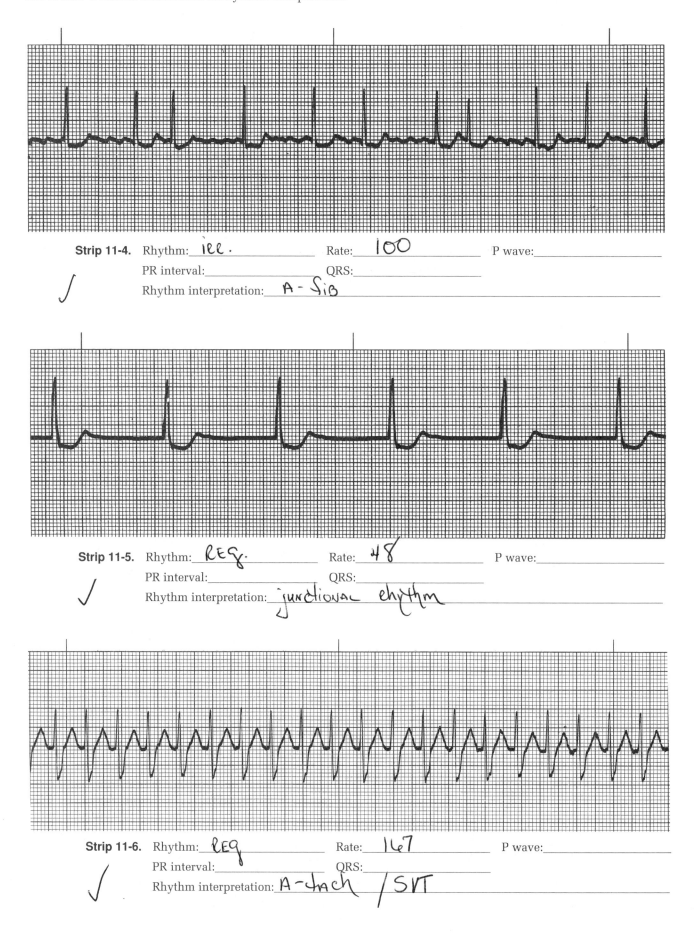

Strip 11-4. Rhythm: _irr._ Rate: _100_ P wave: _____

PR interval: _____ QRS: _____

Rhythm interpretation: _A-fib_

Strip 11-5. Rhythm: _REg._ Rate: _48_ P wave: _____

PR interval: _____ QRS: _____

Rhythm interpretation: _junctional rhythm_

Strip 11-6. Rhythm: _REg_ Rate: _167_ P wave: _____

PR interval: _____ QRS: _____

Rhythm interpretation: _A-tach / SVT_

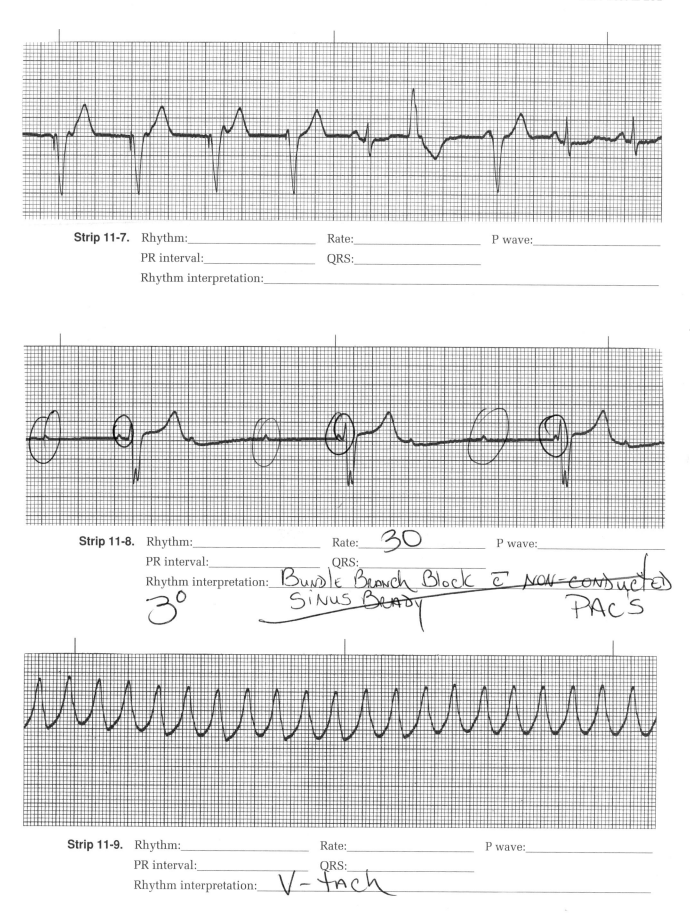

Strip 11-7. Rhythm:_____ Rate:_____ P wave:_____

PR interval:_____ QRS:_____

Rhythm interpretation:_____

Strip 11-8. Rhythm:_____ Rate: 30 P wave:_____

PR interval:_____ QRS:_____

Rhythm interpretation: Bundle Branch Block c̄ NON-CONDUCTED

3° SINUS BRADY PAC's

Strip 11-9. Rhythm:_____ Rate:_____ P wave:_____

PR interval:_____ QRS:_____

Rhythm interpretation: V-tach

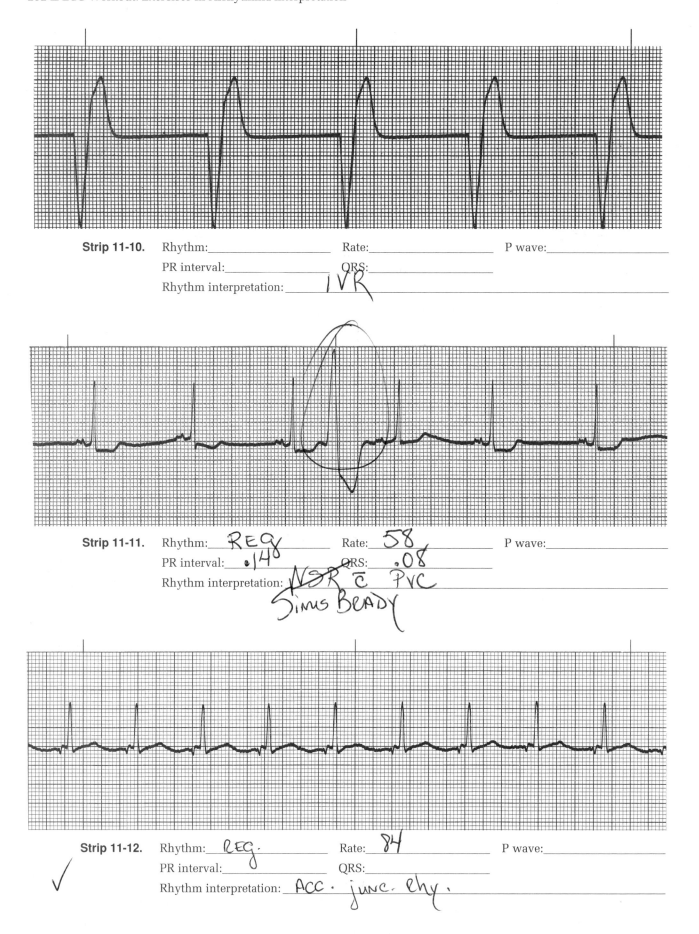

Strip 11-10. Rhythm:_____ Rate:_____ P wave:_____

PR interval:_____ QRS:_____

Rhythm interpretation: _____IVR_____

Strip 11-11. Rhythm:___REG_____ Rate:___58_____ P wave:_____

PR interval:___.14___ QRS:___.08___

Rhythm interpretation: NSR c̄ PVC_____

Sinus Brady

Strip 11-12. Rhythm:___REG.____ Rate:___84___ P wave:_____

PR interval:___0___ QRS:_____

✓ Rhythm interpretation: ___Acc. junc. rhy._____

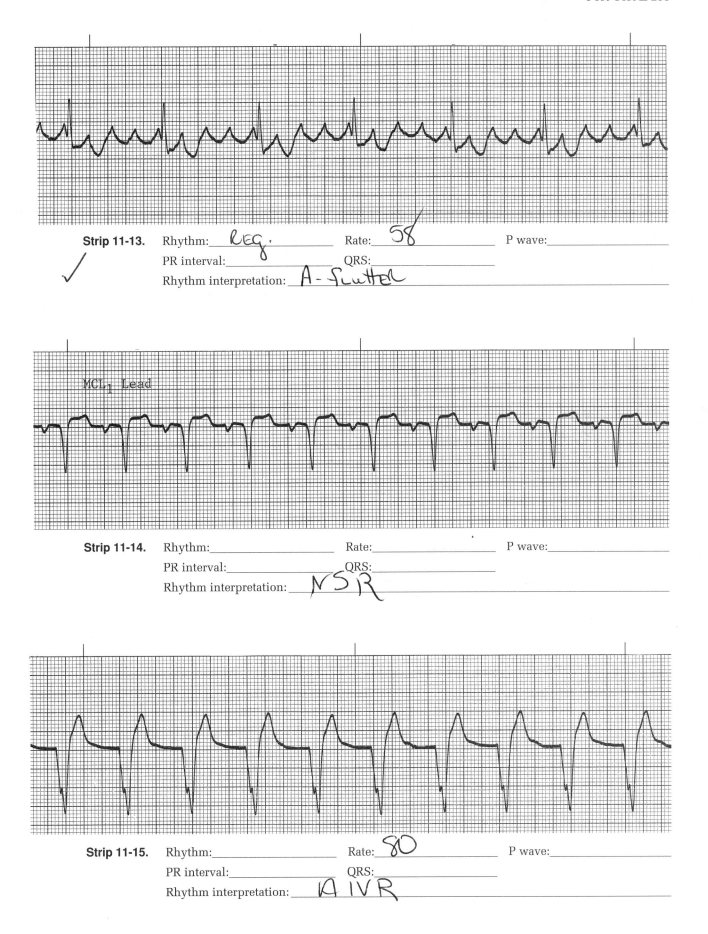

Strip 11-13. Rhythm: ___REG.___ Rate: ___58___ P wave:_____

PR interval:_____ QRS:_____

Rhythm interpretation: ___A-flutter___

✓

Strip 11-14. Rhythm:_____ Rate:_____ P wave:_____

PR interval:_____ QRS:_____

Rhythm interpretation: ___NSR___

MCL₁ Lead

Strip 11-15. Rhythm:_____ Rate: ___80___ P wave:_____

PR interval:_____ QRS:_____

Rhythm interpretation: ___AIVR___

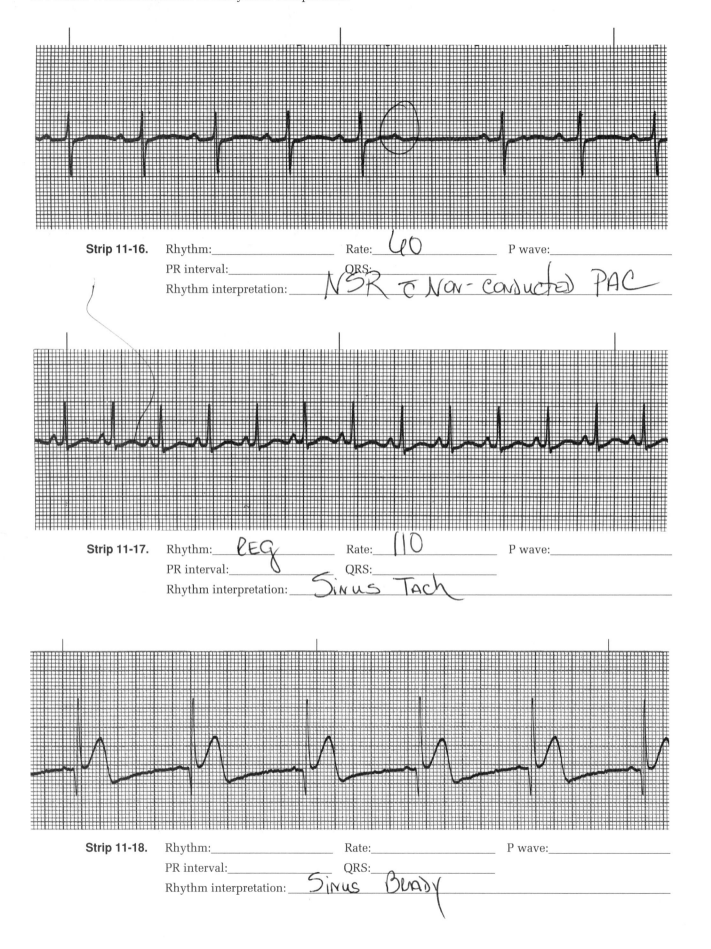

Strip 11-16. Rhythm:_____ Rate: 60 P wave:_____

PR interval:_____ QRS:_____

Rhythm interpretation: NSR c̄ Non-conducted PAC

Strip 11-17. Rhythm: REG Rate: 110 P wave:_____

PR interval:_____ QRS:_____

Rhythm interpretation: Sinus Tach

Strip 11-18. Rhythm:_____ Rate:_____ P wave:_____

PR interval:_____ QRS:_____

Rhythm interpretation: Sinus Brady

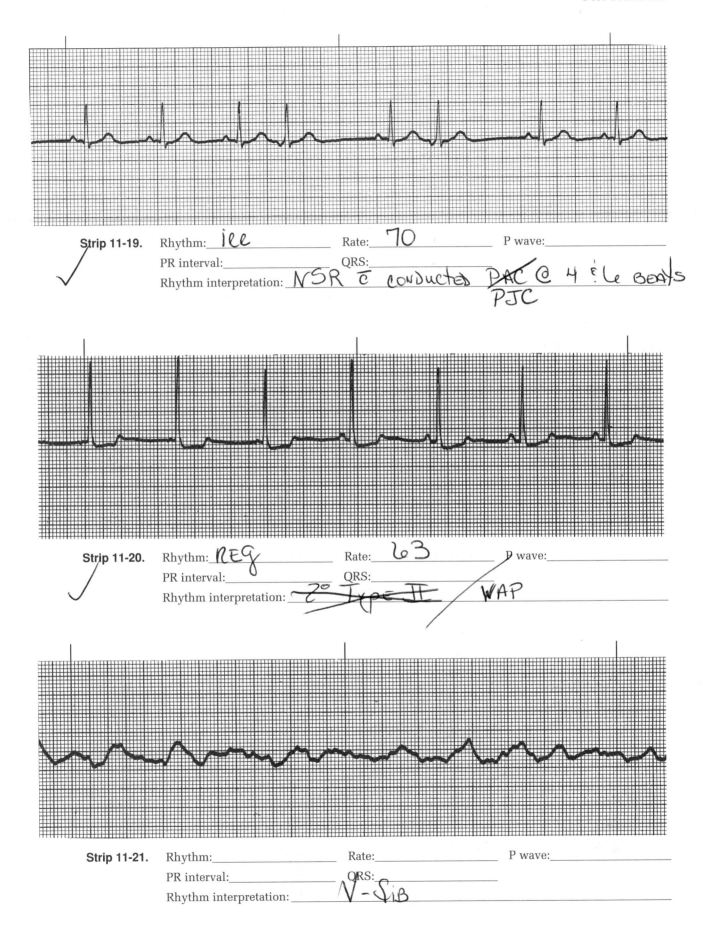

Strip 11-19. Rhythm: _ire_ Rate: _70_ P wave:_____

PR interval:_____ QRS:_____

Rhythm interpretation: _NSR c̄ conducted PAC @ 4 & 6 beats_
PJC

Strip 11-20. Rhythm: _REG_ Rate: _63_ P wave:_____

PR interval:_____ QRS:_____

Rhythm interpretation: _2° Type II / WAP_

Strip 11-21. Rhythm:_____ Rate:_____ P wave:_____

PR interval:_____ QRS:_____

Rhythm interpretation: _V-Fib_

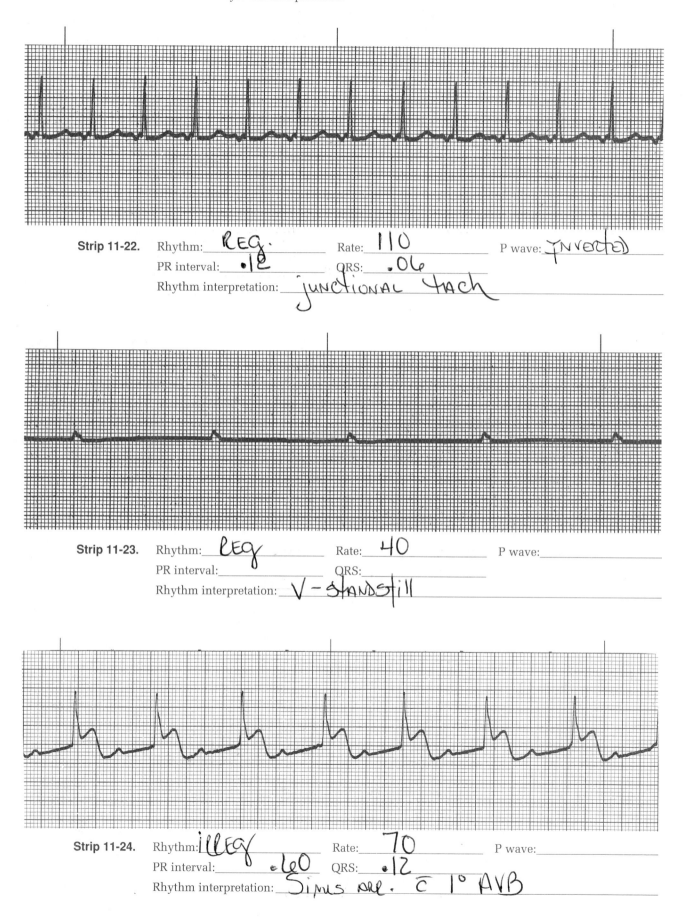

Strip 11-22. Rhythm: REG. Rate: 110 P wave: Inverted
PR interval: .12 QRS: .06
Rhythm interpretation: junctional tach

Strip 11-23. Rhythm: REG Rate: 40 P wave:
PR interval: QRS:
Rhythm interpretation: V-standstill

Strip 11-24. Rhythm: illeg Rate: 70 P wave:
PR interval: .60 QRS: .12
Rhythm interpretation: Sinus arr. c̄ 1° AVB

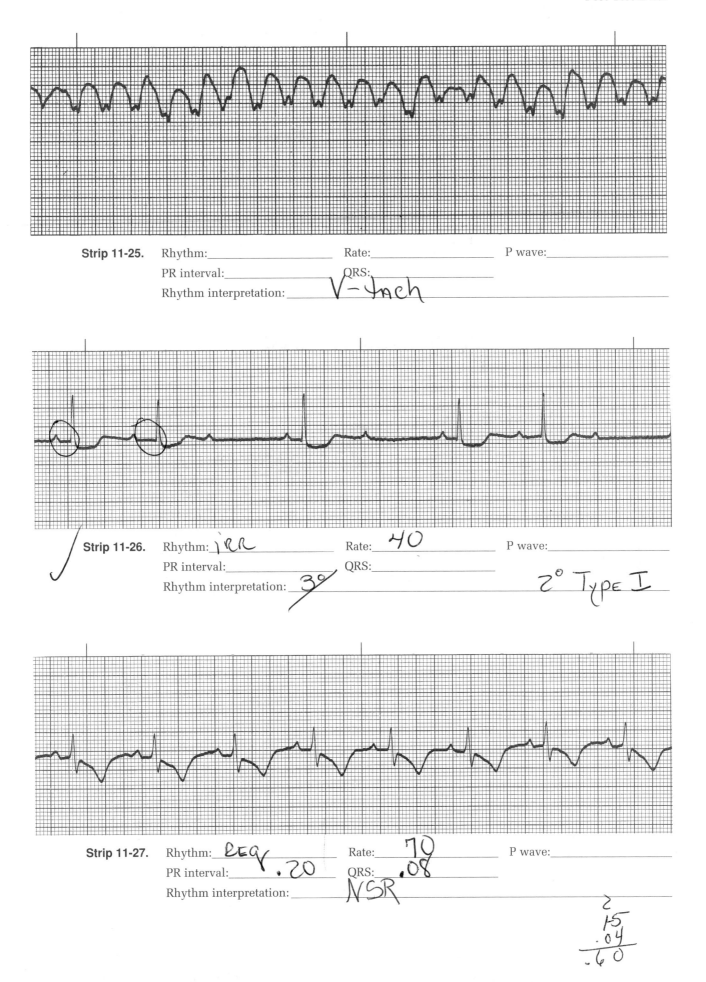

Strip 11-25. Rhythm:_____ Rate:_____ P wave:_____

PR interval:_____ QRS:_____

Rhythm interpretation: ___V-tach_____

Strip 11-26. Rhythm:_irr_____ Rate:___40_____ P wave:_____

PR interval:_____ QRS:_____

Rhythm interpretation: ___3°_____ 2° Type I

Strip 11-27. Rhythm:_Reg_____ Rate:___70_____ P wave:_____

PR interval:___.20_____ QRS:___.08_____

Rhythm interpretation: ___NSR_____

2
15
.04
.60

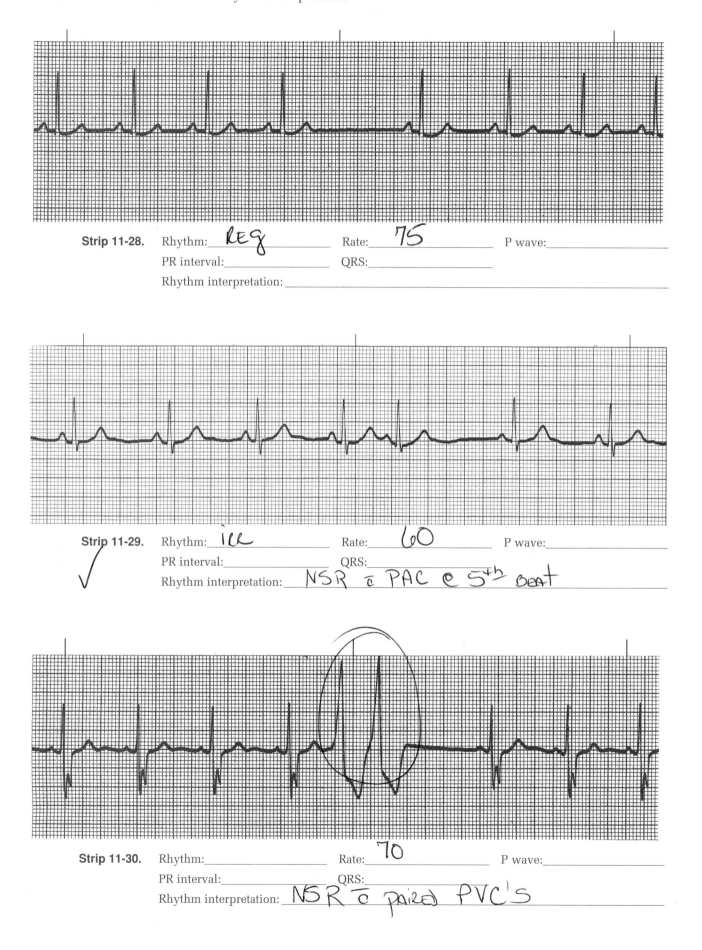

Strip 11-28. Rhythm: REg   Rate: 75   P wave:
PR interval: QRS:
Rhythm interpretation:

Strip 11-29. Rhythm: irr   Rate: 60   P wave:
PR interval: QRS:
Rhythm interpretation: NSR c̄ PAC @ 5th beat

Strip 11-30. Rhythm: Rate: 70   P wave:
PR interval: QRS:
Rhythm interpretation: NSR c̄ paired PVC's

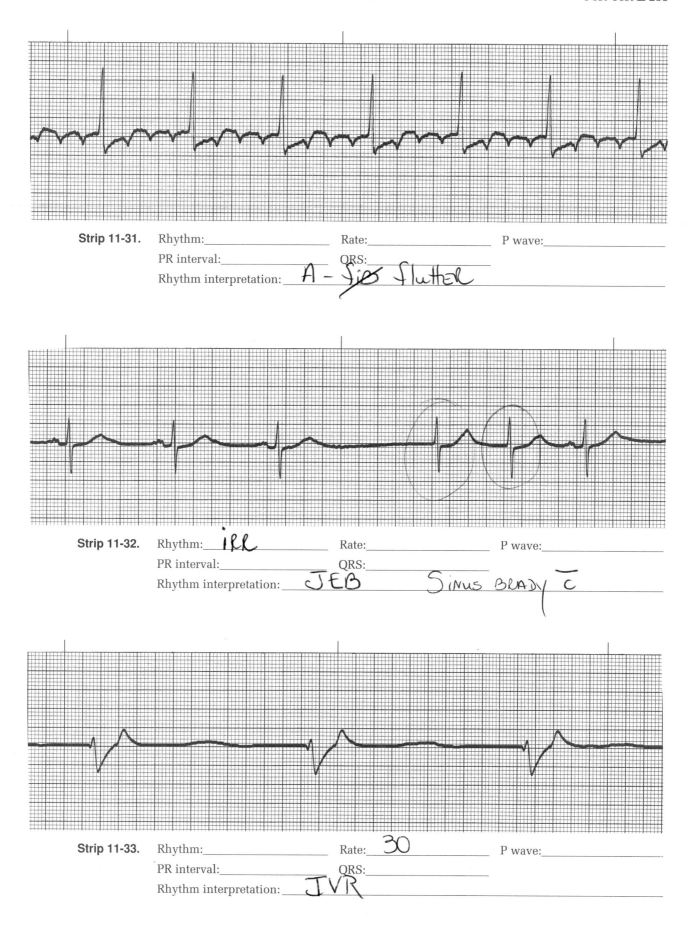

Strip 11-31. Rhythm:_____ Rate:_____ P wave:_____

PR interval:_____ QRS:_____

Rhythm interpretation: _A - Fib Flutter_____

Strip 11-32. Rhythm:_iRR_____ Rate:_____ P wave:_____

PR interval:_____ QRS:_____

Rhythm interpretation: _JEB_____ Sinus Brady c̄_____

Strip 11-33. Rhythm:_____ Rate:_30____ P wave:_____

PR interval:_____ QRS:_____

Rhythm interpretation: _JVR_____

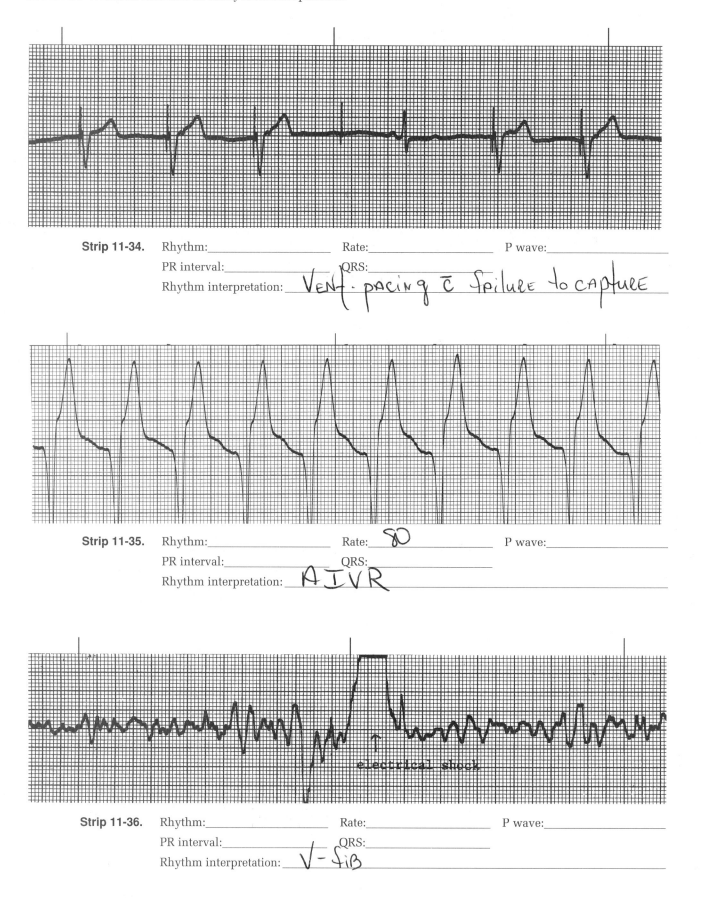

Strip 11-34. Rhythm:_____ Rate:_____ P wave:_____

PR interval:_____ QRS:_____

Rhythm interpretation: _Vent. pacing c̄ failure to capture_

Strip 11-35. Rhythm:_____ Rate: _80_ P wave:_____

PR interval:_____ QRS:_____

Rhythm interpretation: _AIVR_

electrical shock

Strip 11-36. Rhythm:_____ Rate:_____ P wave:_____

PR interval:_____ QRS:_____

Rhythm interpretation: _V-fib_

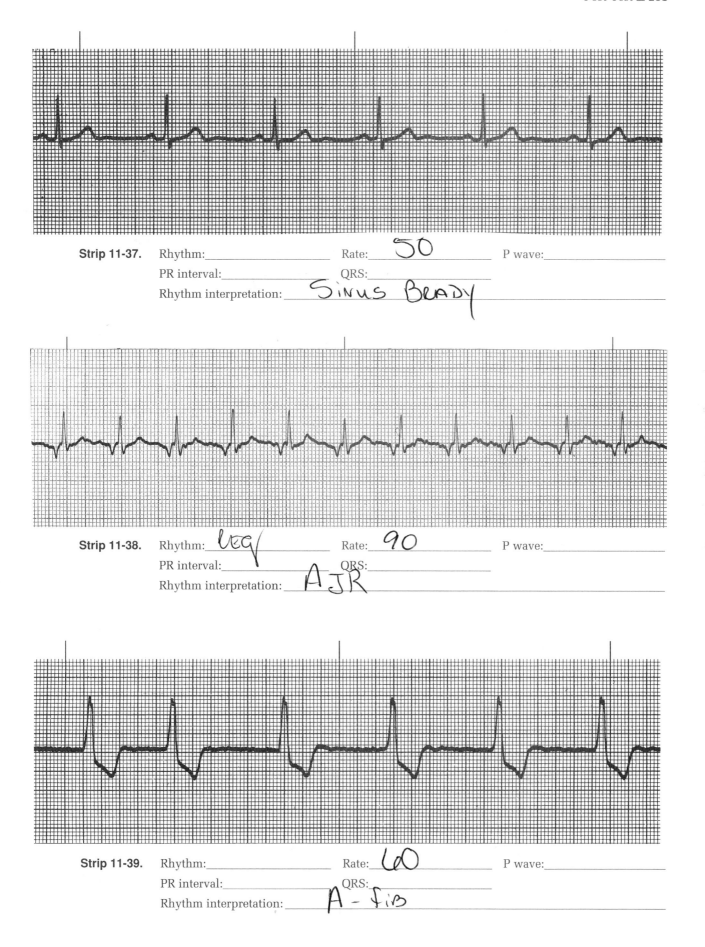

Strip 11-37. Rhythm:_____ Rate: _50_ P wave:_____

PR interval:_____ QRS:_____

Rhythm interpretation: _Sinus Brady_

Strip 11-38. Rhythm: _ECG_ Rate: _90_ P wave:_____

PR interval:_____ QRS:_____

Rhythm interpretation: _AJR_

Strip 11-39. Rhythm:_____ Rate: _60_ P wave:_____

PR interval:_____ QRS:_____

Rhythm interpretation: _A - fib_

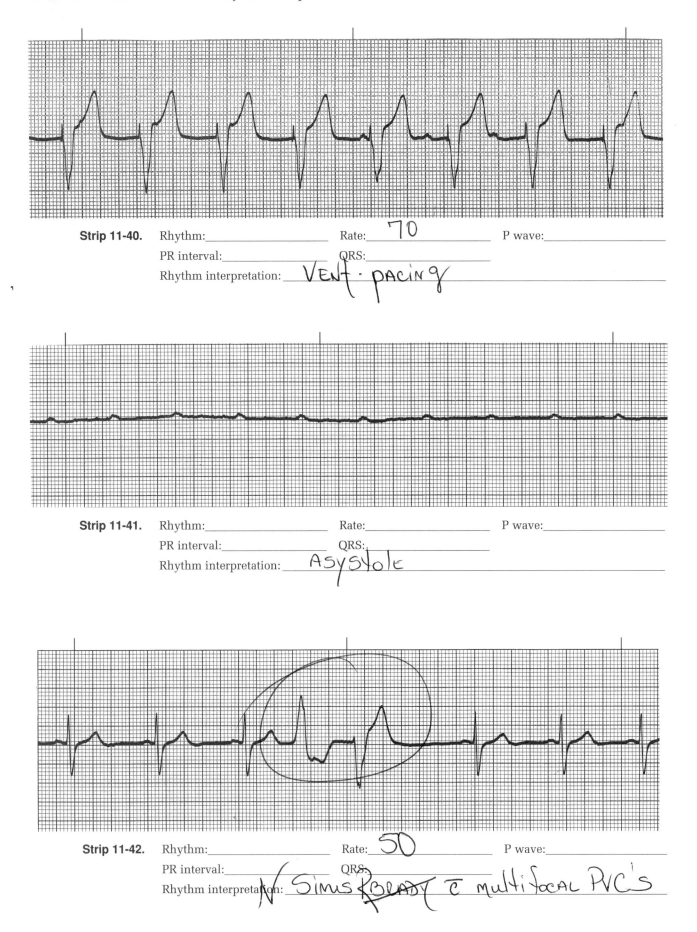

Strip 11-40. Rhythm:_____ Rate:___70_____ P wave:_____

PR interval:_____ QRS:_____

Rhythm interpretation:___Vent · pacing_____

Strip 11-41. Rhythm:_____ Rate:_____ P wave:_____

PR interval:_____ QRS:_____

Rhythm interpretation:___Asystole_____

Strip 11-42. Rhythm:_____ Rate:___50_____ P wave:_____

PR interval:_____ QRS:_____

Rhythm interpretation:___Sinus Brady c̄ multifocal PVC's_____

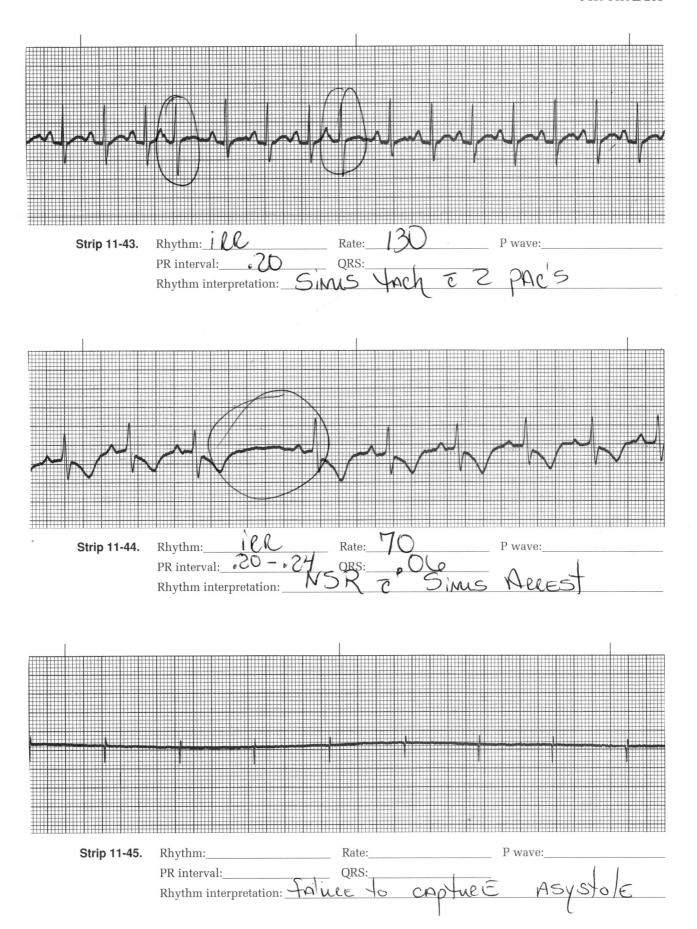

Strip 11-43. Rhythm: _irr_   Rate: _130_   P wave:_____

PR interval: _.20_   QRS:_____

Rhythm interpretation: _Sinus tach c̄ 2 PAC's_

Strip 11-44. Rhythm: _irr_   Rate: _70_   P wave:_____

PR interval: _.20 - .24_   QRS: _.06_

Rhythm interpretation: _NSR c̄ Sinus Arrest_

Strip 11-45. Rhythm:_____   Rate:_____   P wave:_____

PR interval:_____   QRS:_____

Rhythm interpretation: _failure to capture c̄ Asystole_

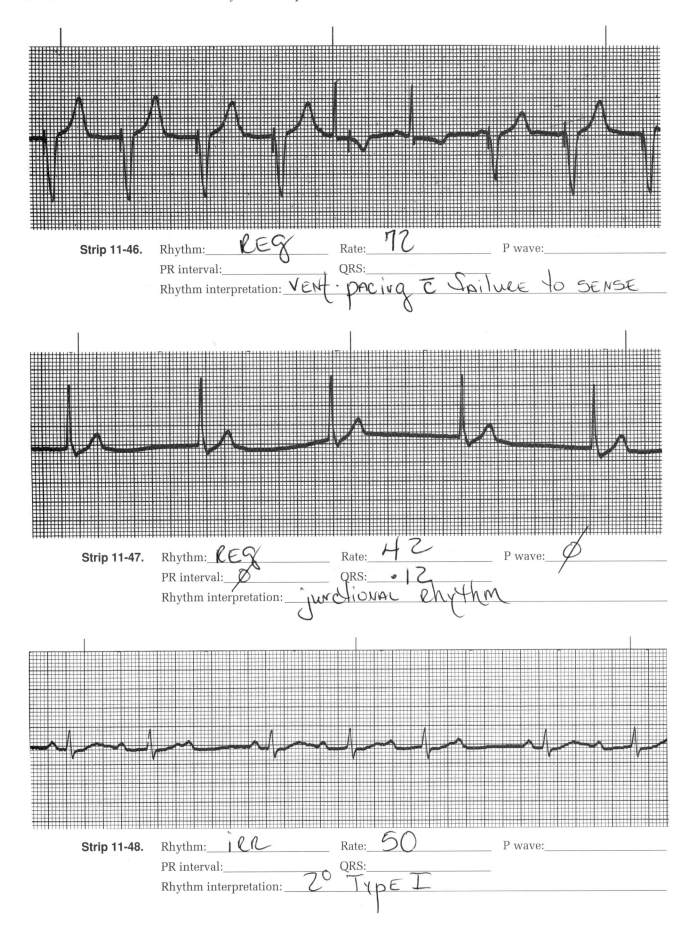

Strip 11-46. Rhythm: REG   Rate: 72   P wave: _____

PR interval: _____   QRS: _____

Rhythm interpretation: VENT. pacing c̄ failure to sense

Strip 11-47. Rhythm: REG   Rate: 42   P wave: ∅

PR interval: ∅   QRS: .12

Rhythm interpretation: junctional rhythm

Strip 11-48. Rhythm: iRR   Rate: 50   P wave: _____

PR interval: _____   QRS: _____

Rhythm interpretation: 2° Type I

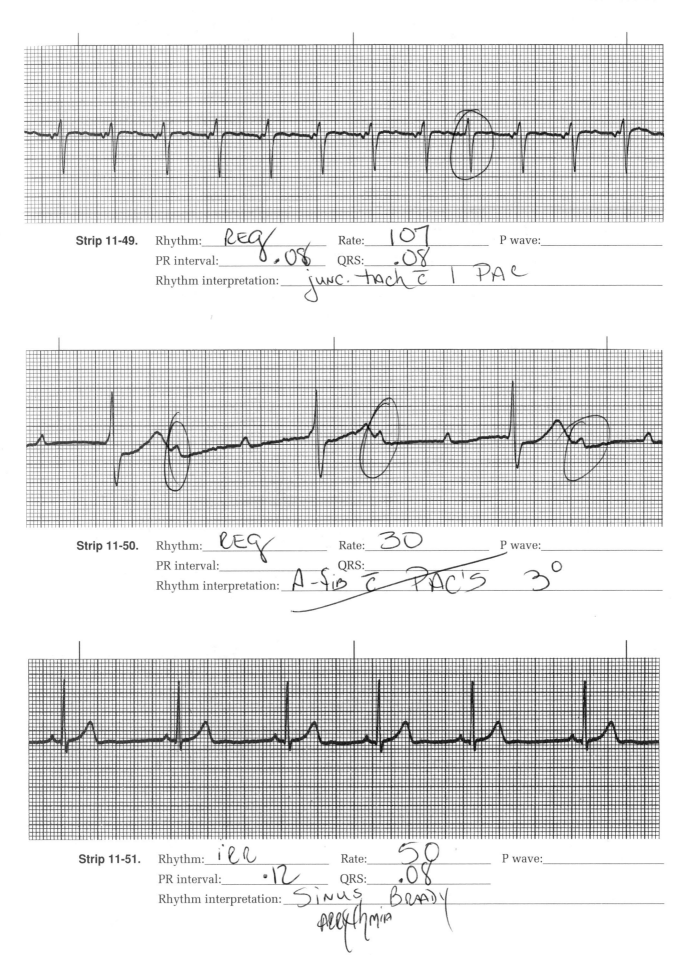

Strip 11-49. Rhythm: REG .08   Rate: 107   P wave:_____

PR interval: .08   QRS: .08

Rhythm interpretation: junc. tach c̄ 1 PAC

Strip 11-50. Rhythm: REG   Rate: 30   P wave:_____

PR interval:_____   QRS:_____

Rhythm interpretation: A-fib c̄ PAC's 3°

Strip 11-51. Rhythm: irr   Rate: 50   P wave:_____

PR interval: .12   QRS: .08

Rhythm interpretation: SINUS BRADY

arrhythmia

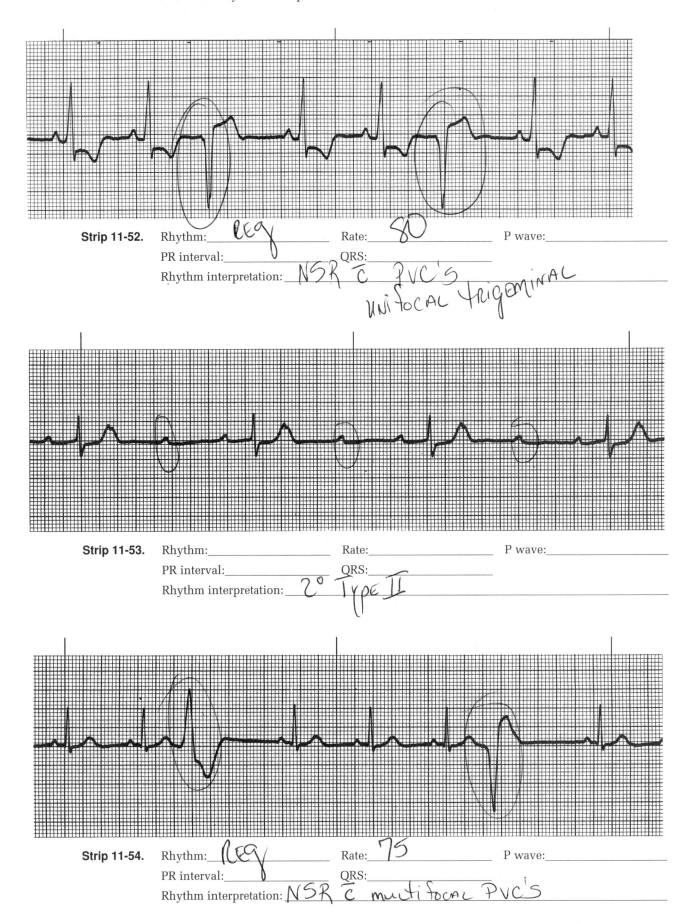

Strip 11-52. Rhythm: _Reg_ Rate: _80_ P wave: _____

PR interval: _____ QRS: _____

Rhythm interpretation: _NSR c̄ PVC's_
unifocal trigeminal

Strip 11-53. Rhythm: _____ Rate: _____ P wave: _____

PR interval: _____ QRS: _____

Rhythm interpretation: _2° Type II_

Strip 11-54. Rhythm: _Reg_ Rate: _75_ P wave: _____

PR interval: _____ QRS: _____

Rhythm interpretation: _NSR c̄ multifocal PVC's_

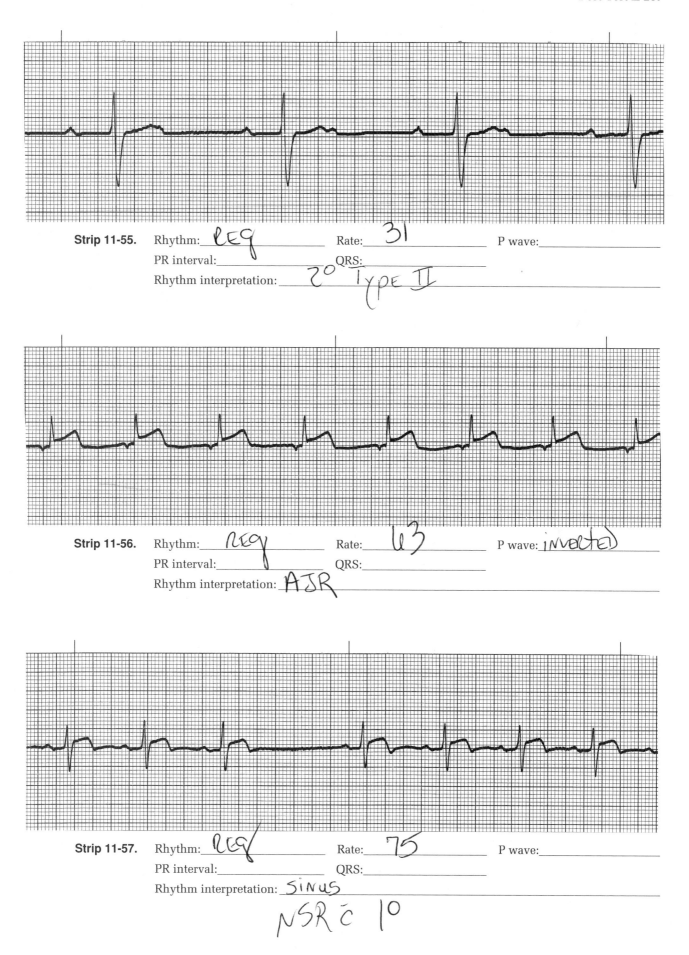

Strip 11-55. Rhythm: REG   Rate: 31   P wave: _____
PR interval: _____ QRS: _____
Rhythm interpretation: 2° TYPE II

Strip 11-56. Rhythm: REG   Rate: 63   P wave: INVERTED
PR interval: _____ QRS: _____
Rhythm interpretation: AJR

Strip 11-57. Rhythm: REG   Rate: 75   P wave: _____
PR interval: _____ QRS: _____
Rhythm interpretation: SINUS
NSR c̄ 1°

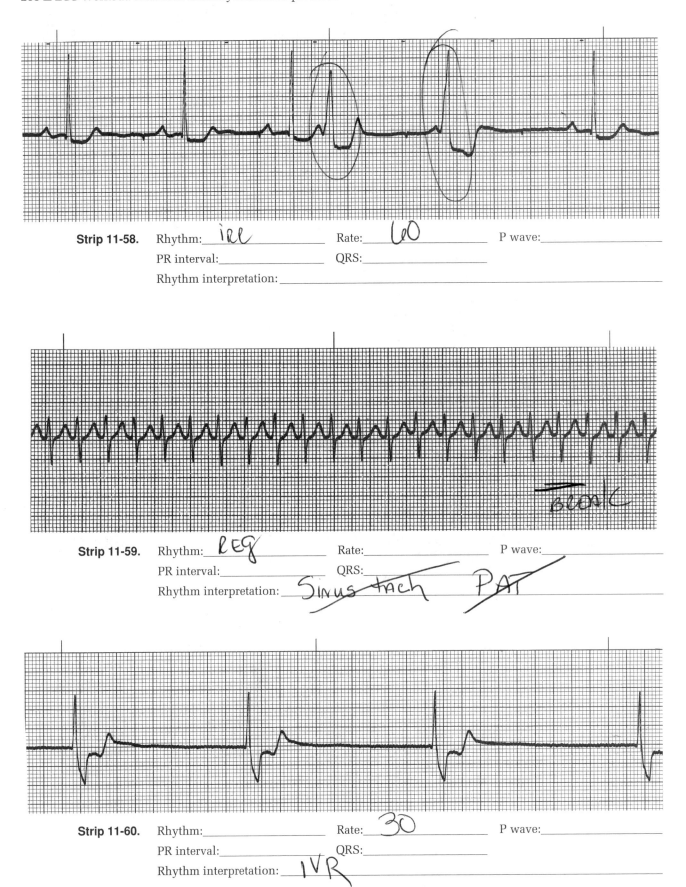

Strip 11-58. Rhythm: _irr_   Rate: _60_   P wave:_____

PR interval:_____   QRS:_____

Rhythm interpretation: _____

Strip 11-59. Rhythm: _REG_   Rate:_____   P wave:_____

PR interval:_____   QRS:_____

Rhythm interpretation: _Sinus tach PAT_

Strip 11-60. Rhythm:_____   Rate: _30_   P wave:_____

PR interval:_____   QRS:_____

Rhythm interpretation: _IVR_

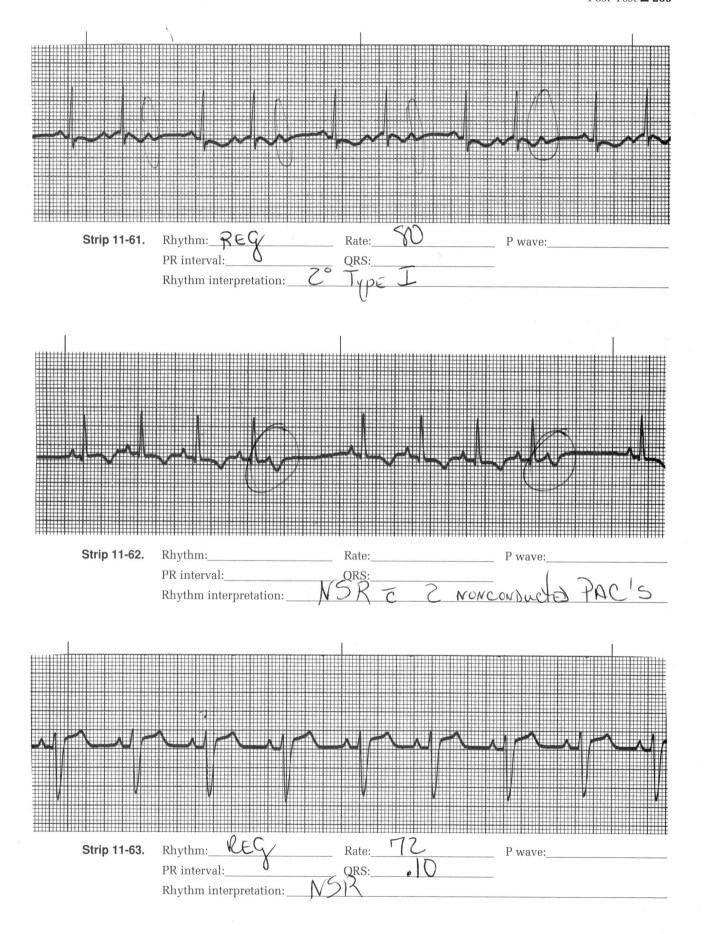

Strip 11-61. Rhythm: REG Rate: 80 P wave: _____
PR interval: _____ QRS: _____
Rhythm interpretation: 2° TYPE I

Strip 11-62. Rhythm: _____ Rate: _____ P wave: _____
PR interval: _____ QRS: _____
Rhythm interpretation: NSR c̄ 2 NONCONDUCTED PAC's

Strip 11-63. Rhythm: REG Rate: 72 P wave: _____
PR interval: _____ QRS: .10
Rhythm interpretation: NSR

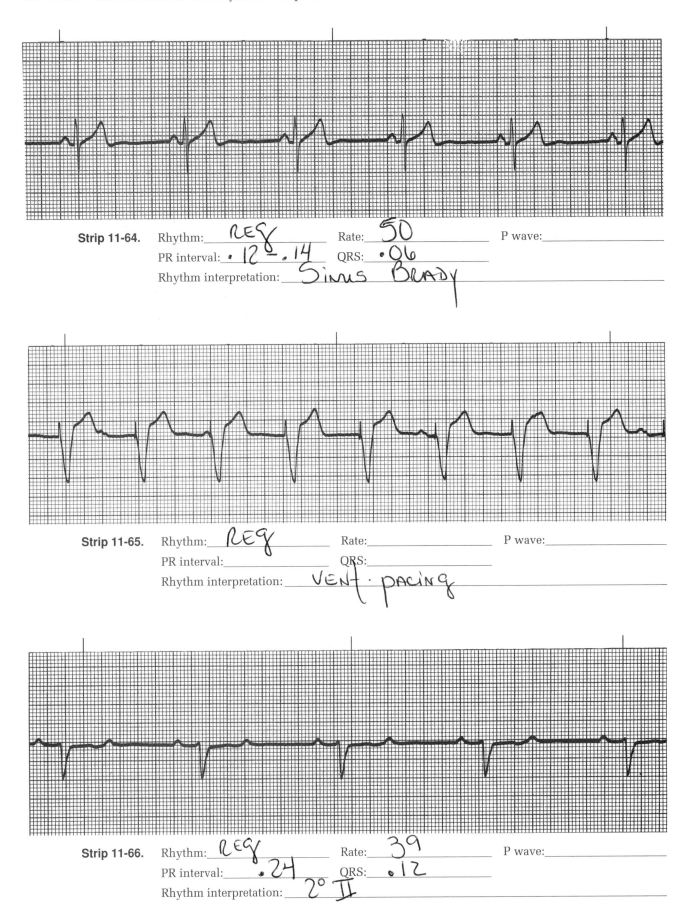

Strip 11-64. Rhythm: REG   Rate: 50   P wave: _____

PR interval: .12 - .14   QRS: .06

Rhythm interpretation: Sinus Brady

Strip 11-65. Rhythm: REG   Rate: _____   P wave: _____

PR interval: _____   QRS: _____

Rhythm interpretation: Vent. pacing

Strip 11-66. Rhythm: REG   Rate: 39   P wave: _____

PR interval: .24   QRS: .12

Rhythm interpretation: 2° II

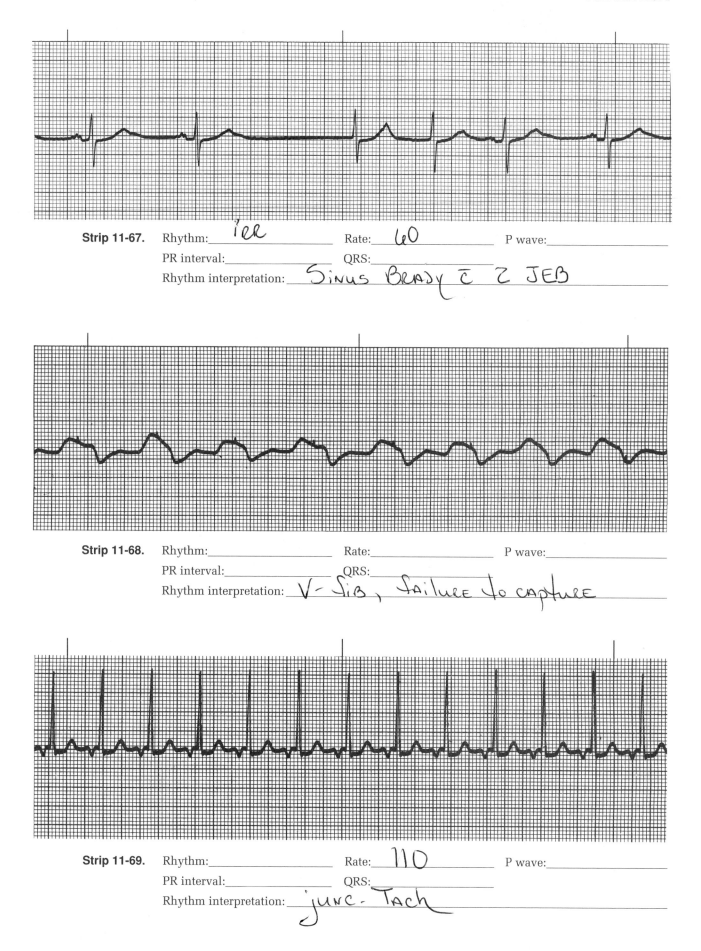

Strip 11-67. Rhythm: _irr_   Rate: _60_   P wave: _____

PR interval: _____   QRS: _____

Rhythm interpretation: _Sinus Brady c̄ 2 JEB_

Strip 11-68. Rhythm: _____   Rate: _____   P wave: _____

PR interval: _____   QRS: _____

Rhythm interpretation: _V-fib, failure to capture_

Strip 11-69. Rhythm: _____   Rate: _110_   P wave: _____

PR interval: _____   QRS: _____

Rhythm interpretation: _junc. Tach_

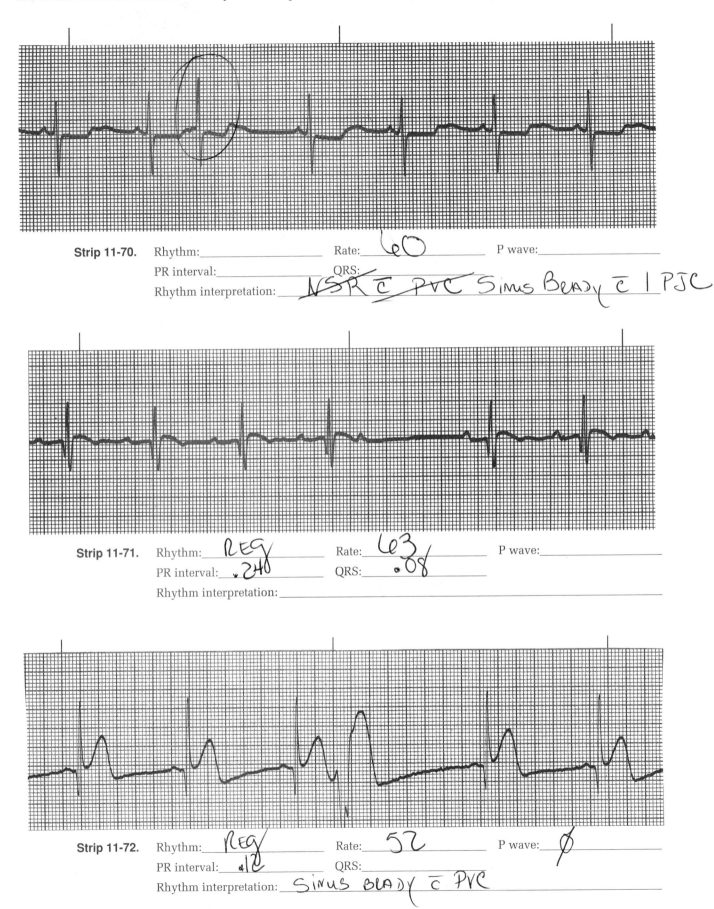

Strip 11-70. Rhythm:_____ Rate: 60 P wave:_____

PR interval:_____ QRS:_____

Rhythm interpretation: NSR c̄ PVC Sinus Brady c̄ 1 PJC

Strip 11-71. Rhythm: REG Rate: 63 P wave:_____

PR interval: .240 QRS: .08

Rhythm interpretation:_____

Strip 11-72. Rhythm: REG Rate: 52 P wave: Ø

PR interval: ∢12 QRS:_____

Rhythm interpretation: SINUS BRADY c̄ PVC

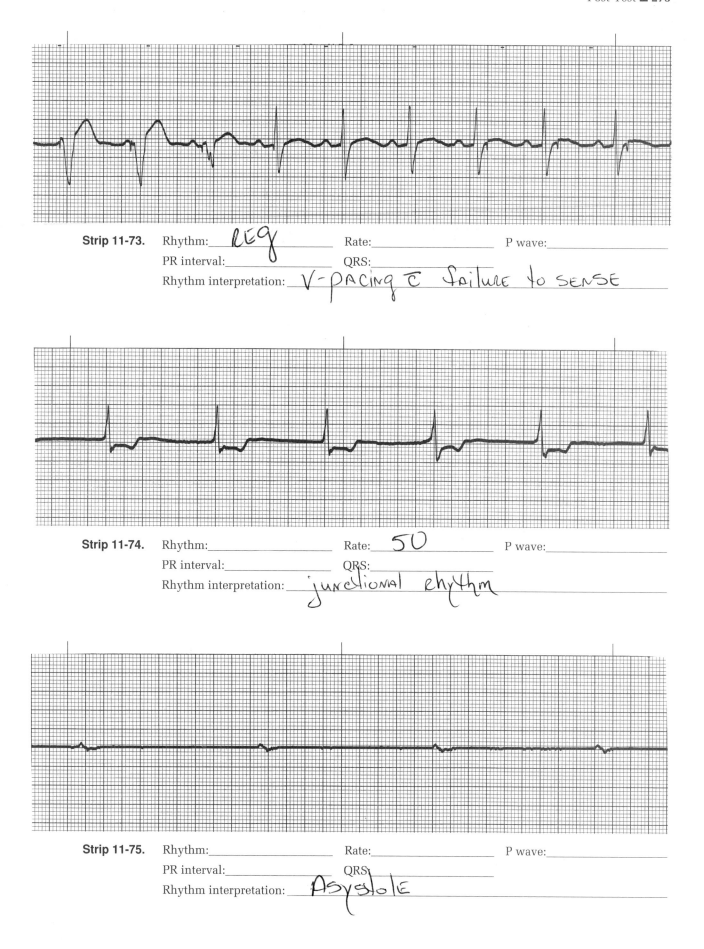

Strip 11-73. Rhythm: REg Rate:_____ P wave:_____
PR interval:_____ QRS:_____
Rhythm interpretation: V-pacing c̄ failure to sense

Strip 11-74. Rhythm:_____ Rate: 50 P wave:_____
PR interval:_____ QRS:_____
Rhythm interpretation: junctional rhythm

Strip 11-75. Rhythm:_____ Rate:_____ P wave:_____
PR interval:_____ QRS:_____
Rhythm interpretation: Asystole

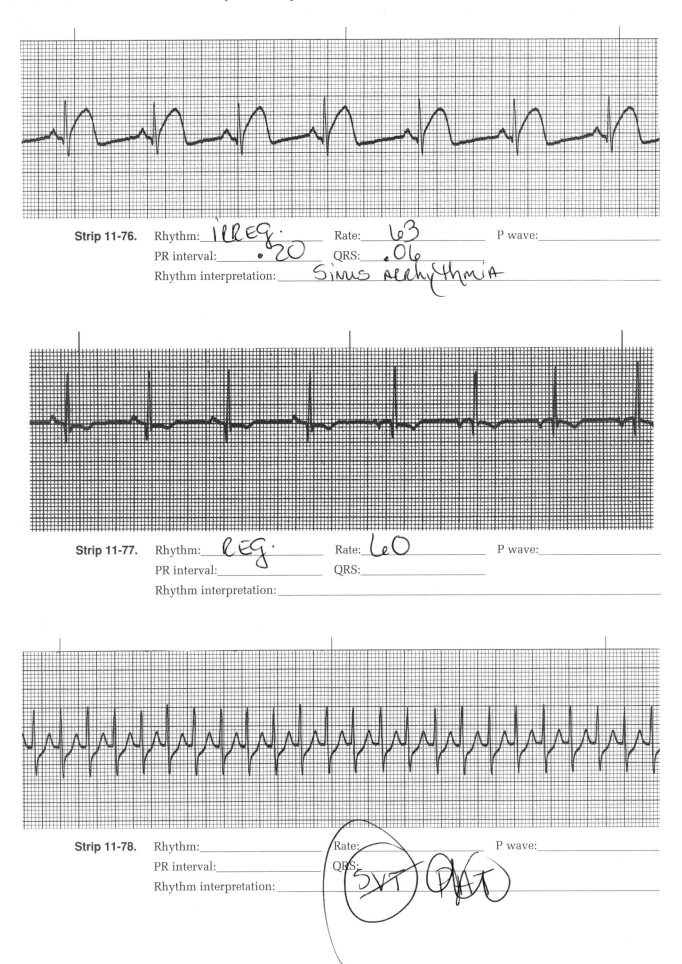

Strip 11-76. Rhythm: IRREG. Rate: 63 P wave: _____
PR interval: .20 QRS: .06
Rhythm interpretation: Sinus Arrhythmia

Strip 11-77. Rhythm: REG. Rate: 60 P wave: _____
PR interval: _____ QRS: _____
Rhythm interpretation: _____

Strip 11-78. Rhythm: _____ Rate: _____ P wave: _____
PR interval: _____ QRS: _____
Rhythm interpretation: SVT PAT

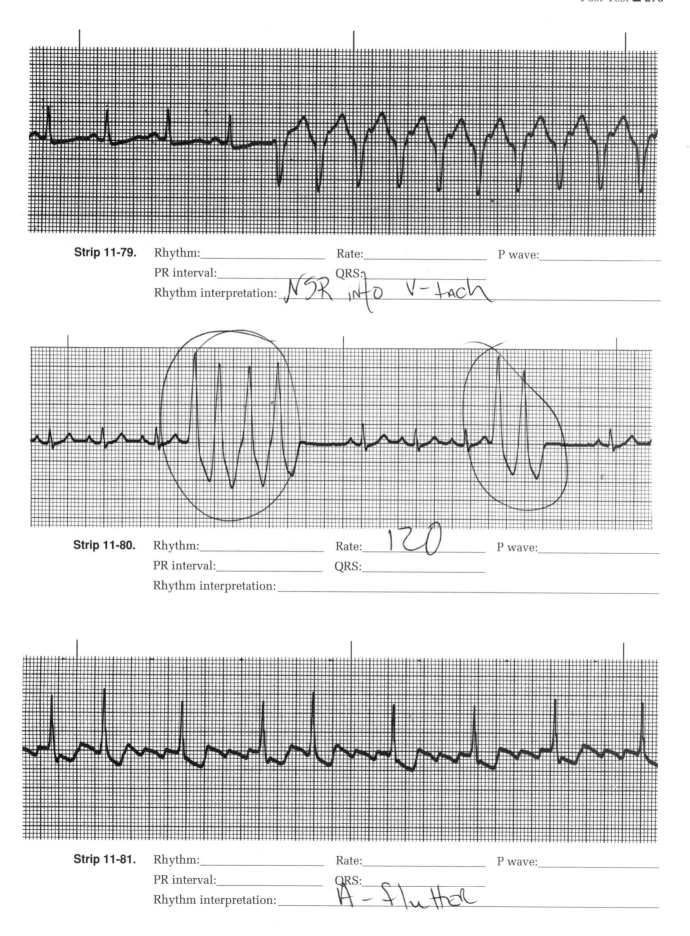

Strip 11-79. Rhythm:_____ Rate:_____ P wave:_____

PR interval:_____ QRS:_____

Rhythm interpretation: NSR into V-tach

Strip 11-80. Rhythm:_____ Rate: 120 P wave:_____

PR interval:_____ QRS:_____

Rhythm interpretation:_____

Strip 11-81. Rhythm:_____ Rate:_____ P wave:_____

PR interval:_____ QRS:_____

Rhythm interpretation: A-flutter

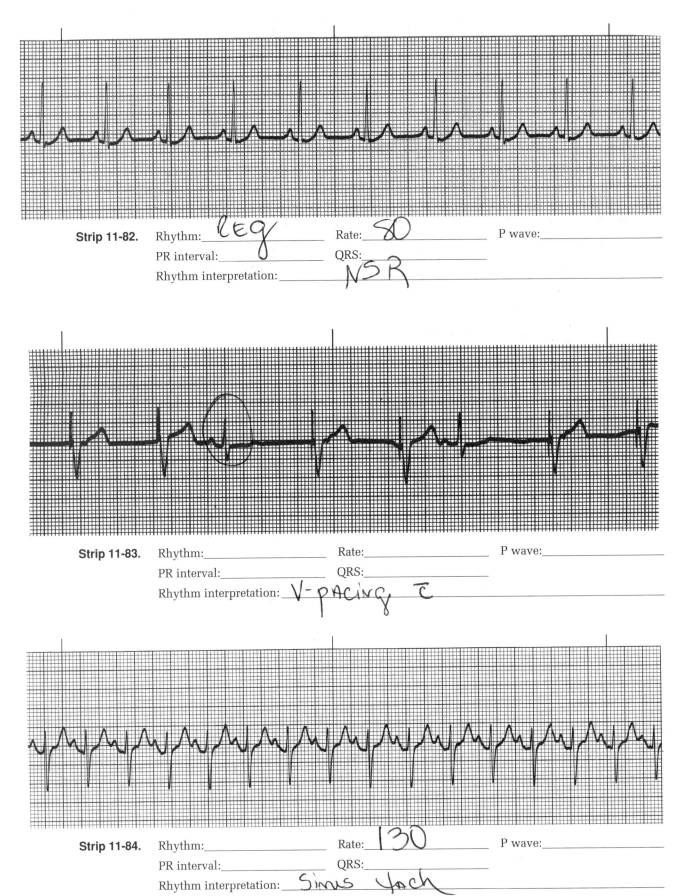

Strip 11-82. Rhythm: _REG_   Rate: _80_   P wave: _____

PR interval: _0_   QRS: _____

Rhythm interpretation: _NSR_

Strip 11-83. Rhythm: _____   Rate: _____   P wave: _____

PR interval: _____   QRS: _____

Rhythm interpretation: _V-pacing, c̄_

Strip 11-84. Rhythm: _____   Rate: _130_   P wave: _____

PR interval: _____   QRS: _____

Rhythm interpretation: _Sinus tach_

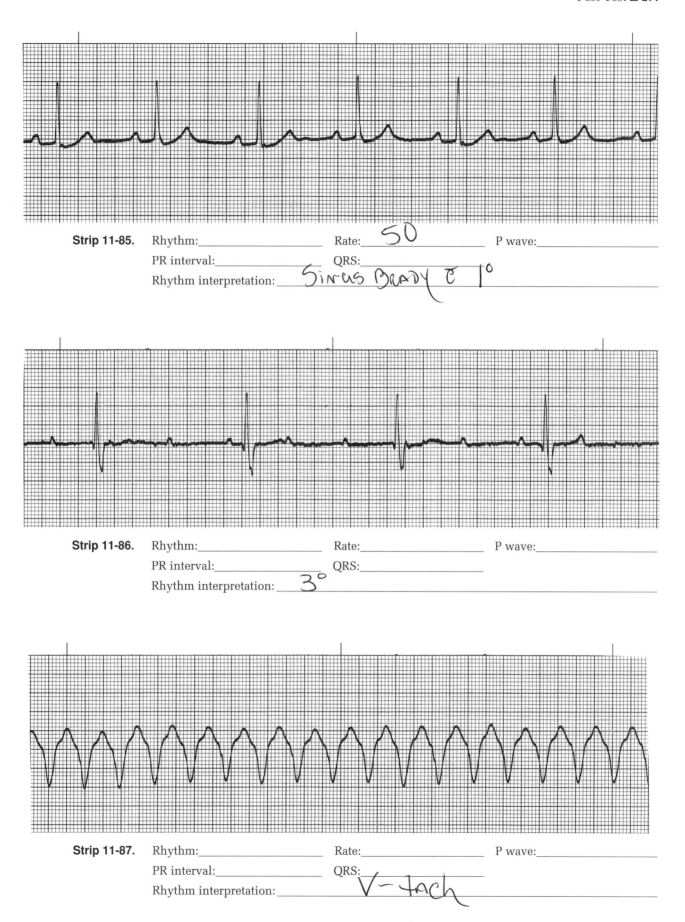

Strip 11-85. Rhythm:_____ Rate:___50___ P wave:_____

PR interval:_____ QRS:_____

Rhythm interpretation:___Sinus Brady c̄ 1°_____

Strip 11-86. Rhythm:_____ Rate:_____ P wave:_____

PR interval:_____ QRS:_____

Rhythm interpretation:___3°_____

Strip 11-87. Rhythm:_____ Rate:_____ P wave:_____

PR interval:_____ QRS:_____

Rhythm interpretation:___V-tach_____

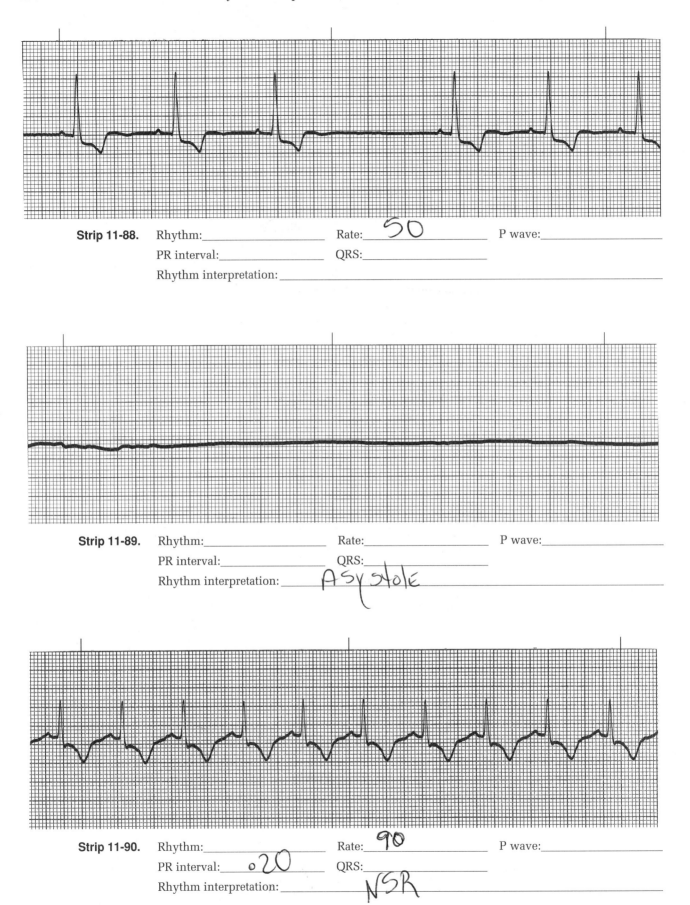

Strip 11-88. Rhythm:_____ Rate:____50____ P wave:_____

PR interval:_____ QRS:_____

Rhythm interpretation:_____

Strip 11-89. Rhythm:_____ Rate:_____ P wave:_____

PR interval:_____ QRS:_____

Rhythm interpretation:____Asystole_____

Strip 11-90. Rhythm:_____ Rate:____90____ P wave:_____

PR interval:____020____ QRS:_____

Rhythm interpretation:_____NSR_____

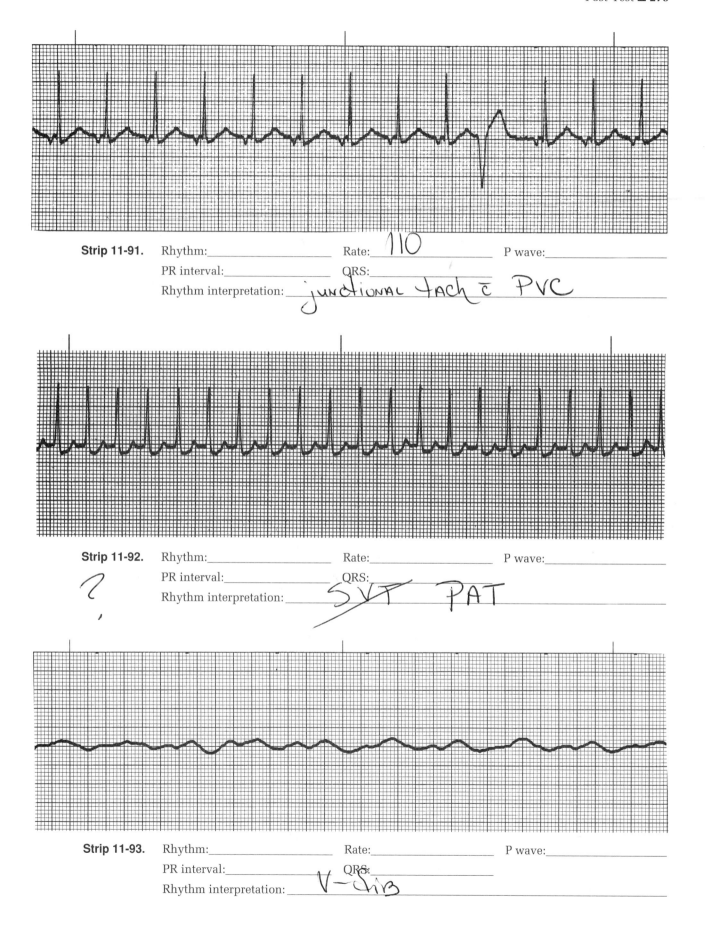

Strip 11-91. Rhythm:_____ Rate:__110__ P wave:_____

PR interval:_____ QRS:_____

Rhythm interpretation:__junctional tach c̄ PVC__

Strip 11-92. Rhythm:_____ Rate:_____ P wave:_____

PR interval:_____ QRS:_____

Rhythm interpretation:__SVT PAT__

Strip 11-93. Rhythm:_____ Rate:_____ P wave:_____

PR interval:_____ QRS:_____

Rhythm interpretation:__V-Fib__

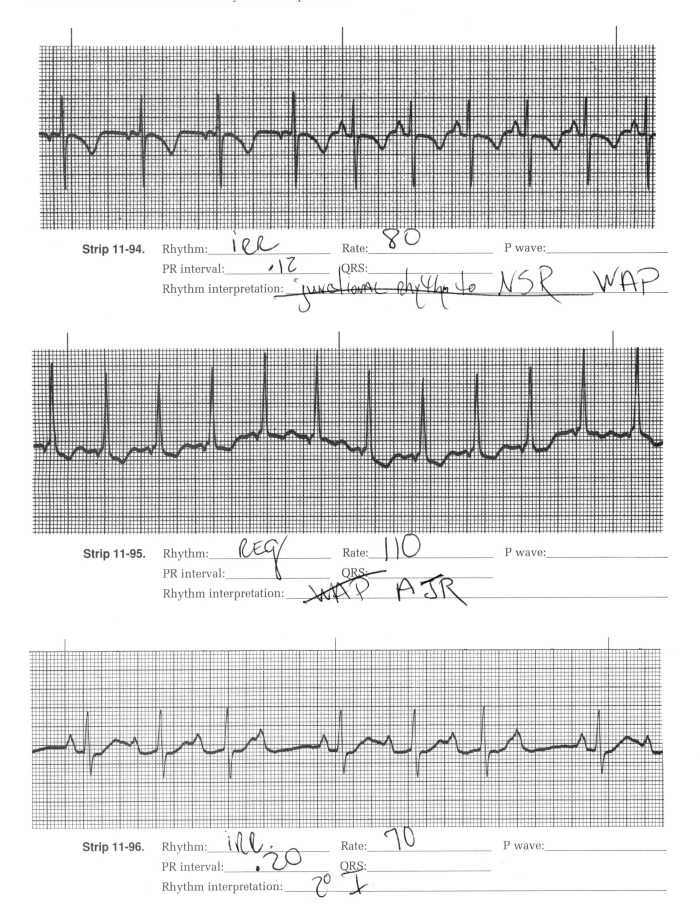

Strip 11-94. Rhythm: _irr_ Rate: _80_ P wave: _____

PR interval: _.12_ QRS: _____

Rhythm interpretation: _junctional rhythm to NSR   WAP_

Strip 11-95. Rhythm: _REG_ Rate: _110_ P wave: _____

PR interval: _____ QRS: _____

Rhythm interpretation: _WAP AJR_

Strip 11-96. Rhythm: _irr .20_ Rate: _70_ P wave: _____

PR interval: _.20_ QRS: _____

Rhythm interpretation: _2° I_

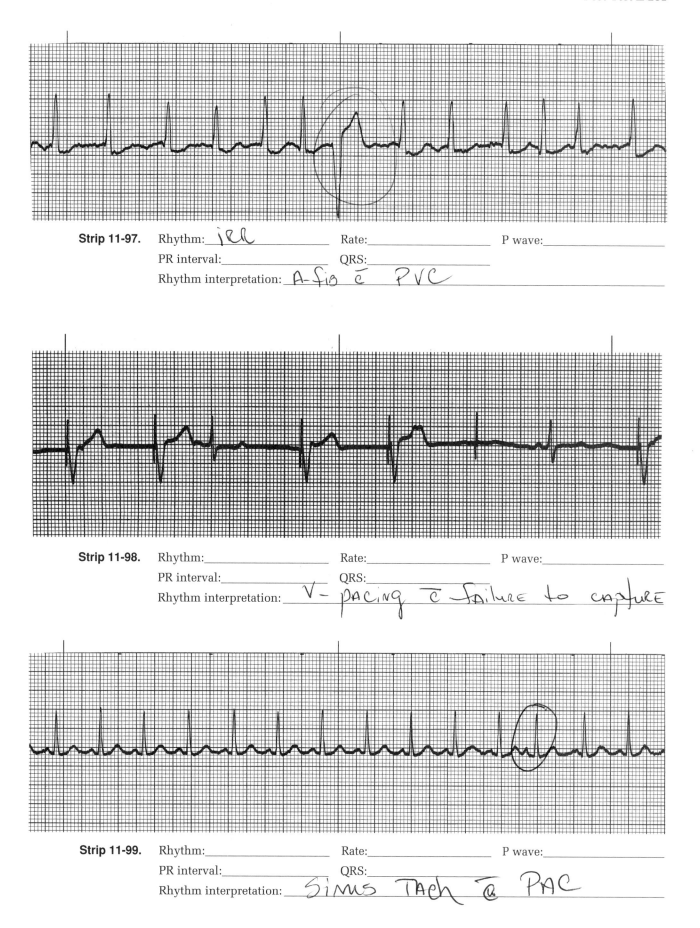

Strip 11-97. Rhythm: _jll_   Rate: _____   P wave: _____

PR interval: _____   QRS: _____

Rhythm interpretation: _A-fib c̄ PVC_

Strip 11-98. Rhythm: _____   Rate: _____   P wave: _____

PR interval: _____   QRS: _____

Rhythm interpretation: _V- pacing c̄ failure to capture_

Strip 11-99. Rhythm: _____   Rate: _____   P wave: _____

PR interval: _____   QRS: _____

Rhythm interpretation: _Sinus Tach c̄ PAC_

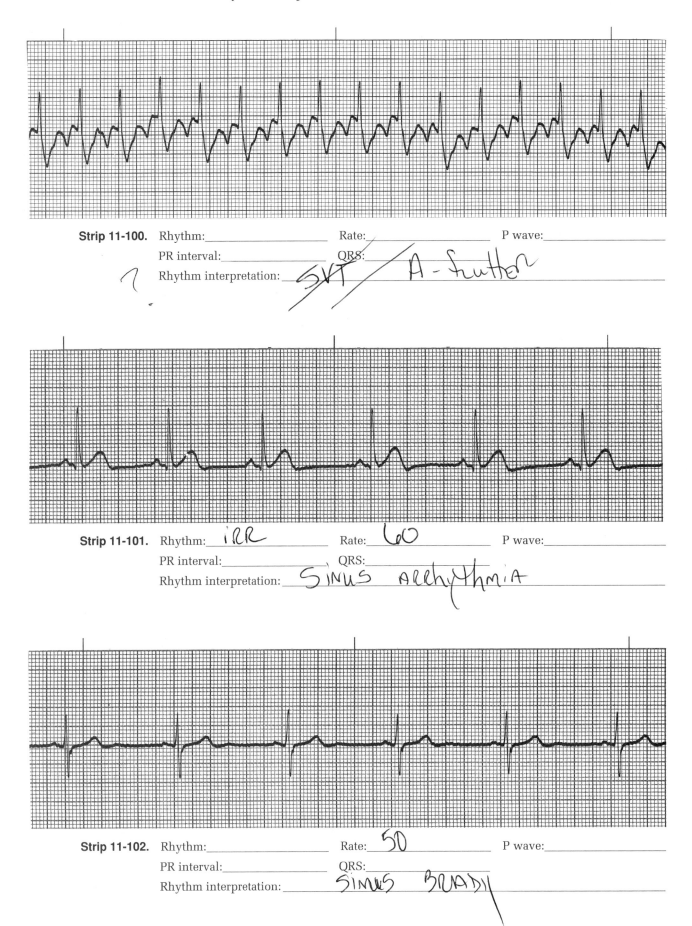

Strip 11-100. Rhythm:_____ Rate:_____ P wave:_____

PR interval:_____ QRS:_____

? Rhythm interpretation: ~~SVT~~ / A-flutter

Strip 11-101. Rhythm: iRR   Rate: 60   P wave:_____

PR interval:_____ QRS:_____

Rhythm interpretation: SINUS ARRhythmiA

Strip 11-102. Rhythm:_____ Rate: 50   P wave:_____

PR interval:_____ QRS:_____

Rhythm interpretation: SINUS BRADY

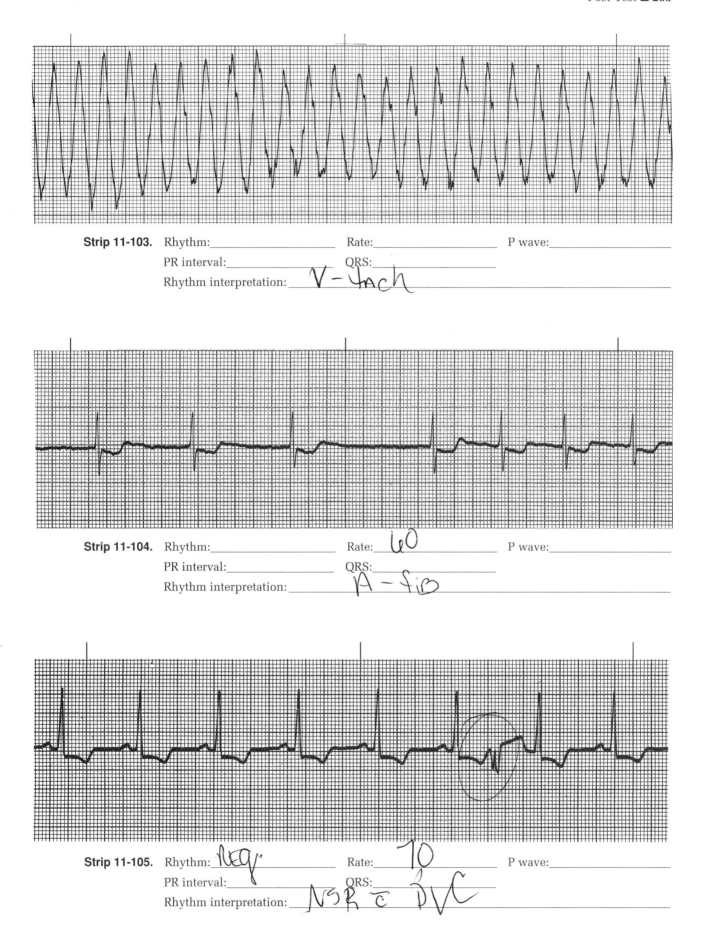

Strip 11-103. Rhythm:_____ Rate:_____ P wave:_____

PR interval:_____ QRS:_____

Rhythm interpretation: __V–Tach_____

Strip 11-104. Rhythm:_____ Rate: _60_____ P wave:_____

PR interval:_____ QRS:_____

Rhythm interpretation: _____A – fib_____

Strip 11-105. Rhythm: _Reg_____ Rate: ___70_____ P wave:_____

PR interval:_____ QRS:_____

Rhythm interpretation: __NSR c̄ PVC_____

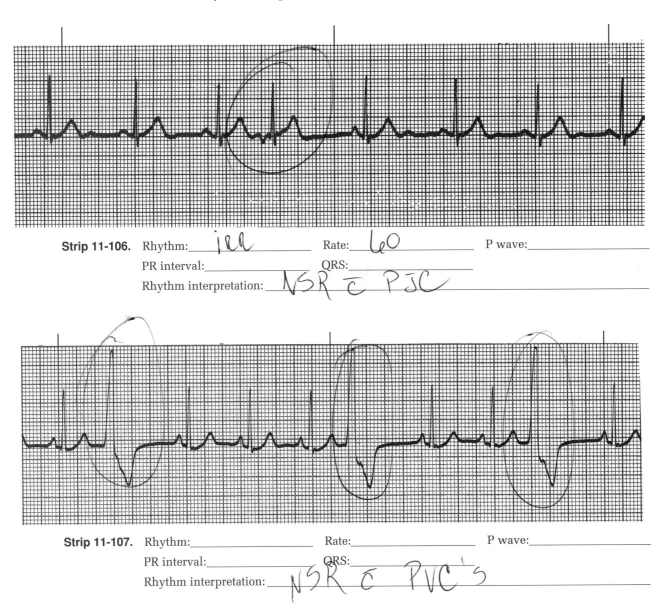

Strip 11-106. Rhythm: irr   Rate: 60   P wave:_____

PR interval:_____ QRS:_____

Rhythm interpretation: NSR c̄ PJC

Strip 11-107. Rhythm:_____ Rate:_____ P wave:_____

PR interval:_____ QRS:_____

Rhythm interpretation: NSR c̄ PVC's

Answer Keys to Chapter 3 and Chapters 5 through 11

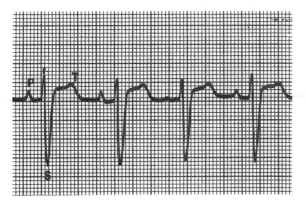

Strip 3-1.

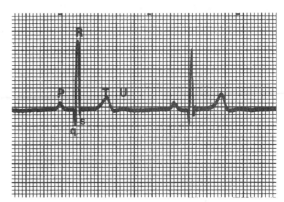

Strip 3-2.

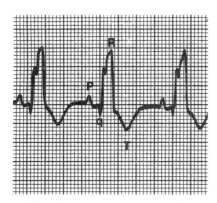

Strip 3-3.

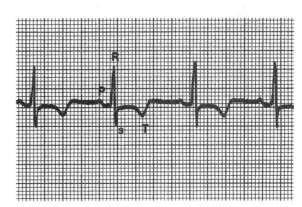

Strip 3-4.

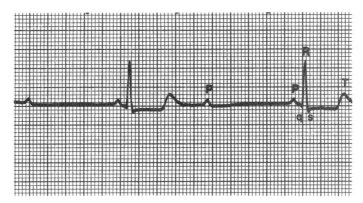

Strip 3-5.

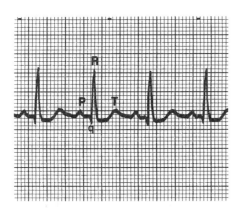

Strip 3-6.

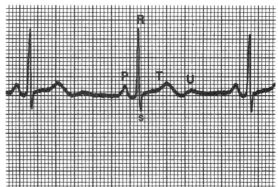

Strip 3-7.

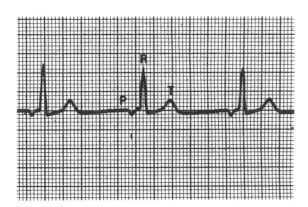

Strip 3-8.

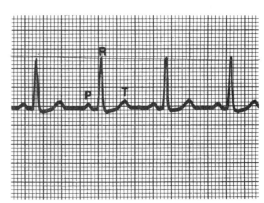

Strip 3-9.

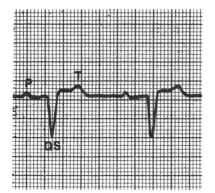

Strip 3-10.

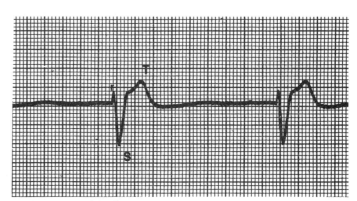

Strip 3-11.

Strip 5-1
Rhythm: Regular
Rate: 79
P waves: Sinus
PR interval: 0.14 to 0.16 seconds
QRS: 0.06 to 0.08 seconds
Comment: An inverted T wave is present

Strip 5-2
Rhythm: Regular
Rate: 45
P waves: Sinus
PR interval: 0.14 to 0.16 seconds
QRS: 0.08 seconds

Strip 5-3
Rhythm: Regular
Rate: 88
P waves: Sinus
PR interval: 0.20 seconds
QRS: 0.08–0.10 seconds
Comment: A depressed ST segment and biphasic
T wave is present

Strip 5-4
Rhythm: Irregular
Rate: 50
P waves: Sinus
PR interval: 0.16 to 0.18 seconds
QRS: 0.04 seconds

Strip 5-5
Rhythm: Regular
Rate: 50
P waves: Sinus
PR interval: 0.16–0.18 seconds
QRS: 0.06–0.08 seconds
Comment: An elevated ST segment is present

Strip 5-6
Rhythm: Regular
Rate: 136
P waves: Sinus
PR interval: 0.14 to 0.16 seconds
QRS: 0.06 to 0.08 seconds

Strip 5-7
Rhythm: Regular
Rate: 68
P waves: Sinus
PR interval: 0.16 to 0.18 seconds
QRS: 0.12 to 0.14 seconds
Comment: A U wave is present

Strip 5-8
Rhythm: Irregular
Rate: 50
P waves: Sinus
PR interval: 0.12 to 0.14 seconds
QRS: 0.06–0.08 seconds
Comment: An elevated ST segment and inverted
T wave are present

Strip 5-9
Rhythm: Regular
Rate: 94
P waves: Sinus
PR interval: 0.14 to 0.16 seconds
QRS: 0.06 to 0.08 seconds
Comment: A depressed ST segment is present

Strip 6-1
Rhythm: Regular
Rate: 44
P waves: Sinus
PR interval: 0.20 seconds
QRS: 0.10 seconds
Rhythm interpretation: Sinus bradycardia; an
elevated ST segment and U wave is present

Strip 6-2
Rhythm: Regular
Rate: 68
P waves: Sinus
PR interval: 0.16–0.18 seconds
QRS: 0.06–0.08 seconds
Rhythm interpretation: Normal sinus rhythm;
ST depression and T wave inversion is present

Strip 6-3
Rhythm: Regular
Rate: 79
P waves: Sinus
PR interval: 0.14–0.16 seconds
QRS: 0.06–0.08 seconds
Rhythm interpretation: Normal sinus rhythm

Strip 6-4
Rhythm: Regular
Rate: 107
P waves: Sinus
PR interval: 0.12–0.16 seconds
QRS: 0.06–0.08 seconds
Rhythm interpretation: Sinus tachycardia;
ST depression and T wave inversion is present

Strip 6-5
Rhythm: Regular
Rate: 58
P waves: Sinus
PR interval: 0.16–0.18 seconds
QRS: 0.06–0.08 seconds
Rhythm interpretation: Sinus bradycardia; a
U wave is present

Strip 6-6
Rhythm: Basic rhythm regular; irregular during
pause
Rate: Basic rhythm 100
P waves: Sinus in basic rhythm; absent during
pause
PR interval: 0.16 to 0.20 seconds
QRS: 0.08 to 0.10 seconds in basic rhythm
Rhythm interpretation: Normal sinus rhythm with
sinus block; ST depression and T wave inversion is
present

Strip 6-7
Rhythm: Regular
Rate: 54
P waves: Sinus (notched P waves usually indicate
left atrial hypertrophy)
PR interval: 0.14–0.16 seconds
QRS: 0.06–0.08 seconds
Rhythm interpretation: Sinus bradycardia; a
U wave is present

Strip 6-8
Rhythm: Irregular
Rate: 50
P waves: Sinus
PR interval: 0.20 seconds
QRS: 0.06–0.08 seconds
Rhythm interpretation: Sinus arrhythmia; sinus
bradycardia (can also be interpreted as sinus
arrhythmia with a bradycardic rate). A U wave is
present

Strip 6-9
Rhythm: Basic rhythm regular; irregular during
pause
Rate: Basic rhythm rate 58
P waves: Sinus in basic rhythm; absent during
pause
PR interval: 0.14–0.18 seconds basic rhythm; absent
during pause
QRS: 0.08–0.10 seconds basic rhythm; absent
during pause
Rhythm interpretation: Sinus bradycardia with
sinus arrest; a depressed ST segment and inverted T
wave is present

Strip 6-10
Rhythm: Regular
Rate: 125
P waves: Sinus
PR interval: 0.12–0.14 seconds
QRS: 0.06–0.08 seconds
Rhythm interpretation: Sinus tachycardia

Strip 6-11
Rhythm: Regular
Rate: 63
P waves: Sinus
PR interval: 0.18–0.20 seconds
QRS: 0.08 seconds
Rhythm interpretation: Normal sinus rhythm; a
U wave is present

Strip 6-12
Rhythm: Regular
Rate: 47
P waves: Sinus
PR interval: 0.18–0.20 seconds
QRS: 0.08 seconds
Rhythm interpretation: Sinus bradycardia; an
elevated ST segment is present

Strip 6-13
Rhythm: Irregular
Rate: 80
P waves: Sinus
PR interval: 0.12–0.14 seconds
QRS: 0.08 seconds
Rhythm interpretation: Sinus arrhythmia

Strip 6-14
Rhythm: Regular
Rate: 63
P waves: Sinus
PR interval: 0.18–0.20 seconds
QRS: 0.08–0.10 seconds
Rhythm interpretation: Normal sinus rhythm; ST
segment depression and T wave inversion is present

Strip 6-15
Rhythm: Basic rhythm irregular
Rate: Basic rhythm rate 60
P waves: Sinus
PR interval: 0.16 to 0.18 seconds
QRS: 0.08 to 0.10 seconds
Rhythm interpretation: Sinus arrhythmia with sinus
arrest/block; ST segment depression and T wave
inversion is present

Strip 6-16
Rhythm: Regular
Rate: 115
P waves: Sinus
PR interval: 0.16 to 0.18 seconds
QRS: 0.06 to 0.08 seconds
Rhythm interpretation: Sinus tachycardia; a
depressed ST segment and an inverted T wave is
present

Strip 6-17
Rhythm: Regular
Rate: 52
P waves: Sinus
PR interval: 0.16–0.18 seconds
QRS: 0.08–0.10 seconds
Rhythm interpretation: Sinus bradycardia

Strip 6-18
Rhythm: Irregular
Rate: 60
P waves: Sinus
PR interval: 0.16–0.18 seconds
QRS: 0.08–0.10 seconds
Rhythm interpretation: Sinus arrhythmia

Strip 6-19
Rhythm: Regular
Rate: 79
P waves: Sinus
PR interval: 0.16 to 0.20 seconds
QRS: 0.06 seconds
Rhythm interpretation: Normal sinus rhythm

Strip 6-20
Rhythm: Basic rhythm regular; irregular during
pause
Rate: Basic rhythm rate 88
P waves: Sinus in basic rhythm; absent during
pause
PR interval: 0.14 to 0.16 seconds in basic rhythm
QRS: 0.08 seconds in basic rhythm
Rhythm interpretation: Normal sinus rhythm with
sinus block; a U wave is present

Strip 6-21
Rhythm: Regular
Rate: 150
P waves: Sinus
PR interval: 0.12 seconds
QRS: 0.06 seconds
Rhythm interpretation: Sinus tachycardia

Strip 6-22
Rhythm: Regular
Rate: 60
P waves: Sinus
PR interval: 0.12 seconds
QRS: 0.08 seconds
Rhythm interpretation: Normal sinus rhythm;
T wave inversion is present

Strip 6-23
Rhythm: Irregular
Rate: 60
P waves: Sinus
PR interval: 0.16 seconds
QRS: 0.08 seconds
Rhythm interpretation: Sinus arrhythmia

Strip 6-24
Rhythm: Basic rhythm regular; irregular during
pause
Rate: Basic rhythm rate 60—rate slows to 47
following pause (temporary rate suppression can
occur following a pause in the basic rhythm)
P waves: Sinus in basic rhythm; absent during
pause
PR interval: 0.16–0.18 seconds in basic rhythm;
absent during pause
QRS: 0.06–0.08 seconds in basic rhythm; absent
during pause
Rhythm interpretation: Normal sinus rhythm with
sinus arrest

Strip 6-25
Rhythm: Regular
Rate: 125
P waves: Sinus
PR interval: 0.12–0.14 seconds
QRS: 0.04–0.06 seconds
Rhythm interpretation: Sinus tachycardia

Strip 6-26
Rhythm: Regular
Rate: 35
P waves: Sinus
PR interval: 0.14–0.16 seconds
QRS: 0.10 seconds
Rhythm interpretation: Marked sinus bradycardia

Strip 6-27

Rhythm: Basic rhythm regular; irregular during pause
Rate: Basic rhythm rate 72
P waves: Sinus in basic rhythm; absent during pause
PR interval: 0.14–0.16 seconds basic rhythm; absent during pause
QRS: 0.08–0.10 seconds basic rhythm; absent during pause
Rhythm interpretation: Normal sinus rhythm with Sinus block

Strip 6-28

Rhythm: Irregular
Rate: 60
P waves: Sinus
PR interval: 0.12–0.14 seconds
QRS: 0.10 seconds
Rhythm interpretation: Sinus arrhythmia; a U wave is present

Strip 6-29

Rhythm: Regular
Rate: 65
P waves: Sinus
PR interval: 0.20 seconds
QRS: 0.08–0.10 seconds
Rhythm interpretation: Normal sinus rhythm; ST segment depression and T wave inversion is present

Strip 6-30

Rhythm: Basic rhythm regular; irregular during pause
Rate: Basic rhythm rate 68; rate slows to 63 following pause; rate suppression can occur following a pause in the basic rhythm; after several cycles the rate returns to the basic rate
P waves: Sinus in basic rhythm; absent during pause
PR interval: 0.16 seconds in basic rhythm; absent during pause
QRS: 0.06 to 0.08 seconds in basic rhythm; absent during pause
Rhythm interpretation: Normal sinus rhythm with sinus arrest; a U wave is present

Strip 6-31

Rhythm: Regular
Rate: 56
P waves: Sinus
PR interval: 0.12 to 0.14 seconds
QRS: 0.08 to 0.10 seconds
Rhythm interpretation: Sinus bradycardia; T wave inversion is present

Strip 6-32

Rhythm: Irregular
Rate: 60
P waves: Sinus
PR interval: 0.14–0.16 seconds
QRS: 0.06–0.08 seconds
Rhythm interpretation: Sinus arrhythmia

Strip 6-33

Rhythm: Regular
Rate: 115
P waves: Sinus
PR interval: 0.16–0.18 seconds
QRS: 0.06–0.08 seconds
Rhythm interpretation: Sinus tachycardia

Strip 6-34

Rhythm: Regular
Rate: 88
P waves: Sinus
PR interval: 0.18–0.20 seconds
QRS: 0.08 seconds
Rhythm interpretation: Normal sinus rhythm; ST segment depression is present

Strip 6-35

Rhythm: Irregular
Rate: 60
P waves: Sinus
PR interval: 0.14–0.16 seconds
QRS: 0.06–0.08 seconds
Rhythm interpretation: Sinus arrhythmia

Strip 6-36

Rhythm: Regular
Rate: 41
P waves: Sinus
PR interval: 0.16–0.18 seconds
QRS: 0.06–0.08 seconds
Rhythm interpretation: Sinus bradycardia; ST segment depression is present

Strip 6-37

Rhythm: Basic rhythm regular; irregular during pause
Rate: Basic rhythm rate 88
P waves: Sinus
PR interval: 0.20 seconds
QRS: 0.06 to 0.08 seconds
Rhythm interpretation: Normal sinus rhythm with sinus arrest; ST segment depression is present

Strip 6-38
Rhythm: Regular
Rate: 107
P waves: Sinus
PR interval: 0.16–0.18 seconds
QRS: 0.06–0.08 seconds
Rhythm interpretation: Sinus tachycardia

Strip 6-39
Rhythm: Regular
Rate: 107
P waves: Sinus
PR interval: 0.16–0.18 seconds
QRS: 0.06–0.08 seconds
Rhythm interpretation: Sinus tachycardia;
ST segment elevation is present

Strip 6-40
Rhythm: Regular
Rate: 54
P waves: Sinus (notched P waves usually indicate left atrial hypertrophy)
PR interval: 0.16–0.20 seconds
QRS: 0.06–0.08 seconds
Rhythm interpretation: Sinus bradycardia

Strip 6-41
Rhythm: Regular
Rate: 94
P waves: Sinus (negative P waves are normal in lead MCL_1)
PR interval: 0.18–0.20 seconds
QRS: 0.08–0.10 seconds (negative QRS complexes are normal in lead MCL_1)
Rhythm interpretation: Normal sinus rhythm

Strip 6-42
Rhythm: Irregular
Rate: 40
P waves: Sinus
PR interval: 0.18 to 0.20 seconds
QRS: 0.06 to 0.08 seconds
Rhythm interpretation: Sinus arrhythmia with sinus bradycardia; (can also be interpreted as sinus arrhythmia with a bradycardic rate); ST segment elevation is present

Strip 6-43
Rhythm: Basic rhythm regular; irregular during pause
Rate: Basic rhythm rate 63
P waves: Sinus in basic rhythm; absent during pause
PR interval: 0.18 to 0.20 seconds in basic rhythm; absent during pause
QRS: 0.04 to 0.06 seconds in basic rhythm; absent during pause
Rhythm interpretation: Normal sinus rhythm with sinus arrest; ST segment depression is present

Strip 6-44
Rhythm: Irregular
Rate: 60
P waves: Sinus
PR interval: 0.12–0.14 seconds
QRS: 0.08–0.10 seconds
Rhythm interpretation: Sinus arrhythmia;
ST segment elevation is present

Strip 6-45
Rhythm: Regular
Rate: 27
P waves: Sinus
PR interval: 0.14 to 0.16 seconds
QRS: 0.08 to 0.10 seconds
Rhythm interpretation: Sinus bradycardia with extremely slow rate; ST segment depression is present

Strip 6-46
Rhythm: Irregular
Rate: 50
P waves: Sinus
PR interval: 0.12–0.14 seconds
QRS: 0.06–0.08 seconds
Rhythm interpretation: Sinus arrhythmia; sinus bradycardia (can also be interpreted as sinus arrhythmia with a bradycardic rate)

Strip 6-47
Rhythm: Regular
Rate: 136
P waves: Sinus
PR interval: 0.12–0.14 seconds
QRS: 0.06–0.08 seconds
Rhythm interpretation: Sinus tachycardia

Strip 6-48
Rhythm: Irregular
Rate: 70
P waves: Sinus
PR interval: 0.16 to 0.20 seconds
QRS: 0.04 to 0.06 seconds
Rhythm interpretation: Sinus arrhythmia; a U wave is present

Strip 6-49
Rhythm: Regular
Rate: 52
P waves: Sinus
PR interval: 0.12 seconds
QRS: 0.08 seconds
Rhythm interpretation: Sinus bradycardia

Strip 6-50
Rhythm: Regular
Rate: 60
P waves: Sinus
PR interval: 0.16–0.18 seconds
QRS: 0.08 seconds
Rhythm interpretation: Normal sinus rhythm; an elevated ST segment is present

Strip 6-51
Rhythm: Regular
Rate: 107
P waves: Sinus
PR interval: 0.12 to 0.14 seconds
QRS: 0.06 to 0.08 seconds
Rhythm interpretation: Sinus tachycardia

Strip 6-52
Rhythm: Basic rhythm regular; irregular during pause
Rate: Basic rhythm rate 60; rate slows to 31 following pause—temporary rate suppression is common following a pause in the basic rhythm
P waves: Sinus
PR interval: 0.16–0.20 seconds
QRS: 0.06–0.08 seconds
Rhythm interpretation: Normal sinus rhythm with sinus arrest; ST segment depression and T wave inversion is present

Strip 6-53
Rhythm: Irregular
Rate: 50
P waves: Sinus
PR interval: 0.14 to 0.16 seconds
QRS: 0.06 to 0.08 seconds
Rhythm interpretation: Sinus arrhythmia; sinus bradycardia; (can also be interpreted as Sinus arrhythmia with a bradycardic rate) a U wave is present

Strip 6-54
Rhythm: Basic rhythm regular; irregular during pause
Rate: Basic rhythm rate 94—rate slows to 54 following pause (rate suppression can occur temporarily following a pause in the basic rhythm)
P waves: Sinus in basic rhythm; absent during pause
PR interval: 0.16–0.18 seconds in basic rhythm; absent during pause
QRS: 0.08–0.10 seconds
Rhythm interpretation: Normal sinus rhythm with sinus block

Strip 6-55
Rhythm: Regular
Rate: 65
P waves: Sinus
PR interval: 0.16–0.18 seconds
QRS: 0.06 seconds
Rhythm interpretation: Normal sinus rhythm

Strip 6-56
Rhythm: Regular
Rate: 125
P waves: Sinus
PR interval: 0.16 seconds
QRS: 0.08 seconds
Rhythm interpretation: Sinus tachycardia; ST segment depression is present

Strip 6-57
Rhythm: Irregular
Rate: 40
P waves: Sinus
PR interval: 0.16–0.18 seconds
QRS: 0.08 seconds
Rhythm interpretation: Sinus arrhythmia/sinus bradycardia (can also be interpreted as sinus arrhythmia with a bradycardic rate) a U wave is present

Strip 6-58
Rhythm: Regular
Rate: 72
P waves: Sinus
PR interval: 0.16 to 0.20 seconds
QRS: 0.06 to 0.08 seconds
Rhythm interpretation: Normal sinus rhythm;
ST segment depression and T wave inversion are
present

Strip 6-59
Rhythm: Regular
Rate: 50
P waves: Sinus
PR interval: 0.20 seconds
QRS: 0.06 to 0.08 seconds
Rhythm interpretation: Sinus bradycardia; ST
segment depression and T wave inversion are
present

Strip 6-60
Rhythm: Basic rhythm regular; irregular during
pause
Rate: Basic rhythm rate 88
P waves: Sinus in basic rhythm; absent during
pause
PR interval: 0.14 to 0.20 seconds in basic rhythm;
absent during pause
QRS: 0.08 to 0.10 seconds in basic rhythm; absent
during pause
Rhythm interpretation: Normal sinus rhythm with
sinus block; ST segment depression is present

Strip 6-61
Rhythm: Regular
Rate: 72
P waves: Sinus
PR interval: 0.12–0.14 seconds
QRS: 0.06–0.08 seconds
Rhythm interpretation: Normal sinus rhythm; an
inverted T wave is present

Strip 6-62
Rhythm: Regular
Rate: 125
P waves: Sinus
PR interval: 0.12 seconds
QRS: 0.04 seconds
Rhythm interpretation: Sinus tachycardia;
ST segment depression is present

Strip 6-63
Rhythm: Regular
Rate: 44
P waves: Sinus
PR interval: 0.18–0.20 seconds
QRS: 0.06–0.08 seconds
Rhythm interpretation: Sinus bradycardia; a
U wave is present

Strip 6-64
Rhythm: Regular
Rate: 79
P waves: Sinus
PR interval: 0.14 to 0.16 seconds
QRS: 0.04 to 0.06 seconds
Rhythm interpretation: Normal sinus rhythm;
T wave inversion is present

Strip 6-65
Rhythm: Regular
Rate: 107
P waves: Sinus
PR interval: 0.18–0.20 seconds
QRS: 0.08–0.10 seconds
Rhythm interpretation: Sinus tachycardia;
an elevated ST segment is present

Strip 6-66
Rhythm: Regular
Rate: 100
P waves: Sinus
PR interval: 0.20 seconds
QRS: 0.08 seconds
Rhythm interpretation: Normal sinus rhythm;
an extremely elevated ST segment is present

Strip 6-67
Rhythm: Regular
Rate: 44
P waves: Sinus
PR interval: 0.14 to 0.16 seconds
QRS: 0.08 seconds
Rhythm interpretation: Sinus bradycardia; a U wave
is present

Strip 6-68
Rhythm: Regular
Rate: 88
P waves: Sinus
PR interval: 0.18–0.20 seconds
QRS: 0.06–0.08 seconds
Rhythm interpretation: Normal sinus rhythm
A depressed ST segment is present

Strip 6-69
Rhythm: Regular
Rate: 136
P waves: Sinus
PR interval: 0.14–0.16 seconds
QRS: 0.08 seconds
Rhythm interpretation: Sinus tachycardia; an
elevated ST segment is present

Strip 6-70
Rhythm: Basic rhythm regular; irregular during
pause
Rate: Basic rhythm rate 56; rate slows to 50 after
pause; rate suppression can occur following a pause
in the basic rhythm; after several cycles the rate
returns to the basic rate
P waves: Sinus in basic rhythm; absent during
pause
PR interval: 0.14 to 0.16 in basic rhythm; absent
during pause
QRS: 0.08 to 0.10 seconds in basic rhythm; absent
during pause
Rhythm interpretation: Sinus bradycardia with
sinus arrest

Strip 6-71
Rhythm: Regular
Rate: 115
P waves: Sinus
PR interval: 0.14–0.16 seconds
QRS: 0.08–0.10 seconds
Rhythm interpretation: Sinus tachycardia;
ST segment depression is present

Strip 6-72
Rhythm: Regular
Rate: 79
P waves: Sinus
PR interval: 0.14–0.16 seconds
QRS: 0.06–0.08 seconds
Rhythm interpretation: Normal sinus rhythm; a
depressed ST segment and a biphasic T wave is
present

Strip 6-73
Rhythm: Regular
Rate: 54
P waves: Sinus
PR interval: 0.14–0.16 seconds
QRS: 0.06–0.08 seconds
Rhythm interpretation: Sinus bradycardia; an
elevated ST segment is present

Strip 6-74
Rhythm: Regular
Rate: 94
P waves: Sinus
PR interval: 0.16 seconds
QRS: 0.08–0.10 seconds
Rhythm interpretation: Normal sinus rhythm;
ST segment depression and a biphasic T wave is
present

Strip 6-75
Rhythm: Regular
Rate: 94
P waves: Sinus
PR interval: 0.16 to 0.20 seconds
QRS: 0.06 to 0.08 seconds
Rhythm interpretation: Normal sinus rhythm

Strip 6-76
Rhythm: Regular
Rate: 125
P waves: Sinus
PR interval: 0.12 seconds
QRS: 0.06 to 0.08 seconds
Rhythm interpretation: Sinus tachycardia

Strip 6-77
Rhythm: Regular
Rate: 79
P waves: Sinus
PR interval: 0.18–0.20 seconds
QRS: 0.06–0.08 seconds
Rhythm interpretation: Normal sinus rhythm; an
elevated ST segment is present

Strip 6-78
Rhythm: Regular
Rate: 58
P waves: Sinus
PR interval: 0.16–0.18 seconds
QRS: 0.06–0.08 seconds
Rhythm interpretation: Sinus bradycardia; an
elevated ST segment and a U wave are present

Strip 6-79
Rhythm: Basic rhythm regular; irregular during pause
Rate: Basic rhythm rate 107—rate slows to 94 for 1 cycle following pause (temporary rate suppression can occur following a pause in the basic rhythm)
P waves: Sinus in basic rhythm; absent during pause
PR interval: 0.16–0.20 seconds in basic rhythm; absent during pause
QRS: 0.10 seconds in basic rhythm; absent during pause
Rhythm interpretation: Sinus tachycardia with sinus block; baseline artifact is present

Strip 6-80
Rhythm: Regular
Rate: 84
P waves: Sinus
PR interval: 0.16 seconds
QRS: 0.06 seconds
Rhythm interpretation: Normal sinus rhythm; T wave inversion is present

Strip 6-81
Rhythm: Regular
Rate: 56
P waves: Sinus
PR interval: 0.16–0.18 seconds
QRS: 0.06–0.08 seconds
Rhythm interpretation: Sinus bradycardia; T wave inversion is present

Strip 6-82
Rhythm: Regular
Rate: 125
P waves: Sinus
PR interval: 0.16–0.18 seconds
QRS: 0.04–0.06 seconds
Rhythm interpretation: Sinus tachycardia

Strip 6-83
Rhythm: Basic rhythm irregular
Rate: Basic rhythm rate 60
P waves: Sinus
PR interval: 0.20 seconds in basic rhythm; absent during pause
QRS: 0.06 to 0.08 seconds in basic rhythm; absent during pause
Rhythm interpretation: Sinus arrhythmia with sinus arrest/block; ST segment depression is present

Strip 6-84
Rhythm: Regular
Rate: 79
P waves: Sinus
PR interval: 0.12 seconds
QRS: 0.06–0.08 seconds
Rhythm interpretation: Normal sinus rhythm; an elevated ST segment is present

Strip 6-85
Rhythm: Regular
Rate: 136
P waves: Sinus
PR interval: 0.14–0.16 seconds
QRS: 0.06–0.08 seconds
Rhythm interpretation: Sinus tachycardia

Strip 6-86
Rhythm: Regular
Rate: 54
P waves: Sinus
PR interval: 0.16 seconds
QRS: 0.06–0.08 seconds
Rhythm interpretation: Sinus bradycardia

Strip 6-87
Rhythm: Basic rhythm regular; irregular during pause
Rate: Basic rhythm rate 84; rate slows to 75 for one cycle following the pause—rate suppression is common following pauses in the basic rhythm
P waves: Sinus in basic rhythm; absent during pause
PR interval: 0.16 to 0.18 seconds in basic rhythm; absent during pause
QRS: 0.06 to 0.08 seconds in basic rhythm; absent during pause
Rhythm interpretation: Normal sinus rhythm with sinus arrest

Strip 6-88
Rhythm: Regular
Rate: 100
P waves: Sinus
PR interval: 0.12–0.14 seconds
QRS: 0.08–0.10 seconds
Rhythm interpretation: Normal sinus rhythm; an elevated ST segment is present

Strip 6-89
Rhythm: Regular
Rate: 54
P waves: Sinus
PR interval: 0.18–0.20 seconds
QRS: 0.06–0.08 seconds
Rhythm interpretation: Sinus bradycardia; an elevated ST segment and T wave inversion is present

Strip 6-90
Rhythm: Basic rhythm regular; irregular during pause
Rate: Basic rhythm rate 72- rate slows to 68 for two cycles following pause (temporary rate suppression can occur following a pause in the basic rhythm)
P waves: Sinus in basic rhythm; absent during pause
PR interval: 0.12–0.14 seconds in basic rhythm; absent during pause
QRS: 0.06–0.08 seconds in basic rhythm; absent during pause
Rhythm interpretation: Normal sinus rhythm with sinus arrest; T wave inversion is present

Strip 6-91
Rhythm: Regular
Rate: 65
P waves: Sinus
PR interval: 0.14–0.16 seconds
QRS: 0.06–0.08 seconds
Rhythm interpretation: Normal sinus rhythm; a U wave is present

Strip 6-92
Rhythm: Regular
Rate: 63
P waves: Sinus
PR interval: 0.18–0.20 seconds
QRS: 0.08–0.10 seconds
Rhythm interpretation: Normal sinus rhythm; ST segment depression and T wave inversion is present

Strip 6-93
Rhythm: Basic rhythm regular; irregular during pause
Rate: Basic rhythm rate 79- rate slows to 72 following pause (temporary rate suppression can occur following a pause in the basic rhythm).
P waves: Sinus in basic rhythm; absent during pause
PR interval: 0.20 seconds in basic rhythm; absent during pause
QRS: 0.08–0.10 seconds in basic rhythm; absent during pause
Rhythm interpretation: Normal sinus rhythm with sinus arrest; ST segment depression and T wave inversion is present

Strip 6-94
Rhythm: Regular
Rate: 150
P waves: Sinus
PR interval: 0.12 seconds
QRS: 0.04 to 0.06 seconds
Rhythm interpretation: Sinus tachycardia

Strip 6-95
Rhythm: Regular
Rate: 136
P waves: Sinus
PR interval: 0.12 seconds
QRS: 0.06–0.08 seconds
Rhythm interpretation: Sinus tachycardia

Strip 7-1
Rhythm: Irregular
Rate: Ventricular rate 60; atrial rate not measurable
P waves: fibrillation waves present
PR interval: not measurable
QRS: 0.06–0.08 seconds
Rhythm interpretation: Atrial fibrillation; ST segment depression is present

Strip 7-2
Rhythm: Regular
Rate: 188
P waves: Hidden in T waves
PR interval: Not measurable
QRS: 0.06–0.08 seconds
Rhythm interpretation: Paroxysmal atrial tachycardia

Strip 7-3

Rhythm: Basic rhythm regular; irregular with PACs
Rate: Basic rhythm rate 94
P waves: Sinus P waves with basic rhythm; Premature, abnormal P waves with PACs
PR interval: 0.12 seconds (basic rhythm) 0.14 seconds (PACs)
QRS: 0.08–0.10 seconds (basic rhythm and PACs)
Rhythm interpretation: Normal sinus rhythm with 2 PACs (4th and 8th complex) ST segment depression is present

Strip 7-4

Rhythm: Irregular
Rate: 100
P waves: Vary in size, shape, position
PR interval: 0.12 seconds
QRS: 0.06 to 0.08 seconds
Rhythm interpretation: Wandering atrial pacemaker

Strip 7-5

Rhythm: Basic rhythm regular; irregular with PAC
Rate: Basic rhythm rate 125
P waves: Sinus P waves with basic rhythm; premature, pointed P wave with PAC
PR interval: 0.12 seconds (basic rhythm)
QRS: 0.04–0.06 seconds (basic rhythm)
Rhythm interpretation: Sinus tachycardia with one PAC (8th complex)

Strip 7-6

Rhythm: Regular
Rate: 167
P waves: Pointed, abnormal
PR interval: 0.14 to 0.16 seconds
QRS: 0.06 to 0.08 seconds
Rhythm interpretation: Paroxysmal atrial tachycardia; ST segment depression is present

Strip 7-7

Rhythm: Basic rhythm regular; irregular with nonconducted PAC
Rate: Basic rhythm rate 88
P waves: Sinus P waves with basic rhythm; premature, abnormal P wave with nonconducted PAC
PR interval: 0.16 seconds
QRS: 0.06 to 0.08 seconds
Rhythm interpretation: Normal sinus rhythm with nonconducted PAC (following 7th QRS) ST segment depression is present

Strip 7-8

Rhythm: Irregular
Rate: Atrial, 320; ventricular, 80
P waves: Flutter waves are present (varying ratios)
PR interval: Not measurable
QRS: 0.06–0.08 seconds
Rhythm interpretation: Atrial flutter with variable block

Strip 7-9

Rhythm: Irregular
Rate: 50
P waves: Changing morphology across strip (1st three P waves are upright; last three P waves are inverted)
PR interval: 0.18–0.20 seconds (1st three PR intervals) 0.12 seconds (last three PR intervals)
QRS: 0.08–0.10 seconds
Rhythm interpretation: Wandering atrial pacemaker with bradycardic rate

Strip 7-10

Rhythm: Irregular
Rate: Ventricular rate 60; Atrial rate not measurable
P waves: fibrillatory waves are present
PR interval: not measurable
QRS: 0.04–0.06 seconds
Rhythm interpretation: Atrial fibrillation

Strip 7-11

Rhythm: Basic rhythm regular; irregular with PAC
Rate: Basic rate 72
P waves: Sinus with basic rhythm; premature, pointed with PAC
PR interval: 0.18–0.20 seconds (basic rhythm)
QRS: 0.06–0.08 seconds (basic rhythm)
Rhythm interpretation: Normal sinus rhythm with 1 PAC (6th complex)

Strip 7-12

Rhythm: Regular
Rate: Atrial: 237 Ventricular: 79
P waves: 3 flutter waves to each QRS
PR interval: not necessary to measure
QRS: 0.04 seconds
Rhythm interpretation: Atrial flutter with 3:1 AV conduction

Strip 7-13

Rhythm: Basic rhythm regular; irregular with PAC
Rate: Basic rate 107
P waves: Sinus with basic rhythm; premature, pointed P wave without QRS complex follows 5th QRS
PR interval: 0.18–0.20 seconds
QRS: 0.04–0.06 seconds
Rhythm interpretation: Sinus tachycardia with 1 non-conducted PAC (following 5th QRS)

Strip 7-14

Rhythm: Irregular
Rate: Ventricular rate 110; Atrial rate not measurable
P waves: Fibrillatory waves are present
PR interval: Not measurable
QRS: 0.06 to 0.08 seconds
Rhythm interpretation: Atrial fibrillation; some flutter waves are noted

Strip 7-15

Rhythm: First rhythm regular; second rhythm regular
Rate: 167 first rhythm; 100 second rhythm
P waves: Obscured in T waves in first rhythm; sinus P waves in second rhythm
PR interval: Not measurable in first rhythm; 0.16–0.18 seconds in second rhythm
QRS: 0.08 seconds (both rhythms)
Rhythm interpretation: Paroxysmal atrial tachycardia converting to normal sinus rhythm

Strip 7-16

Rhythm: Regular
Rate: Atrial, 300; ventricular, 100
P waves: Three flutter waves before each QRS
PR interval: Not measurable
QRS: 0.08 seconds
Rhythm interpretation: Atrial flutter with 3:1 AV conduction

Strip 7-17

Rhythm: Irregular
Rate: 40
P waves: Fibrillatory waves
PR interval: Not measurable
QRS: 0.08 seconds
Rhythm interpretation: Atrial fibrillation

Strip 7-18

Rhythm: Irregular
Rate: Atrial, 320; ventricular, 90
P waves: Flutter waves (varying ratios)
PR interval: Not discernible
QRS: 0.04 to 0.06 seconds
Rhythm interpretation: Atrial flutter with variable AV conduction

Strip 7-19

Rhythm: Basic rhythm regular; irregular following nonconducted PACs
Rate: 79 in basic rhythm
P waves: Vary in morphology across strip; P wave following 5th and 8th QRS is premature, abnormal without associated QRS
PR interval: 0.18–0.22 seconds
QRS: 0.06–0.08 seconds
Rhythm interpretation: Wandering atrial pacemaker with 2 nonconducted PACs (following 5th and 8th QRS)

Strip 7-20

Rhythm: 1st rhythm regular; not enough complexes to measure 2nd rhythm
Rate: 1st rhythm: 136, 2nd rhythm: 58
P waves: 1st rhythm: obscured; 2nd rhythm: sinus
PR interval: 1st rhythm: not measurable; 2nd rhythm: 0.16 seconds
QRS: 0.08 seconds both rhythms
Rhythm interpretation: Paroxysmal atrial tachycardia converting to sinus bradycardia (9th complex is an atrial escape beat)

Strip 7-21

Rhythm: Basic rhythm regular; irregular with nonconducted PAC
Rate: Basic rhythm 75—rate slows to 72 for 2 cycles following pause; temporary rate suppression is common following a pause in the underlying rhythm
P waves: Sinus in basic rhythm; premature, pointed P wave without QRS complex follows 3rd QRS
PR interval: 0.16 seconds
QRS: 0.08 seconds
Rhythm interpretation: Normal sinus rhythm with one non-conducted PAC (following 3rd QRS); a U wave is present

Strip 7-22
Rhythm: Regular
Rate: Atrial: 290 Ventricular: 58
P waves: 5 flutter waves to each QRS
PR interval: Not measurable
QRS: 0.06–0.08 seconds
Rhythm interpretation: Atrial flutter with 5:1
AV conduction

Strip 7-23
Rhythm: Basic rhythm regular; irregular with pause
Rate: Basic rhythm rate 79
P waves: Sinus with basic rhythm; premature abnormal P wave without QRS follows 4th QRS
PR interval: 0.16–0.18 seconds basic rhythm
QRS: 0.06–0.08 seconds basic rhythm
Rhythm interpretation: Normal sinus rhythm with 1 nonconducted PAC (follows 4th QRS) ST segment depression and T wave inversion is present

Strip 7-24
Rhythm: Irregular
Rate: Ventricular rate: 170; atrial rate not measurable
P waves: Fibrillatory waves present
PR interval: Not measurable
QRS: 0.06–0.08 seconds
Rhythm interpretation: Atrial fibrillation

Strip 7-25
Rhythm: Regular
Rate: 84
P waves: Vary in size, shape, and position
PR interval: 0.12 to 0.14 seconds
QRS: 0.06 to 0.08 seconds
Rhythm interpretation: Wandering atrial pacemaker; T wave inversion is present

Strip 7-26
Rhythm: Basic rhythm regular; irregular with PACs
Rate: Basic rhythm rate 68
P waves: Sinus with basic rhythm; premature, inverted P wave with PAC
PR interval: 0.12–0.14 seconds (basic rhythm); 0.12 seconds (PAC)
QRS: 0.06–0.08 seconds (basic rhythm); 0.08 seconds (PAC)
Rhythm interpretation: Normal sinus rhythm with 1 PAC (4th complex) a U wave is present

Strip 7-27
Rhythm: Regular
Rate: Atrial: 232 Ventricular: 58
P waves: 4 flutter waves to each QRS
PR interval: Not measurable
QRS: 0.06–0.08 seconds
Rhythm interpretation: Atrial flutter with 4:1
AV conduction

Strip 7-28
Rhythm: Basic rhythm regular; irregular with PACs
Rate: Basic rhythm 42
P waves: Sinus P waves with basic rhythm; premature, abnormal P waves with PACs
PR interval: 0.12 to 0.14 seconds (basic rhythm); 0.16 seconds (PACs)
QRS: 0.08 to 0.10 seconds
Rhythm interpretation: Sinus bradycardia with four PACs (2nd, 4th, 7th and 9th complexes)

Strip 7-29
Rhythm: Regular
Rate: 150
P waves: Obscured in preceding T wave
PR interval: Not measurable
QRS: 0.08 seconds
Rhythm interpretation: Paroxysmal atrial tachycardia

Strip 7-30
Rhythm: Regular
Rate: Atrial: 272 Ventricular: 136
P waves: 2 flutter waves to each QRS
PR interval: Not measurable
QRS: 0.06 seconds
Rhythm interpretation: Atrial flutter with 2:1
AV conduction

Strip 7-31
Rhythm: Basic rhythm regular; irregular with PACs and atrial fibrillation
Rate: Basic rhythm rate 68; Atrial fibrillation rate 140
P waves: Sinus P waves are present with basic rhythm; premature, abnormal P waves with PACs; fibrillation waves with atrial fibrillation
PR interval: 0.12 to 0.14 seconds (basic rhythm)
QRS: 0.08 to 0.10 seconds
Rhythm interpretation: Normal sinus rhythm with two PACs, (2nd and 5th complex); last PAC initiates atrial fibrillation; ST segment depression is present

Strip 7-32

Rhythm: Basic rhythm regular; irregular with nonconducted PAC

Rate: Basic rate 94—rate slows to 84 for one cycle following pause (temporary rate suppression can occur following a pause in the basic rhythm)

P waves: Sinus P waves in basic rhythm; premature, abnormal P wave without a QRS is hidden in T wave following 7th QRS complex

PR interval: 0.16–0.18 seconds

QRS: 0.06–0.08 seconds

Rhythm interpretation: Normal sinus rhythm with one nonconducted PAC (following 7th QRS)

Strip 7-33

Rhythm: Basic rhythm regular; irregular with PAC

Rate: Basic rhythm rate 47

P waves: Sinus with basic rhythm; premature, pointed P wave associated with PAC

PR interval: 0.18–0.20 seconds

QRS: 0.08 seconds

Rhythm interpretation: Sinus bradycardia with one PAC (5th complex); a U wave is present

Strip 7-34

Rhythm: Irregular

Rate: Ventricular rate: 50; Atrial rate not measurable

P waves: Fibrillatory waves are present

PR interval: Not measurable

QRS: 0.06 to 0.08 seconds

Rhythm interpretation: Atrial fibrillation; ST segment depression and T wave inversion are present

Strip 7-35

Rhythm: Regular

Rate: 188

P waves: Obscured in T waves

PR interval: Unmeasurable

QRS: 0.04–0.08 seconds

Rhythm interpretation: Paroxysmal atrial tachycardia; ST segment depression is present

Strip 7-36

Rhythm: Irregular

Rate: 60

P waves: Vary in size, shape, direction across strip

PR interval: Varies (0.14–0.20 seconds)

QRS: 0.10 seconds

Rhythm interpretation: Wandering atrial pacemaker

Strip 7-37

Rhythm: Irregular

Rate: Atrial, 260; ventricular, 70

P waves: Flutter waves (varying ratios)

PR interval: Not measurable

QRS: 0.08 seconds

Rhythm interpretation: Atrial flutter with variable AV conduction

Strip 7-38

Rhythm: Regular

Rate: 150

P waves: Obscured in T wave

PR interval: Not measurable

QRS: 0.04–0.06 seconds

Rhythm interpretation: Paroxysmal atrial tachycardia; ST segment depression is present

Strip 7-39

Rhythm: Basic rhythm regular; irregular with PAC

Rate: Basic rhythm rate 136

P waves: Sinus with basic rhythm; premature, pointed P wave with PAC

PR interval: 0.16–0.18 (basic rhythm); 0.18 seconds (PAC)

QRS: 0.06–0.08 seconds (basic rhythm); 0.06 seconds (PAC)

Rhythm interpretation: Sinus tachycardia with 1 PAC (11th complex)

Strip 7-40

Rhythm: Irregular

Rate: Ventricular rate: 130; Atrial rate not measurable

P waves: Fibrillatory waves present

PR interval: Not measurable

QRS: 0.04–0.06 seconds

Rhythm interpretation: Atrial fibrillation (uncontrolled rate)

Strip 7-41

Rhythm: Basic rhythm regular; irregular with nonconducted PAC

Rate: Basic rhythm rate 79

P waves: Sinus P waves with basic rhythm; premature, abnormal P waves hidden in T wave following 7th QRS

PR interval: 0.20 seconds

QRS: 0.08–0.10 seconds

Rhythm interpretation: Normal sinus rhythm with one nonconducted PAC (hidden in T wave following 7th QRS) a U wave is present

Strip 7-42

Rhythm: Basic rhythm regular; irregular with nonconducted PAC

Rate: 72

P waves: Sinus P waves are present; one premature, abnormal P wave without a QRS (follows 5th QRS)

PR interval: 0.16 seconds

QRS: 0.08 seconds

Rhythm interpretation: Normal sinus rhythm with one nonconducted PAC (follows 5th QRS); T wave inversion is present

Strip 7-43

Rhythm: Regular

Rate: 68

P waves: Vary in size, shape, and position

PR interval: 0.12 seconds

QRS: 0.06–0.08 seconds

Rhythm interpretation: Wandering atrial pacemaker; ST segment depression is present

Strip 7-44

Rhythm: Regular

Rate: Atrial: 428 Ventricular: 214

P waves: 2 flutter waves to each QRS

PR interval: Not measurable

QRS: 0.06–0.08 seconds

Rhythm interpretation: Atrial flutter with 2:1 AV conduction

Strip 7-45

Rhythm: Regular

Rate: 188

P waves: Hidden in T waves

PR interval: Not measurable

QRS: 0.04 to 0.06 seconds

Rhythm interpretation: Paroxysmal atrial tachycardia; ST segment depression is present

Strip 7-46

Rhythm: Basic rhythm regular; irregular with premature beat

Rate: Basic rhythm rate 79

P waves: Sinus with basic rhythm; premature pointed P wave with PAC

PR interval: 0.14–0.16 seconds (basic rhythm); 0.12 seconds (PAC)

QRS: 0.06–0.08 seconds

Rhythm interpretation: Normal sinus rhythm with 1 PAC (5th complex)

Strip 7-47

Rhythm: Basic rhythm regular; irregular with PAC

Rate: Basic rhythm rate 84

P waves: Sinus P waves present; premature, pointed P wave with PAC

PR interval: 0.14 to 0.16 (basic rhythm); 0.16 seconds (PAC)

QRS: 0.06 to 0.08 seconds (basic rhythm) 0.08 seconds (PAC)

Rhythm interpretation: Normal sinus rhythm with one PAC (7th complex); ST segment depression is present

Strip 7-48

Rhythm: Irregular

Rate: 40

P waves: Fibrillatory waves are present

PR interval: Not measurable

QRS: 0.08 seconds

Rhythm interpretation: Atrial fibrillation (controlled rate)

Strip 7-49

Rhythm: Irregular

Rate: Atrial, 280; ventricular, 50

P waves: Flutter waves present (varying ratios)

PR interval: Not measurable

QRS: 0.06 to 0.08 seconds

Rhythm interpretation: Atrial flutter with variable AV conduction

Strip 7-50

Rhythm: Irregular

Rate: Atrial, 300; ventribular, 100

P waves: Flutter waves (varying ratios)

PR interval: Not measurable

QRS: 0.04–0.06 seconds

Rhythm interpretation: Atrial flutter with variable AV conduction

Strip 7-51

Rhythm: Regular

Rate: 150

P waves: Hidden in T waves

PR interval: Not measurable

QRS: 0.08 to 0.10 seconds

Rhythm interpretation: Paroxysmal atrial tachycardia

Strip 7-52

Rhythm: Basic rhythm regular; irregular with nonconducted PAC

Rate: Basic rhythm rate 88—rate slows to 79 following each nonconducted PAC (temporary rate suppression is common following a pause in the basic rhythm)

P waves: Sinus with basic rhythm; two premature abnormal P waves without a QRS complex follows 5th QRS and 7th QRS

PR interval: 0.18–0.20 seconds

QRS: 0.06–0.08 seconds

Rhythm interpretation: Normal sinus rhythm with two nonconducted PACs (following 5th and 7th QRS)

Strip 7-53

Rhythm: Irregular

Rate: 70

P waves: Fibrillatory waves

PR interval: Not measurable

QRS: 0.06–0.08 seconds

Rhythm interpretation: Atrial fibrillation; ST segment depression is present

Strip 7-54

Rhythm: Basic rhythm regular; irregular with PAC

Rate: Basic rhythm rate 94

P waves: Sinus in basic rhythm; premature pointed P wave with PAC

PR interval: 0.12–0.16 seconds

QRS: 0.06–0.08 seconds

Rhythm interpretation: Normal sinus rhythm with one PAC (8th complex); ST segment depression is present

Strip 7-55

Rhythm: Irregular

Rate: Ventricular: 140 Atrial: not measurable

P waves: Fibrillatory waves 1st part of strip; sinus P waves last part of strip

PR interval: Not measurable 1st part of strip; 0.14 seconds (with the two sinus beats last part of strip)

QRS: 0.04–0.06 seconds

Rhythm interpretation: Atrial fibrillation converting to a sinus rhythm (one PAC follows 1st sinus beat)

Strip 7-56

Rhythm: Basic rhythm regular; irregular with PAC

Rate: Basic rhythm rate 84

P waves: Sinus in basic rhythm; premature, pointed P wave with PAC

PR interval: 0.12–0.14 seconds (basic rhythm); 0.12 seconds (PAC)

QRS: 0.06–0.08 seconds (basic rhythm) 0.08 seconds (PAC)

Rhythm interpretation: Normal sinus rhythm with 1 PAC (5th complex); baseline artifact is present (baseline artifact should not be confused with atrial fibrillation)

Strip 7-57

Rhythm: Regular

Rate: Atrial, 300; ventricular, 75

P waves: Four flutter waves to each QRS

PR interval: Not measurable

QRS: 0.04 seconds

Rhythm interpretation: Atrial flutter with 4:1 AV conduction

Strip 7-58

Rhythm: Basic rhythm regular; irregular with nonconducted PAC

Rate: Basic rhythm rate 88—rate slows to 72 following pause (temporary rate suppression is common following a pause in the basic rhythm)

P waves: Sinus with basic rhythm; premature abnormal P wave (without associated QRS) hidden in T wave following 7th QRS

PR interval: 0.12–0.14 seconds (basic rhythm)

QRS: 0.08–0.10 seconds

Rhythm interpretation: Normal sinus rhythm with one nonconducted PAC (follows 7th QRS)

Strip 7-59

Rhythm: Irregular

Rate: 70

P waves: Vary in size, shape, direction

PR interval: 0.14–0.16 seconds

QRS: 0.06–0.08 seconds

Rhythm interpretation: Wandering atrial pacemaker; T wave inversion is present

Strip 7-60

Rhythm: Irregular

Rate: Atrial: 300 Ventricular: 80

P waves: Flutter waves are present before each QRS in varying ratios

PR interval: Not measurable

QRS: 0.04–0.06 seconds

Rhythm interpretation: Atrial flutter with variable AV conduction

Strip 7-61
Rhythm: Irregular
Rate: 50
P waves: Fibrillatory waves are present
PR interval: Not measurable
QRS: 0.06–0.08 seconds
Rhythm interpretation: Atrial fibrillation; some
flutter waves are present

Strip 7-62
Rhythm: Regular with basic rhythm; irregular with
PAC
Rate: Basic rhythm rate 58
P waves: Sinus with basic rhythm; premature,
abnormal P wave with PAC
PR interval: 0.16–0.18 seconds (basic rhythm)
QRS: 0.06–0.08 seconds
Rhythm interpretation: Sinus bradycardia with one
PAC (5th complex); a U wave is present

Strip 7-63
Rhythm: Irregular
Rate: Ventricular rate: 80 Atrial rate not measurable
P waves: Fibrillatory waves present
PR interval: Not measurable
QRS: 0.04 to 0.06 seconds
Rhythm interpretation: Atrial fibrillation;
ST segment depression is present

Strip 7-64
Rhythm: Regular
Rate: 214
P waves: Hidden in T waves
PR interval: Not measurable
QRS: 0.08 seconds
Rhythm interpretation: Paroxysmal atrial
tachycardia

Strip 7-65
Rhythm: Basic rhythm regular; irregular with PAC
Rate: Basic rhythm rate 52
P waves: Sinus with basic rhythm; premature
pointed P wave associated with PAC (abnormal P
wave hidden in T wave following 4th QRS)
PR interval: 0.16–0.18 seconds
QRS: 0.06–0.08 seconds
Rhythm interpretation: Sinus bradycardia with one
PAC (5th complex); a U wave is present

Strip 7-66
Rhythm: Basic rhythm regular; irregular with
nonconducted PAC
Rate: Basic rhythm rate 75
P waves: Sinus with basic rhythm; premature,
abnormal P wave hidden in T wave following 4th
QRS
PR interval: 0.20 seconds
QRS: 0.06–0.08 seconds
Rhythm interpretation: Normal sinus rhythm with
one nonconducted PAC (follows 4th QRS) a U wave
is present

Strip 7-67
Rhythm: Regular
Rate: 84
P waves: Vary in size, shape, direction
PR interval: 0.16 seconds
QRS: 0.04–0.06 seconds
Rhythm interpretation: Wandering atrial
pacemaker

Strip 7-68
Rhythm: Regular
Rate: 150
P waves: Hidden (possibly in preceding T waves)
PR interval: Not measurable
QRS: 0.04–0.06 seconds
Rhythm interpretation: Paroxysmal atrial
tachycardia; ST segment depression is present

Strip 7-69
Rhythm: Irregular
Rate: Atrial: 250 Ventricular: 70
P waves: Flutter waves before each QRS in varying
ratios
PR interval: Not measurable
QRS: 0.06–0.08 seconds
Rhythm interpretation: Atrial flutter with variable
AV conduction

Strip 7-70
Rhythm: Irregular
Rate: Ventricular rate: 130; Atrial rate not
measurable
P waves: Fibrillatory waves; some flutter waves are
seen
PR interval: Not measurable
QRS: 0.04 seconds
Rhythm interpretation: Atrial fibrillation; some
flutter waves are noted; ST segment depression is
present

Strip 7-71
Rhythm: Basic rhythm regular; irregular with PACs
Rate: Basic rhythm rate 88
P waves: Sinus P waves with basic rhythm;
premature, abnormal P waves with PACs
PR interval: 0.14 to 0.16 seconds (basic rhythm)
QRS: 0.06 to 0.08 seconds
Rhythm interpretation: Normal sinus rhythm with
paired PACs (3rd and 4th complexes)

Strip 7-72
Rhythm: Regular
Rate: 54
P waves: Varying in size and shape
PR interval: 0.12
QRS: 0.08 to 0.10 seconds
Rhythm interpretation: Wandering atrial
pacemaker; ST segment depression is present

Strip 7-73
Rhythm: Regular
Rate: Atrial: 272; Ventricular: 136
P waves: 2 flutter wave to each QRS
PR interval: Not measurable
QRS: 0.08 seconds
Rhythm interpretation: Atrial flutter with 2:1
AV conduction

Strip 7-74
Rhythm: Basic rhythm regular; irregular with PAC
Rate: Basic rhythm rate 63
P waves: Sinus in basic rhythm; premature,
abnormal P wave with PAC
PR interval: 0.12–0.14 seconds (basic rhythm);
0.14 seconds (PAC)
QRS: 0.06–0.08 seconds (basic rhythm) 0.08
seconds (PAC)
Rhythm interpretation: Normal sinus rhythm with 1
PAC (4th complex); a small U wave is present

Strip 7-75
Rhythm: Regular
Rate: 150
P waves: Hidden in T waves
PR interval: Not measurable
QRS: 0.06 to 0.08 seconds
Rhythm interpretation: Paroxysmal atrial
tachycardia; ST segment depression is present

Strip 7-76
Rhythm: Irregular
Rate: Ventricular rate: 80; Atrial rate not measurable
P waves: Fibrillatory waves present
PR interval: Not measurable
QRS: 0.04 seconds
Rhythm interpretation: Atrial fibrillation; ST
segment depression and T wave inversion are
present

Strip 7-77
Rhythm: Regular
Rate: 88
P waves: Vary in size, shape, position
PR interval: 0.12 to 0.14 seconds
QRS: 0.06 to 0.08 seconds
Rhythm interpretation: Wandering atrial
pacemaker; T wave inversion is present

Strip 7-78
Rhythm: Irregular
Rate: 50
P waves: Vary in size, shape, and position
PR interval: 0.12 to 0.16 seconds
QRS: 0.08 seconds
Rhythm interpretation: Wandering atrial
pacemaker; ST segment depression is present

Strip 7-79
Rhythm: Regular
Rate: Atrial: 232; Ventricular: 58
P waves: 4 flutter waves to each QRS
PR interval: Not measurable
QRS: 0.08 seconds
Rhythm interpretation: Atrial flutter with 4:1 AV
conduction

Strip 7-80
Rhythm: Basic rhythm regular; irregular with PAC
and nonconducted PAC
Rate: Basic rhythm rate 79
P waves: Sinus with basic rhythm; premature
pointed P waves with PAC and nonconducted PAC
PR interval: 0.14–0.16 seconds (basic rhythm)
QRS: 0.04–0.06 seconds
Rhythm interpretation: Normal sinus rhythm with
one PAC (4th complex) and one nonconducted PAC
(following 5th QRS); T wave inversion is present

Strip 7-81
Rhythm: Regular
Rate: 68
P waves: Vary in size, shape, direction
PR interval: 0.12–0.16 seconds
QRS: 0.08 seconds
Rhythm interpretation: Wandering atrial
pacemaker; a U wave is present

Strip 7-82
Rhythm: Regular
Rate: Atrial: 240; Ventricular: 60
P waves: 4 flutter waves to each QRS
PR interval: Not measurable
QRS: 0.06 seconds
Rhythm interpretation: Atrial flutter with 4:1 AV
conduction

Strip 7-83
Rhythm: Regular
Rate: 167
P waves: Hidden in preceding T wave
PR interval: Not measurable
QRS: 0.08–0.10 seconds
Rhythm interpretation: Paroxysmal atrial
tachycardia

Strip 7-84
Rhythm: Irregular
Rate: 50
P waves: Fibrillatory waves
PR interval: Not measurable
QRS: 0.08–0.10 seconds
Rhythm interpretation: Atrial fibrillation

Strip 7-85
Rhythm: Irregular
Rate: 40
P waves: Vary in size, shape, direction
PR interval: 0.14–0.16 seconds
QRS: 0.08 seconds
Rhythm interpretation: Wandering atrial
pacemaker

Strip 7-86
Rhythm: Basic rhythm regular; irregular with PACs
Rate: Basic rhythm rate 107
P waves: Sinus with basic rhythm; premature,
pointed P waves with PACs
PR interval: 0.16 seconds (basic rhythm)
QRS: 0.06 seconds
Rhythm interpretation: Sinus tachycardia with 3
PACs (4th, 9th, 11th complex)

Strip 7-87
Rhythm: Irregular
Rate: Atrial: 250; Ventricular: 40
P waves: Flutter waves before each QRS in varying
ratios
PR interval: Not measuable
QRS: 0.06–0.08 seconds
Rhythm interpretation: Atrial flutter with variable
AV conduction

Strip 7-88
Rhythm: Irregular
Rate: Ventricular rate: 40; atrial rate not measurable
P waves: Fibrillatory waves present
PR interval: Not measurable
QRS: 0.04–0.06 seconds
Rhythm interpretation: Atrial fibrillation;
ST segment depression is present

Strip 7-89
Rhythm: Basic rhythm regular; irregular with
nonconducted PAC
Rate: Basic rhythm rate 84
P waves: Sinus in basic rhythm; premature, pointed
P wave with nonconducted PAC
PR interval: 0.16–0.20 seconds
QRS: 0.06–0.08 seconds
Rhythm interpretation: Normal sinus rhythm with
one nonconducted PAC (follows 5th QRS) ST
segment depression is present

Strip 7-90
Rhythm: Basic rhythm regular; irregular with PAC
Rate: Basic rhythm rate: 54
P waves: Sinus with basic rhythm; premature
abnormal P wave with PAC
PR interval: 0.16–0.18 seconds
QRS: 0.06 seconds
Rhythm interpretation: Sinus bradycardia with one
PAC (4th complex)

Strip 7-91
Rhythm: Basic rhythm regular; irregular with PAC
Rate: Basic rhythm 63
P waves: Sinus P waves with basic rhythm;
premature, abnormal P waves with PAC
PR interval: 0.14 to 0.16 seconds
QRS: 0.06 seconds
Rhythm interpretation: Normal sinus rhythm with
one PAC (5th complex); a U wave is present

Strip 7-92
Rhythm: Regular
Rate: Atrial, 235; ventricular, 47
P waves: Five flutter waves to each QRS
PR interval: Not discernible
QRS: 0.08 seconds
Rhythm interpretation: Atrial flutter with 5:1 block;
T wave inversion is present

Strip 8-1
Rhythm: Basic rhythm regular; irregular with PJC
Rate: Basic rhythm rate 58
P waves: Sinus with basic rhythm; premature
inverted P wave with PJC
PR interval: 0.14–0.16 (basic rhythm); 0.08 (PJC)
QRS: 0.06 seconds (basic rhythm and PJC)
Rhythm interpretation: Sinus bradycardia with 1
PJC (5th complex); a U wave is present

Strip 8-2
Rhythm: Regular
Rate: 60
P waves: Sinus P waves present
PR interval: 0.24
QRS: 0.06 to 0.08 seconds
Rhythm interpretation: Normal sinus rhythm with
first-degress AV block; ST segment elevation and
T wave inversion are present

Strip 8-3
Rhythm: Regular atrial and ventricular rhythm
Rate: Atrial: 46 Ventricular: 23
P waves: 2 Sinus P waves before each QRS
PR interval: 0.22–0.24 seconds (remains constant)
QRS: 0.08–0.10 seconds
Rhythm interpretation: Second-degree AV block,
Mobitz II; clinical correlation is suggested to
diagnose Mobitz II when 2:1 conduction is present;
ST segment elevation is present

Strip 8-4
Rhythm: Basic rhythm regular; irregular with
junctional beat
Rate: Basic rhythm rate 58
P waves: Sinus P waves with basic rhythm; hidden
P wave with junctional beat
PR interval: 0.16 to 0.18 seconds (basic rhythm)
QRS: 0.08 to 0.10 seconds (basic rhythm and
junctional beat)
Rhythm interpretation: Sinus bradycardia with
junctional escape beat (4th complex) following
pause in basic rhythm; ST segment depression is
present

Strip 8-5
Rhythm: Regular
Rate: 115
P waves: Inverted
PR interval: 0.08 seconds
QRS: 0.04–0.06 seconds
Rhythm interpretation: Junctional tachycardia

Strip 8-6
Rhythm: Regular
Rate: 84
P waves: Sinus
PR interval: 0.22–0.24 seconds
QRS: 0.08–0.10 seconds
Rhythm interpretation: Normal sinus rhythm with
first-degree AV block

Strip 8-7
Rhythm: Regular
Rate: 65
P waves: Inverted before each QRS
PR interval: 0.08 seconds
QRS: 0.06 to 0.08 seconds
Rhythm interpretation: Accelerated junctional
rhythm; ST segment elevation and T wave inversion
are present

Strip 8-8
Rhythm: Regular atrial rhythm; irregular ventricular
rhythm
Rate: Atrial, 75; ventricular, 70
P waves: Sinus P waves present; one P wave
without QRS
PR interval: Progresses from 0.28 to 0.32 seconds
QRS: 0.04 to 0.08 seconds
Rhythm interpretation: Second-degree AV block,
Mobitz I; ST segment depression and T wave
inversion are present

Strip 8-9
Rhythm: Regular
Rate: 47
P waves: Hidden in QRS
PR interval: Not measurable
QRS: 0.08 seconds
Rhythm interpretation: Junctional rhythm; ST
segment depression is present

Strip 8-10

Rhythm: Atrial rhythm regular; Ventricular rhythm irregular

Rate: Atrial: 75; Ventricular: 30

P waves: 2 Sinus P waves before each QRS

PR interval: 0.20–0.22 seconds

QRS: 0.08–0.10 seconds

Rhythm interpretation: Second-degree AV block, Mobitz II (clinical correlation is suggested to diagnose Mobitz II when 2:1 conduction is present) ST segment depression is present

Strip 8-11

Rhythm: Atrial rhythm regular; ventricular rhythm regular

Rate: Atrial 63; Ventricular: 33

P waves: Sinus P waves are present; P waves have no relationship to QRS (found hidden in QRS and T waves)

PR interval: Varies greatly

QRS: 0.12 seconds

Rhythm interpretation: Third-degree AV block; ST segment depression and T wave inversion are present

Strip 8-12

Rhythm: Regular

Rate: 84

P waves: Hidden in QRS

PR interval: Not measurable

QRS: 0.06–0.08 seconds

Rhythm interpretation: Accelerated junctional rhythm; ST segment depression is present

Strip 8-13

Rhythm: Regular

Rate: 65

P waves: Sinus

PR interval: 0.44–0.48 seconds

QRS: 0.08–0.10 seconds

Rhythm interpretation: Normal sinus rhythm with first-degree AV block; an elevated ST segment is present

Strip 8-14

Rhythm: Basic rhythm regular; irregular with PJC

Rate: Basic rhythm rate 136

P waves: Sinus P waves with basic rhythm; hidden P wave with PJC

PR interval: 0.12 to 0.14 seconds

QRS: 0.04–0.06 seconds

Rhythm interpretation: Sinus tachycardia with PJC (13th complex)

Strip 8-15

Rhythm: Regular

Rate: 94

P waves: Sinus

PR interval: 0.26–0.28 seconds

QRS: 0.06 seconds

Rhythm interpretation: Normal sinus rhythm with first-degree AV block

Strip 8-16

Rhythm: Basic rhythm regular; irregular with premature beat

Rate: Basic rate 58

P waves: Sinus with basic rhythm; inverted P wave with premature beat

PR interval: Basic rhythm 0.16–0.18 seconds; PJC 0.08 seconds

QRS: 0.06–0.08 seconds

Rhythm interpretation: Sinus bradycardia with 1 PJC (4th complex); ST segment depression is present

Strip 8-17

Rhythm: Regular atrial and ventricular rhythm

Rate: Atrial: 108; ventricular: 54

P waves: Two P waves to each QRS complex

PR interval: 0.20 and constant

QRS: 0.08 to 0.10 seconds

Rhythm interpretation: Second-degree AV block Mobitz II. Clinical correlation is suggested to diagnose Mobitz II when 2:1 conduction is present; ST segment elevation and T wave inversion are present

Strip 8-18

Rhythm: Irregular ventricular rhythm; regular atrial rhythm

Rate: Atrial: 65; ventricular: 50

P waves: Sinus P waves present; one P wave without QRS

PR interval: Progresses from 0.20 to 0.48 seconds

QRS: 0.04 seconds

Rhythm interpretation: Second-degree AV block, Mobitz I

Strip 8-19

Rhythm: Regular

Rate: 125

P waves: Inverted before each QRS

PR interval: 0.08 to 0.10 seconds

QRS: 0.06 seconds

Rhythm interpretation: Junctional tachycardia

Strip 8-20

Rhythm: Regular atrial and ventricular rhythm
Rate: Atrial: 100 Ventricular: 38
P waves: Sinus P waves present; bear no relationship to QRS (found hidden in QRS and T waves)
PR interval: Varies greatly
QRS: 0.06–0.08 seconds
Rhythm interpretation: Third-degree AV block; ST segment depression is present

Strip 8-21

Rhythm: Basic rhythm regular; irregular with PJC
Rate: Basic rhythm rate 60
P waves: Sinus P waves with basic rhythm; premature, inverted P wave with PJC
PR interval: 0.12 to 0.14 seconds (basic rhythm); 0.08 seconds (PJC)
QRS: 0.08 seconds (basic rhythm and PJC)
Rhythm interpretation: Normal sinus rhythm with one PJC (4th complex)

Strip 8-22

Rhythm: Regular atrial and ventricular rhythm
Rate: Atrial, 100; ventricular, 50
P waves: Two sinus P waves before each QRS complex
PR interval: 0.16 and constant
QRS: 0.08 seconds
Rhythm interpretation: Second-degree AV block, Mobitz II. Clinical correlation is suggested to diagnose Mobitz II when 2:1 conduction is present

Strip 8-23

Rhythm: Regular
Rate: 35
P waves: Sinus
PR interval: 0.60–0.62 seconds (remains constant)
QRS: 0.06 seconds
Rhythm interpretation: Sinus bradycardia with first-degree AV block

Strip 8-24

Rhythm: Irregular ventricular rhythm; regular atrial rhythm
Rate: Atrial, 68; ventricular, 60
P waves: Sinus P waves present; one without a QRS
PR interval: Progresses from 0.28 to 0.36 seconds
QRS: 0.08 seconds
Rhythm interpretation: Second-degree AV block, Mobitz I; a U wave is present

Strip 8-25

Rhythm: Regular
Rate: 75
P waves: Sinus P waves
PR interval: 0.28
QRS: 0.08 seconds
Rhythm interpretation: Sinus rhythm with first-degree AV block

Strip 8-26

Rhythm: Basic rhythm regular; irregular with PJCs
Rate: Basic rhythm rate 100
P waves: Sinus P waves with basic rhythm; premature, inverted P waves with PJCs
PR interval: 0.20 seconds (basic rhythm); 0.06 seconds (PJC)
QRS: 0.06 to 0.08 seconds (basic rhythm and PJC)
Rhythm interpretation: Normal sinus rhythm with paired PJCs; (8th and 9th complexes); ST segment depression is present

Strip 8-27

Rhythm: Regular
Rate: 65
P waves: Inverted before each QRS
PR interval: 0.08 seconds
QRS: 0.08 seconds
Rhythm interpretation: Accelerated junctional rhythm; ST segment is present

Strip 8-28

Rhythm: Basic rhythm regular; irregular with nonconducted PAC
Rate: Basic rhythm rate 56
P waves: Sinus P waves with basic rhythm; premature, abnormal P wave without QRS
PR interval: 0.24–0.26 seconds (remains constant)
QRS: 0.08 seconds
Rhythm interpretation: Sinus bradycardia with first-degree AV block and nonconducted PAC (follows 4th QRS); ST segment depression is present

Strip 8-29

Rhythm: Regular atrial rhythm; irregular ventricular rhythm
Rate: Atrial: 63; Ventricular: 50
P waves: Sinus P waves are present
PR interval: Progressively lengthens from 0.28–0.32 seconds
QRS: 0.06–0.08 seconds
Rhythm interpretation: Second degree AV block, Mobitz I; ST segment depression is present

Strip 8-30
Rhythm: Regular atrial and ventricular rhythm
Rate: Atrial: 79; Ventricular: 32
P waves: Sinus P waves which have no constant relationship to QRS (found hidden in QRS complexes and T waves)
PR interval: Varies greatly
QRS: 0.12 seconds
Rhythm interpretation: Third-degree AV block

Strip 8-31
Rhythm: Regular atrial and ventricular rhythm
Rate: Atrial, 84; ventricular, 28
P waves: Three sinus P waves to each QRS
PR interval: 0.28 to 0.32 (remains constant)
QRS: 0.08 seconds
Rhythm interpretation: Second-degree AV block, Mobitz II

Strip 8-32
Rhythm: Regular atrial and ventricular rhythm
Rate: Atrial: 75; Ventricular: 34
P waves: Sinus P waves present with no relationship to QRS complexes (found hidden in QRS and T waves)
PR interval: Varies greatly
QRS: 0.12–0.14 seconds
Rhythm interpretation: Third-degree AV block; ST segment elevation is present

Strip 8-33
Rhythm: Basic rhythm regular; irregular with PAC
Rate: Basic rhythm rate 100
P waves: Inverted before QRS in basic rhythm; upright and premature with PAC
PR interval: 0.08 seconds (basic rhythm); 0.12 seconds (PAC)
QRS: 0.08 seconds (basic rhythm and PAC)
Rhythm interpretation: Accelerated junctional rhythm with one PAC (6th complex); ST segment depression is present

Strip 8-34
Rhythm: Irregular ventricular rhythm; regular atrial rhythm
Rate: Atrial: 75; ventricular: 50
P waves: Sinus P waves present; two P waves without QRS
PR interval: Progresses from 0.28 to 0.40 seconds
QRS: 0.08 to 0.10 seconds
Rhythm interpretation: Second-degree AV block, Mobitz I

Strip 8-35
Rhythm: Regular
Rate: 60
P waves: Sinus
PR interval: 0.24–0.26 seconds
QRS: 0.06–0.08 seconds
Rhythm interpretation: Normal sinus rhythm with first-degree AV block

Strip 8-36
Rhythm: Regular
Rate: 41
P waves: Inverted after QRS
PR interval: 0.04 to 0.06 seconds
QRS: 0.06 to 0.08 seconds
Rhythm interpretation: Junctional rhythm

Strip 8-37
Rhythm: Basic rhythm regular; irregular with PJC
Rate: Basic rhythm rate 58
P waves: Sinus P waves with basic rhythm; premature, inverted P waves with PJCs
PR interval: 0.16 seconds (basic rhythm); 0.08 to 0.10 seconds (PJC)
QRS: 0.08 seconds (basic rhythm and PJC)
Rhythm interpretation: Sinus bradycardia with two PJCs (4th complex and 6th complex); a U wave is present

Strip 8-38
Rhythm: Regular atrial and ventricular rhythm
Rate: Atrial: 66; Ventricular: 33
P waves: 2 Sinus P waves to each QRS
PR interval: 0.44 seconds (remains constant)
QRS: 0.14–0.16 seconds
Rhythm interpretation: Second-degree AV block, Mobitz II; clinical correlation is suggested to diagnose Mobitz II when 2:1 conduction is present

Strip 8-39
Rhythm: Regular atrial and ventricular rhythm
Rate: Atrial: 52; ventricular: 26
P waves: Two sinus P waves present before each QRS complex
PR interval: 0.22 (remains constant)
QRS: 0.12 seconds
Rhythm interpretation: Second-degree AV block, Mobitz II. Clinical correlation is suggested to diagnose Mobitz II when 2:1 conduction is present

Strip 8-40
Rhythm: Regular atrial rhythm; irregular ventricular rhythm
Rate: Atrial: 107; Ventricular: 50
P waves: Sinus P waves present—bear no relationship to QRS complexes (found hidden in QRS and T waves)
PR interval: Varies greatly
QRS: 0.08 seconds
Rhythm interpretation: Third-degree AV block

Strip 8-41
Rhythm: Regular
Rate: 68
P waves: Inverted before each QRS
PR interval: 0.08 seconds
QRS: 0.06–0.08 seconds
Rhythm interpretation: Accelerated junctional rhythm

Strip 8-42
Rhythm: Regular atrial and ventricular rhythm
Rate: Atrial: 104; Ventricular: 52
P waves: Two sinus P waves to each QRS complex
PR interval: 0.24 and constant
QRS: 0.06 to 0.08 seconds
Rhythm interpretation: Second-degree AV block, Mobitz II. Clinical correlation is suggested to diagnose Mobitz II when 2:1 conduction is present; ST segment elevation and T wave inversion are present

Strip 8-43
Rhythm: First rhythm irregular; second rhythm regular
Rate: First rhythm about 80; second rhythm 42
P waves: Fibrillatory waves in first rhythm; hidden P waves in second rhythm
PR interval: Not measurable in either rhythm
QRS: 0.06–0.08 seconds
Rhythm interpretation: Atrial fibrillation to junctional rhythm; ST segment depression is present

Strip 8-44
Rhythm: Basic rhythm regular; irregular with premature beats
Rate: Basic rhythm rate 60
P waves: Sinus P waves with basic rhythm; premature, abnormal P waves with premature beats
PR interval: 0.12 to 0.16 seconds (basic rhythm); 0.12 seconds (PAC); 0.08 sec (PJC)
QRS: 0.06 to 0.08 seconds
Rhythm interpretation: Normal sinus rhythm with one PAC (4th complex) and one PJC (5th complex); ST segment depression and T wave inversion are present

Strip 8-45
Rhythm: Regular atrial and ventricular rhythm
Rate: Atrial: 72; Ventricular: 32
P waves: Sinus P waves present; bear no relationship to QRS complexes (hidden in QRS and T waves)
PR interval: Varies greatly
QRS: 0.12 seconds
Rhythm interpretation: Third-degree AV block; ST segment elevation is present

Strip 8-46
Rhythm: Irregular
Rate: 40
P waves: Sinus P waves are present
PR interval: 0.28 seconds (remains constant)
QRS: 0.08 to 0.10 seconds
Rhythm interpretation: Sinus arrhythmia with first-degree AV block; a U wave is present

Strip 8-47
Rhythm: Regular atrial rhythm; irregular ventricular rhythm
Rate: Atrial: 79; Ventricular: 50
P waves: Sinus P waves present
PR interval: Lengthens 0.24–0.40 seconds
QRS: 0.08–0.10 seconds
Rhythm interpretation: Second-degree AV block, Mobitz I

Strip 8-48
Rhythm: Regular atrial and ventricular rhythm
Rate: Atrial: 108; ventricular: 54
P waves: Two sinus P waves before each QRS complex
PR interval: 0.18 to 0.20 seconds (remains constant)
QRS: 0.08 seconds
Rhythm interpretation: Second-degree AV block Mobitz II. Clinical correlation is suggested to diagnose Mobitz II when 2:1 conduction is present. ST segment elevation and T wave inversion are present

Strip 8-49
Rhythm: Irregular
Rate: 40
P waves: Inverted before each QRS
PR interval: 0.04 to 0.06 seconds
QRS: 0.08 to 0.10 seconds
Rhythm interpretation: Junctional rhythm; ST segment depression is present

Strip 8-50

Rhythm: Basic rhythm regular; irregular with escape beat

Rate: Basic rhythm rate 84; rate slows to 75 after escape beat; rate suppression can occur following premature or escape beats; after several cycles rate will return to basic rate

P waves: Sinus P waves present; P wave hidden with escape beat

PR interval: 0.14 to 0.16 seconds

QRS: 0.06 to 0.08 seconds

Rhythm interpretation: Normal sinus rhythm with junctional escape beat (5th complex) following a pause in the basic rhythm; a U wave is present

Strip 8-51

Rhythm: Regular ventricular rhythm; irregular atrial rhythm

Rate: Atrial: 70; ventricular: 25

P waves: Sinus P waves present; bear no relationship to QRS

PR interval: Varies greatly

QRS: 0.12 seconds

Rhythm interpretation: Third-degree AV block

Strip 8-52

Rhythm: Regular

Rate: 63

P waves: Hidden in QRS

PR interval: Not measurable

QRS: 0.08 seconds

Rhythm interpretation: Accelerated junctional rhythm

Strip 8-53

Rhythm: Regular atrial and ventricular rhythm

Rate: Atrial: 76; ventricular: 38

P waves: Two sinus P waves before each QRS complex

PR interval: 0.24–0.26 seconds

QRS: 0.12–0.14 seconds

Rhythm interpretation: Second-degree AV block, Mobitz II. Clinical correlation is suggested to diagnose Mobitz II when 2:1 conduction is present

Strip 8-54

Rhythm: Regular

Rate: 94

P waves: Inverted before QRS

PR interval: 0.08 seconds

QRS: 0.06 to 0.08 seconds

Rhythm interpretation: Accelerated junctional rhythm

Strip 8-55

Rhythm: Basic rhythm regular

Rate: 55 (basic rhythm)

P waves: Sinus P waves with basic rhythm (notched P waves usually indicate left atrial hypertropy); no P wave seen with 4th complex; 5th complex has P wave on top of preceding T wave

PR interval: 0.20 seconds (basic rhythm); 0.40 seconds (PAC)

QRS: 0.06–0.08 seconds

Rhythm interpretation: Sinus bradycardia with 1 junctional escape beat (4th complex) and 1 PAC (5th complex) (Both follow a pause in the basic rhythm)

Strip 8-56

Rhythm: Both rhythms regular

Rate: 72 (first rhythm) about 140 (second rhythm)

P waves: Sinus P waves (first rhythm); inverted P waves (second rhythm)

PR interval: 0.12 seconds (first rhythm); 0.08 to 0.10 seconds (second rhythm)

QRS: 0.08 seconds

Rhythm interpretation: Normal sinus rhythm changing to junctional tachycardia; ST segment depression is present

Strip 8-57

Rhythm: Regular

Rate: 84

P waves: Sinus P waves present

PR interval: 0.30 to 0.32 seconds (remains constant)

QRS: 0.04–0.06 seconds

Rhythm interpretation: Normal sinus rhythm with first-degree AV block; ST segment elevation is present

Strip 8-58

Rhythm: Regular atrial and ventricular rhythm

Rate: Atrial: 75; ventricular: 30

P waves: Sinus P waves present; bear no relationship to QRS

PR interval: Varies greatly

QRS: 0.12 to 0.14 seconds

Rhythm interpretation: Third-degree AV block

Strip 8-59

Rhythm: Regular atrial and ventricular rhythm

Rate: Atrial: 93; ventricular: 31

P waves: 3 Sinus P waves to each QRS (one hidden in T-wave)

PR interval: 0.32 to 0.36 seconds

QRS: 0.08 seconds

Rhythm interpretation: Second-degree AV block, Mobitz II; ST segment depression is present

Strip 8-60

Rhythm: Basic rhythm regular; irregular with premature beats
Rate: Basic rhythm rate 60
P waves: Sinus P waves present with basic rhythm; premature, abnormal P waves with premature beats
PR interval: 0.12 seconds (basic rhythm); 0.12 seconds (PAC); 0.08 to 0.10 seconds (PJCs)
QRS: 0.08 seconds
Rhythm interpretation: Normal sinus rhythm with one PAC (3rd complex) and paired PJCs (6th and 7th complexes)

Strip 8-61

Rhythm: Regular
Rate: 47
P waves: Hidden in QRS
PR interval: Not measurable
QRS: 0.08 seconds
Rhythm interpretation: Junctional rhythm

Strip 8-62

Rhythm: Basic rhythm regular; irregular with nonconducted PAC
Rate: Basic rhythm rate 79—rate slows to 63 following pause (temporary rate suppression is common following a pause in the basic rhythm
P waves: Sinus with basic rhythm; premature, pointed P wave distorting T wave following 6th QRS
PR interval: 0.24 seconds (remains constant)
QRS: 0.08 seconds
Rhythm interpretation: Normal sinus rhythm with first degree AV block; a nonconducted PAC is present following 6th QRS

Strip 8-63

Rhythm: Irregular ventricular rhythm; regular atrial rhythm
Rate: Atrial: 75; ventricular: 50
P waves: Sinus P waves are present
PR interval: Progresses from 0.24 to 0.32 seconds
QRS: 0.08 seconds
Rhythm interpretation: Second-degree AV block, Mobitz I

Strip 8-64

Rhythm: Regular atrial and ventricular rhythm
Rate: Atrial: 72; ventricular: 31
P waves: Sinus P waves present; bear no relationship to QRS (hidden in QRS complexes and T waves)
PR interval: Varies greatly
QRS: 0.12 seconds
Rhythm interpretation: Third-degree AV block

Strip 8-65

Rhythm: Regular atrial and ventricular rhythm
Rate: Atrial: 90; ventricular: 45
P waves: Two sinus P waves to each QRS
PR interval: 0.26–0.28 seconds (remains constant)
QRS: 0.12 seconds
Rhythm interpretation: Second-degree AV block, Mobitz II; clinical correlation is suggested to diagnose Mobitz II when 2:1 conduction is present; ST segment elevation is present

Strip 8-66

Rhythm: Regular
Rate: 79
P waves: Inverted P waves before each QRS
PR interval: 0.08–0.10 seconds
QRS: 0.06–0.08 seconds
Rhythm interpretation: Accelerated junctional rhythm

Strip 8-67

Rhythm: Regular
Rate: 94
P waves: Sinus
PR interval: 0.24 seconds
QRS: 0.08 seconds
Rhythm interpretation: Normal sinus rhythm with first-degree AV block

Strip 8-68

Rhythm: Basic rhythm regular; irregular with premature beats
Rate: Basic rhythm rate 72
P waves: Sinus P waves with basic rhythm; premature, abnormal P waves with premature beats
PR interval: 0.14 to 0.16 seconds (basic rhythm); 0.12 seconds (PACs); 0.10 seconds (PJCs)
QRS: 0.06 to 0.08 seconds
Rhythm interpretation: Normal sinus rhythm with two PACs (3rd and 8th complex) and one PJC (5th complex); a U wave is present

Strip 8-69

Rhythm: Basic rhythm regular; irregular with premature beats
Rate: Basic rhythm rate 52
P waves: Hidden with basic rhythm; premature, abnormal with premature beats
PR interval: Not measurable in basic rhythm; 0.12–0.14 seconds (PACs)
QRS: 0.06 to 0.08 seconds
Rhythm interpretation: Junctional rhythm with two PACs (2nd and 5th complex); ST segment depression is present

Strip 8-70

Rhythm: Irregular ventricular rhythm; regular atrial rhythm

Rate: Atrial: 79; ventricular: 70

P waves: Sinus P waves present

PR interval: Progresses from 0.24 to 0.28 seconds

QRS: 0.08 seconds

Rhythm interpretation: Second-degree AV block Mobitz I

Strip 8-71

Rhythm: Regular atrial and ventricular rhythm

Rate: Atrial: 80; ventricular: 40

P waves: Two sinus P waves to each QRS

PR interval: 0.24 seconds (remain constant)

QRS: 0.04 to 0.06 seconds

Rhythm interpretation: Second-degree AV block, Mobitz II; clinical correlation is suggested to diagnose Mobitz II when 2:1 conduction is present; ST segment depression is present

Strip 8-72

Rhythm: Regular atrial and ventricular rhythm

Rate: Atrial: 94; ventricular: 40

P waves: Sinus P waves are present; bear no relationship to QRS (hidden in QRS complexes and T waves)

PR interval: Varies greatly

QRS: 0.10 seconds

Rhythm interpretation: Third-degree AV block

Strip 8-73

Rhythm: Regular

Rate: 84

P waves: Hidden in QRS complexes

PR interval: Not measurable

QRS: 0.06 seconds

Rhythm interpretation: Accelerated junctional rhythm; ST segment depression and T wave inversion are present

Strip 8-74

Rhythm: Regular atrial rhythm; irregular ventricular rhythm

Rate: Atrial: 54 Ventricular: 50

P waves: Sinus P waves are present

PR interval: Lengthens from 0.34–0.44 seconds

QRS: 0.08 seconds

Rhythm interpretation: Second-degree AV block, Mobitz I

Strip 8-75

Rhythm: Basic rhythm regular; irregular with escape beat

Rate: Basic rhythm rate 58

P waves: Sinus P waves with basic rhythm; hidden P wave with escape beat

PR interval: 0.16 to 0.18 seconds

QRS: 0.08 to 0.10 seconds

Rhythm interpretation: Sinus bradycardia with junctional escape beat (4th complex) following a pause in the basic rhythm

Strip 8-76

Rhythm: Regular

Rate: 47

P waves: Hidden in QRS

PR interval: Not measurable

QRS: 0.06–0.08 seconds

Rhythm interpretation: Junctional rhythm; ST segment depression is present

Strip 8-77

Rhythm: Regular atrial and ventricular rhythm

Rate: Atrial: 94; ventricular: 44

P waves: Sinus P waves are present; P waves bear no relationship to QRS (found hidden in QRS complexes and T waves)

PR interval: Varies greatly

QRS: 0.14–0.16 seconds

Rhythm interpretation: Third-degree AV block; ST segment elevation is present

Strip 8-78

Rhythm: Basic rhythm regular; irregular with premature beats

Rate: Basic rhythm rate 68

P waves: Sinus with basic rhythm; premature abnormal P waves with premature beats

PR interval: 0.12–0.14 seconds (basic rhythm); 0.14 seconds (PAC); 0.10 seconds (PJC)

QRS: 0.06–0.08 seconds

Rhythm interpretation: Normal sinus rhythm with 1 PAC (3rd complex) and 1 PJC (7th complex) a U wave is present

Strip 8-79

Rhythm: Regular atrial and ventricular rhythm

Rate: Atrial: 80; ventricular: 40

P waves: Two P waves to each QRS

PR interval: 0.12 to 0.14 seconds (remain constant)

QRS: 0.06–0.08 seconds

Rhythm interpretation: Second-degree AV block, Mobitz II; clinical correlation is suggested to diagnose Mobitz II when 2:1 conduction is present

Strip 8-80
Rhythm: Basic rhythm regular; irregular with nonconducted PAC
Rate: Basic rhythm rate 72
P waves: Sinus with basic rhythm; premature, pointed P wave without QRS follows 6th QRS
PR interval: 0.22–0.24 seconds (remains constant)
QRS: 0.04–0.06 seconds
Rhythm interpretation: Normal sinus rhythm with first-degree AV block and 1 nonconducted PAC (follows 6th QRS); ST segment depression and T wave inversion are present

Strip 8-81
Rhythm: Regular
Rate: 88
P waves: Inverted before each QRS
PR interval: 0.08 seconds
QRS: 0.06–0.08 seconds
Rhythm interpretation: Accelerated junctional rhythm

Strip 8-82
Rhythm: Irregular ventricular rhythm; regular atrial rhythm
Rate: Atrial: 75; ventricular: 50
P waves: Sinus P waves are present
PR interval: Progresses from 0.26 to 0.40 seconds
QRS: 0.06 to 0.08 seconds
Rhythm interpretation: Second-degree AV block, Mobitz I; ST depression is present

Strip 8-83
Rhythm: Regular
Rate: 107
P waves: Inverted before each QRS
PR interval: 0.08 seconds
QRS: 0.08–0.10 seconds
Rhythm interpretation: Junctional tachycardia

Strip 8-84
Rhythm: There are two separate rhythms, both regular
Rate: 79 (1st rhythm); 84 (2nd rhythm)
P waves: Sinus (1st rhythm); inverted (2nd rhythm)
PR interval: 0.14–0.16 seconds (1st rhythm); 0.08 seconds (2nd rhythm)
QRS: 0.06–0.08 seconds (both rhythms)
Rhythm interpretation: Normal sinus rhythm changing to accelerated junctional rhythm

Strip 8-85
Rhythm: Regular atrial and ventricular rhythm
Rate: Atrial: 79; ventricular: 31
P waves: Sinus P waves present; bear no relationship to QRS; hidden in QRS complexes and T waves
PR interval: Varies greatly
QRS: 0.12 seconds
Rhythm interpretation: Third-degree AV block

Strip 8-86
Rhythm: Regular
Rate: 60
P waves: Sinus P waves present
PR interval: 0.24 seconds
QRS: 0.08 seconds
Rhythm interpretation: Normal sinus rhythm with first-degree AV block; ST segment depression and T wave inversion are present

Strip 8-87
Rhythm: Regular atrial and ventricular rhythm
Rate: Atrial: 88; ventricular: 33
P waves: Sinus P waves present—bear no relationship to QRS (found hidden in QRS and T waves)
PR interval: Varies greatly
QRS: 0.12–0.14 seconds
Rhythm interpretation: Third-degree AV block

Strip 8-88
Rhythm: Basic rhythm regular; irregular with premature and escape beats
Rate: Basic rate is 60
P waves: Sinus P waves with basic rhythm; pointed P wave with atrial beat and inverted P wave with junctional beats
PR interval: 0.12–0.14 seconds (basic rhythm); 0.14 seconds (atrial beat); 0.08–0.10 seconds (junctional beats)
QRS: 0.06 to 0.08 seconds
Rhythm interpretation: Normal sinus rhythm with one PJC (3rd complex), one atrial escape beat (4th complex), and one junctional escape beat (5th complex)

Strip 8-89
Rhythm: Irregular ventricular rhythm; regular atrial rhythm
Rate: Atrial, 65; ventricular, 50
P waves: Sinus P waves present
PR interval: Progresses from 0.32 to 0.40 seconds
QRS: 0.08–0.10 seconds
Rhythm interpretation: Second-degree AV block, Mobitz I

Strip 8-90
Rhythm: Regular
Rate: 107
P waves: Inverted before each QRS
PR interval: 0.08 to 0.10 seconds
QRS: 0.06 seconds
Rhythm interpretation: Junctional tachycardia

Strip 8-91
Rhythm: Basic rhythm regular; irregular with nonconducted PAC
Rate: Basic rhythm rate 88
P waves: Sinus with basic rhythm; premature pointed P wave deforming T wave following 6th QRS; pointed abnormal P wave with 7th QRS
PR interval: 0.22–0.24 seconds (remains constant)
QRS: 0.06–0.08 seconds
Rhythm interpretation: Normal sinus rhythm with First-Degree AV Block; Nonconducted PAC (following 6th QRS); an atrial escape beat (7th complex) occurs during the pause following the nonconducted PAC (note different P wave when compared with that of underlying rhythm

Strip 8-92
Rhythm: Irregular ventricular rhythm; regular atrial rhythm
Rate: Atrial: 75; ventricular: 30
P waves: Sinus P waves present (two to three P waves before each QRS)
PR interval: 0.16 seconds (remains constant)
QRS: 0.12 seconds
Rhythm interpretation: Second-degree AV block, Mobitz II; ST segment depression is present

Strip 8-93
Rhythm: Regular
Rate: 65
P waves: Inverted before each QRS
PR interval: 0.08–0.10 seconds
QRS: 0.06 seconds
Rhythm interpretation: Accelerated junctional rhythm; ST segment elevation is present

Strip 8-94
Rhythm: Regular with basic rhythm; irregular with PJCs
Rate: Basic rhythm rate 72
P waves: Sinus P waves with basic rhythm; inverted P waves with PJCs
PR interval: 0.14 seconds (basic rhythm); 0.08 seconds (PJCs)
QRS: 0.08 seconds
Rhythm interpretation: Normal sinus rhythm with 2 PJCs (4th and 6th complex)

Strip 8-95
Rhythm: Regular atrial and ventricular rhythm
Rate: Atrial: 90; ventricular: 45
P waves: Two sinus P waves before each QRS complex
PR interval: 0.16 seconds (remains constant)
QRS: 0.12 seconds
Rhythm interpretation: Second-degree AV block Mobitz II. Clinical correlation is suggested to diagnose Mobitz II when 2:1 conduction is present. T wave inversion is present

Strip 8-96
Rhythm: Regular atrial rhythm; irregular ventricular rhythm
Rate: Atrial: 75 Ventricular: 70
P waves: Sinus P waves present
PR interval: Lengthens from 0.32–0.40 seconds
QRS: 0.04–0.06 seconds
Rhythm interpretation: Second-degree AV block, Mobitz I

Strip 8-97
Rhythm: Regular
Rate: 40
P waves: Hidden in QRS
PR interval: Not measurable
QRS: 0.10 seconds
Rhythm interpretation: Junctional rhythm; ST segment elevation is present

Strip 8-98
Rhythm: Regular atrial and ventricular rhythm
Rate: Atrial; 80; Ventricular: 40
P waves: 2 sinus P waves to each QRS
PR interval: 0.22–0.24 seconds (remain constant)
QRS: 0.10 seconds
Rhythm interpretation: Second-degree AV block, Mobitz II; clinical correlation is suggested to diagnose Mobitz II when 2:1 conduction is present; ST segment elevation is present

Strip 8-99
Rhythm: Basic rhythm regular; irregular with PJC
Rate: Basic rhythm rate 84
P waves: Sinus P waves with basic rhythm; inverted P waves with PJC
PR interval: 0.12 seconds (basic rhythm); 0.08 seconds (PJC)
QRS: 0.06 to 0.08 seconds
Rhythm interpretation: Normal sinus rhythm with one PJC

Strip 9-1
Rhythm: Regular
Rate: 167
P waves: Absent
PR interval: Not measurable
QRS: 0.12–0.14 seconds
Rhythm interpretation: Ventricular tachycardia

Strip 9-2
Rhythm: Regular
Rate: 65
P waves: Sinus; notched P waves usually indicate left atrial hypertrophy
PR interval: 0.14–0.16 seconds
QRS: 0.12–0.14 seconds
Rhythm interpretation: Normal sinus rhythm with bundle branch block; an elevated ST segment is present

Strip 9-3
Rhythm: Basic rhythm regular; irregular with PVCs
Rate: Basic rhythm rate 75
P waves: Sinus P waves with basic rhythm; no P waves associated with PVCs; sinus P waves can be seen after the PVCs
PR interval: 0.18 to 0.20 seconds
QRS: 0.08 seconds (basic rhythm); 0.12 seconds (PVCs)
Rhythm interpretation: Normal sinus rhythm with two unifocal PVCs (5th complex and 8th complex)

Strip 9-4
Rhythm: Irregular
Rate: 30
P waves: Absent
PR interval: Not measurable
QRS: 0.16 seconds
Rhythm interpretation: Idioventricular rhythm

Strip 9-5
Rhythm: 0
Rate: Not measurable
P waves: Chaotic wave deflection of varying height, size, and shape
PR interval: Not measurable
QRS: Absent
Rhythm interpretation: Ventricular fibrillation

Strip 9-6
Rhythm: Basic rhythm regular; irregular with PVCs
Rate: Basic rhythm 100
P waves: Sinus P waves present with basic rhythm
PR interval: 0.14 to 0.16 seconds (basic rhythm)
QRS: 0.08 seconds (basic rhythm); 0.12 seconds (PVCs)
Rhythm interpretation: Normal sinus rhythm with unifocal PVCs in a bigeminal pattern (2nd, 4th, 6th, 8th complex)

Strip 9-7
Rhythm: First rhythm (cannot be determined for sure; only one cardiac cycle); second rhythm irregular
Rate: First rhythm 54; second rhythm 80
P waves: Sinus P waves present with basic rhythm
PR interval: 0.16 seconds (basic rhythm)
QRS: 0.08 seconds (basic rhythm); 0.12 seconds (ventricular beats)
Rhythm interpretation: Sinus bradycardia changing to accelerated idioventricular rhythm; ST segment depression is present (basic rhythm)

Strip 9-8
Rhythm: 1st rhythm: irregular; 2nd rhythm: irregular
Rate: 1st rhythm: 60; 2nd rhythm: about 200
P waves: 1st rhythm: fibrillation waves; 2nd rhythm: none identified
PR interval: Not measurable
QRS: 1st rhythm: 0.06–0.08 seconds; 2nd rhythm: 0.12–0.14 seconds
Rhythm interpretation: Atrial fibrillation with burst of ventricular tachycardia; ST segment depression is noted with basic rhythm

Strip 9-9
Rhythm: Ventricular rhythm regular; atrial rhythm slightly irregular
Rate: Atrial, about 36; ventricular, 38
P waves: Sinus P waves present; bear no relationship to QRS
PR interval: Varies
QRS: 0.12 seconds
Rhythm interpretation: Third-degree AV block changing to ventricular standstill, ST segment elevation is present

Strip 9-10
Rhythm: Basic rhythm regular; irregular with PVCs
Rate: Basic rhythm rate 79
P waves: Sinus P waves present with basic rhythm
PR interval: 0.16 seconds
QRS: 0.06 seconds (basic rhythm); 0.14 to 0.16 seconds (PVCs)
Rhythm interpretation: Normal sinus rhythm with paired unifocal PVCs (6th and 7th complex)

Strip 9-11
Rhythm: Regular
Rate: 42
P waves: Absent
PR interval: Not measurable
QRS: 0.12 to 0.14 seconds
Rhythm interpretation: Idioventricular rhythm

Strip 9-12
Rhythm: Regular
Rate: 125
P waves: Sinus
PR interval: 0.12 seconds
QRS: 0.12 seconds
Rhythm interpretation: Sinus tachycardia with bundle branch block; an elevated ST segment is present

Strip 9-13
Rhythm: Cannot be determined
Rate: 0
P waves: None identified
PR interval: Not measurable
QRS: 0.12 seconds
Rhythm interpretation: One QRS complex followed by ventricular standstill

Strip 9-14
Rhythm: Regular
Rate: 214
P waves: None identified
PR interval: Not measurable
QRS: 0.16 seconds
Rhythm interpretation: Ventricular tachycardia

Strip 9-15
Rhythm: Basic rhythm regular
Rate: Basic rhythm 50
P waves: Sinus in basic rhythm
PR interval: 0.16–0.18 seconds
QRS: 0.08 seconds (basic rhythm) 0.14 seconds (PVC)
Rhythm interpretation: Sinus bradycardia with one PVC (3rd complex); ST segment depression is present

Strip 9-16
Rhythm: Chaotic
Rate: 0
P waves: Absent; wave deflections are irregular and vary in height, size, and shape
PR interval: Not measurable
QRS: Absent
Rhythm interpretation: Ventricular fibrillation

Strip 9-17
Rhythm: Chaotic
Rate: 0
P waves: Wave deflections are chaotic and vary in height, size, and shape
PR interval: Not measurable
QRS: Absent
Rhythm interpretation: Ventricular fibrillation followed by electrical shock and return to ventricular fibrillation

Strip 9-18
Rhythm: Regular
Rate: 107
P waves: Sinus
PR interval: 0.16–0.18 seconds
QRS: 0.12 seconds
Rhythm interpretation: Sinus tachycardia with bundle branch block

Strip 9-19
Rhythm: Irregular
Rate: Atrial: 300; Ventricular: 50
P waves: Flutter waves before each QRS
PR interval: Not measurable
QRS: 0.06–0.08 seconds (basic rhythm) 0.12 seconds (PVC)
Rhythm interpretation: Atrial flutter with variable AV conduction and 1 PVC (5th complex)

Strip 9-20
Rhythm: Regular atrial rhythm
Rate: Atrial, 136; ventricular, 0 (no QRS complexes)
P waves: Sinus P waves are present
PR interval: Not measurable
QRS: Absent
Rhythm interpretation: Ventricular standstill

Strip 9-21
Rhythm: Irregular
Rate: 40
P waves: Absent
PR interval: Not measurable
QRS: 0.16 seconds
Rhythm interpretation: Idioventricular rhythm

Strip 9-22
Rhythm: Chaotic
Rate: 0 (no QRS complexes)
P waves: None identified
PR interval: No measurable
QRS: Absent
Rhythm interpretation: Ventricular fibrillation

Strip 9-23
Rhythm: Regular
Rate: 100
P waves: Absent
PR interval: Not measurable
QRS: 0.12 seconds
Rhythm interpretation: Accelerated idioventricular rhythm

Strip 9-24
Rhythm: Irregular
Rate: 60
P waves: Fibrillation waves present
PR interval: Not measurable
QRS: 0.12 seconds
Rhythm interpretation: Atrial fibrillation with bundle branch block; ST segment depression and T wave inversion are present

Strip 9-25
Rhythm: Basic rhythm regular
Rate: 1st rhythm (100); 2nd rhythm (188)
P waves: Sinus with basic rhythm
PR interval: 0.14–0.16 seconds
QRS: 0.08 seconds (basic rhythm); 0.12–0.16 seconds (ventricular beats)
Rhythm interpretation: Normal sinus rhythm with burst of ventricular tachycardia and paired PVCs

Strip 9-26
Rhythm: Basic rhythm regular; irregular with PVC
Rate: Basic rhythm rate 107
P waves: Sinus with basic rhythm
PR interval: 0.18–0.20 seconds
QRS: 0.08–0.10 seconds (basic rhythm); 0.16 seconds (PVC)
Rhythm interpretation: Sinus tachycardia with 1 PVC (R-on-T pattern); an elevated ST segment is present

Strip 9-27
Rhythm: Regular
Rate: 43
P waves: Absent
PR interval: Not measurable
QRS: 0.16 to 0.18 seconds
Rhythm interpretation: Idioventricular rhythm

Strip 9-28
Rhythm: Regular
Rate: 250
P waves: None identified
PR interval: Not measurable
QRS: 0.12–0.16 seconds (QRS complexes change in polarity from negative to positive across strip)
Rhythm interpretation: Ventricular tachycardia (torsades de pointes)

Strip 9-29
Rhythm: Regular
Rate: 84
P waves: None identified
PR interval: Not measurable
QRS: 0.14–0.16 seconds
Rhythm interpretation: Accelerated idioventricular rhythm

Strip 9-30
Rhythm: Chaotic
Rate: 0
P waves: Absent; wave deflections are irregular and vary in height, size, and shape
PR interval: Not measurable
QRS: Absent
Rhythm interpretation: Ventricular fibrillation

Strip 9-31
Rhythm: Basic rhythm regular; irregular with PVCs
Rate: Basic rhythm rate 115
P waves: Sinus P waves with basic rhythm
PR interval: 0.14 to 0.16 seconds
QRS: 0.04 to 0.06 seconds (basic rhythm); 0.12 seconds (PVCs)
Rhythm interpretation: Sinus tachycardia with two unifocal PVCs (4th complex and 12th complex)

Strip 9-32
Rhythm: Basic rhythm regular; irregular with PVCs
Rate: Basic rhythm rate 125
P waves: Sinus with basic rhythm
PR interval: 0.14–0.16 seconds
QRS: 0.08–0.10 seconds (basic rhythm); 0.12 seconds (PVCs)
Rhythm interpretation: Sinus tachycardia with multifocal paired PVCs (8th and 9th complex)

Strip 9-33

Rhythm: Basic rhythm regular
Rate: Basic rate 37
P waves: Sinus with basic rhythm
PR interval: 0.14–0.16 seconds
QRS: 0.06–0.08 seconds (basic rhythm); 0.12 seconds (PVC)
Rhythm interpretation: Sinus bradycardia with 1 ventricular escape beat (3rd complex)

Strip 9-34

Rhythm: 1st rhythm regular; 2nd rhythm regular
Rate: 1st rhythm (72); 2nd rhythm (150)
P waves: Sinus with basic rhythm
PR interval: 0.18–0.20 seconds
QRS: 0.08 seconds (basic rhythm); 0.12 seconds (ventricular beats)
Rhythm interpretation: Normal sinus rhythm with burst of ventricular tachycardia; an inverted T wave is present in basic rhythm

Strip 9-35

Rhythm: Chaotic
Rate: 0
P waves: Absent; wave deflections vary in height, size, and shape
PR interval: Not measurable
QRS: Absent
Rhythm interpretation: Ventricular fibrillation

Strip 9-36

Rhythm: Irregular
Rate: About 30
P waves: Absent
PR interval: Not measurable
QRS: 0.12 seconds
Rhythm interpretation: Idioventricular rhythm; ST segment elevation is present

Strip 9-37

Rhythm: Not measurable
Rate: Not measurable (1 complex present)
P waves: None identified
PR interval: Not measurable
QRS: 0.28 seconds or wider
Rhythm interpretation: One ventricular complex followed by ventricular standstill

Strip 9-38

Rhythm: Regular
Rate: 84
P waves: None identified
PR interval: Not measurable
QRS: 0.14–0.16 seconds
Rhythm interpretation: Accelerated idioventricular rhythm

Strip 9-39

Rhythm: Basic rhythm regular
Rate: Basic rhythm rate 115
P waves: Inverted before each QRS in basic rhythm
PR interval: 0.08 seconds (basic rhythm)
QRS: 0.06 to 0.08 seconds (basic rhythm); 0.12 seconds (PVC)
Rhythm interpretation: Junctional tachycardia with one PVC (10th complex)

Strip 9-40

Rhythm: Regular atrial rhythm
Rate: Atrial, 30; ventricular, 0 (no QRS complexes)
P waves: Sinus P waves present
PR interval: No measurable
QRS: Absent
Rhythm interpretation: Ventricular standstill

Strip 9-41

Rhythm: Basic rhythm regular; irregular with PVCs
Rate: Basic rhythm rate 65
P waves: Sinus P waves present with basic rhythm
PR interval: 0.16 seconds
QRS: 0.06 to 0.08 seconds (basic rhythm); 0.12 seconds (PVC)
Rhythm interpretation: Normal sinus rhythm with two unifocal PVCs (3rd and 6th complex); ST segment depression is present

Strip 9-42

Rhythm: Basic rhythm irregular
Rate: Basic rhythm rate 100
P waves: Basic rhythm (fibrillation waves)
PR interval: Not measurable
QRS: 0.08 seconds (basic rhythm); 0.12 seconds (PVCs)
Rhythm interpretation: Atrial fibrillation with a burst of ventricular tachycardia

Strip 9-43

Rhythm: 1st rhythm (regular); 2nd rhythm (irregular)
Rate: 1st rhythm (100); 2nd rhythm (100)
P waves: Sinus with basic rhythm
PR interval: 0.12 seconds
QRS: 1st rhythm (0.12–0.14 seconds); 2nd rhythm (0.12 seconds)
Rhythm interpretation: Normal sinus rhythm with bundle branch block with transient episode of accelerated idioventricular rhythm

Strip 9-44
Rhythm: First rhythm (cannot be determined for sure; only one cardiac cycle present); second rhythm (regular)
Rate: First rhythm 50; second rhythm 41
P waves: Sinus P waves with first rhythm
PR interval: 0.12 seconds (first rhythm)
QRS: 0.06 to 0.08 seconds (first rhythm); 0.12 to 0.14 seconds (second rhythm)
Rhythm interpretation: Sinus bradycardia changing to idioventricular rhythm; a U wave is present

Strip 9-45
Rhythm: Regular
Rate: 214
P waves: Not identified
PR interval: Not measurable
QRS: 0.16–0.18 seconds or wider
Rhythm interpretation: Ventricular tachycardia

Strip 9-46
Rhythm: Basic rhythm slightly irregular; irregular with ventricular beats
Rate: Basic rhythm is about 58
P waves: Sinus P waves with basic rhythm
PR interval: 0.20 seconds
QRS: 0.06 seconds (basic rhythm); 0.16 seconds (1st ventricular beat); 0.12 seconds (2nd ventricular beat)
Rhythm interpretation: Sinus bradycardia, with one PVC (4th complex) and 1 ventricular escape beat (5th complex); ST segment depression is present

Strip 9-47
Rhythm: Basic rhythm regular; irregular with PVC
Rate: Basic rhythm rate 94
P waves: Sinus with basic rhythm
PR interval: 0.20 seconds
QRS: 0.08 seconds (basic rhythm); 0.12 seconds (PVC)
Rhythm interpretation: Normal sinus rhythm with 1 PVC (5th complex)

Strip 9-48
Rhythm: Not measurable
Rate: Not measurable (1 complex present)
P waves: None identified
PR interval: Not measurable
QRS: 0.12 seconds
Rhythm interpretation: 1 ventricular complex followed by ventricular standstill

Strip 9-49
Rhythm: Regular
Rate: 56
P waves: Sinus P waves present
PR interval: 0.12 to 0.16 seconds
QRS: 0.12 seconds
Rhythm interpretation: Sinus bradycardia with bundle branch block; ST segment depression is present

Strip 9-50
Rhythm: Regular
Rate: 188
P waves: Not identified
PR interval: Not measurable
QRS: 0.12 seconds
Rhythm interpretation: Ventricular tachycardia

Strip 9-51
Rhythm: Regular atrial rhythm; irregular ventricular rhythm
Rate: Atrial, 58; ventricular, about 40
P waves: Sinus P waves present
PR interval: Progresses from 0.30 to 0.36 seconds
QRS: 0.08 seconds (basic rhythm); 0.12 seconds (escape beat)
Rhythm interpretation: Second-degree AV block, Mobitz I with one ventricular escape beat

Strip 9-52
Rhythm: 1st rhythm regular; 2nd rhythm regular
Rate: 1st rhythm: 72; 2nd rhythm: 72
P waves: Sinus in 1st rhythm
PR interval: 0.12–0.14 seconds (1st rhythm)
QRS: 0.08 seconds (1st rhythm); 0.12–0.14 seconds (2nd rhythm)
Rhythm interpretation: Normal sinus rhythm with a transient episode of accelerated idioventricular rhythm

Strip 9-53
Rhythm: Slightly irregular atrial rhythm
Rate: Atrial: about 40 ventricular: 0 (no QRS complexes)
P waves: Sinus P waves present
PR interval: Not measurable
QRS: Absent
Rhythm interpretation: Ventricular standstill

Strip 9-54

Rhythm: Regular
Rate: 84
P waves: Sinus
PR interval: 0.16 seconds
QRS: 0.12–0.14 seconds
Rhythm interpretation: Normal sinus rhythm with bundle branch block; a depressed ST segment is present

Strip 9-55

Rhythm: Regular
Rate: 41
P waves: Absent
PR interval: Not measurable
QRS: 0.16 seconds
Rhythm interpretation: Idioventricular rhythm

Strip 9-56

Rhythm: Regular
Rate: 75
P waves: Sinus P waves present
PR interval: 0.12 seconds
QRS: 0.16–0.18 seconds
Rhythm interpretation: Normal sinus rhythm with bundle branch block. T wave inversion is present

Strip 9-57

Rhythm: Basic rhythm regular; irregular with PVCs
Rate: Basic rhythm rate 72
P waves: Sinus with basic rhythm
PR interval: 0.12 seconds
QRS: 0.08 seconds (basic rhythm); 0.12–0.14 seconds (PVCs)
Rhythm interpretation: Normal sinus rhythm with unifocal PVCs (4th, 8th complex) in a quadrigeminal pattern

Strip 9-58

Rhythm: Atrial: regular P waves; Ventricular: not measurable—only 1 QRS complex present
Rate: Atrial: 29; Ventricular: not measurable—only 1 QRS complex
P waves: Sinus P waves present
PR interval: Not measurable
QRS: 0.08 seconds
Rhythm interpretation: One QRS complex followed by ventricular standstill

Strip 9-59

Rhythm: Chaotic
Rate: 0
P waves: Absent; wave deflections are irregular and chaotic and vary in size, shape, height
PR interval: Not measurable
QRS: Absent
Rhythm interpretation: Ventricular fibrillation

Strip 9-60

Rhythm: Not measurable (only 1 QRS)
Rate: Not measurable (only 1 QRS)
P waves: None identified
PR interval: Not measurable
QRS: 0.12 seconds or greater
Rhythm interpretation: One QRS complex followed by ventricular standstill

Strip 9-61

Rhythm: Regular (first rhythm); regular (second rhythm)
Rate: 100 (first rhythm); 100 (second rhythm)
P waves: Sinus P waves with first rhythm; no P waves with second rhythm
PR interval: 0.14 to 0.16 seconds (first rhythm)
QRS: 0.06 to 0.08 seconds (first rhythm); 0.12 seconds (second rhythm)
Rhythm interpretation: Normal sinus rhythm changing to accelerated idioventricular rhythm

Strip 9-62

Rhythm: Regular
Rate: 40
P waves: Absent
PR interval: Not measurable
QRS: 0.16 seconds
Rhythm interpretation: Idioventricular rhythm

Strip 9-63

Rhythm: Regular
Rate: 167
P waves: Not identified
PR interval: Not measurable
QRS: 0.16–0.18 seconds
Rhythm interpretation: Ventricular tachycardia

Strip 9-64

Rhythm: Regular
Rate: 88
P waves: Sinus
PR interval: 0.22–0.24 seconds
QRS: 0.12 seconds
Rhythm interpretation: Normal sinus rhythm with bundle branch block and first-degree AV block

Strip 9-65
Rhythm: Irregular
Rate: Basic rhythm rate 80
P waves: Fibrillation waves present
PR interval: Not measurable
QRS: 0.06–0.08 seconds (basic rhythm); 0.12
seconds (PVCs)
Rhythm interpretation: Atrial fibrillation with
paired PVCs

Strip 9-66
Rhythm: Basic rhythm regular
Rate: Basic rhythm rate 84
P waves: Sinus P waves present
PR interval: 0.24 seconds
QRS: 0.08 seconds
Rhythm interpretation: Normal sinus rhythm with
first-degree AV block changing to ventricular standstill

Strip 9-67
Rhythm: Chaotic
Rate: 0
P waves: None identified
PR interval: Not measurable
QRS: Absent
Rhythm interpretation: Ventricular fibrillation

Strip 9-68
Rhythm: Regular
Rate: 167
P waves: None identified
PR interval: Not measurable
QRS: 0.14–0.16 seconds
Rhythm interpretation: Ventricular tachycardia

Strip 9-69
Rhythm: 1st rhythm regular; 2nd rhythm slightly
irregular
Rate: 1st rhythm (115); 2nd rhythm (about 214)
P waves: Sinus in first rhythm; none identified in
2nd rhythm
PR interval: 0.12–0.14 seconds (1st rhythm)
QRS: 0.10 seconds (1st rhythm); 0.12–0.16 seconds
(2nd rhythm)
Rhythm interpretation: Sinus tachycardia with
burst of ventricular tachycardia returning to sinus
tachycardia; an inverted T wave is present

Strip 9-70
Rhythm: Regular
Rate: 40
P waves: Absent
PR interval: Not measurable
QRS: 0.16 seconds
Rhythm interpretation: Idioventricular rhythm

Strip 9-71
Rhythm: Regular
Rate: 100
P waves: Absent
PR interval: Not measurable
QRS: 0.12 seconds
Rhythm interpretation: Accelerated idioventricular
rhythm

Strip 9-72
Rhythm: 0 (only 1 QRS complex)
Rate: 0 (only 1 QRS complex)
P waves: None identified
PR interval: Not measurable
QRS: 0.24–0.26 seconds
Rhythm interpretation: One QRS complex followed
by ventricular standstill

Strip 9-73
Rhythm: Regular
Rate: 188
P waves: Not identified
PR interval: Not measurable
QRS: 0.16–0.20 seconds or wider
Rhythm interpretation: Ventricular tachycardia
followed by electrical shock and return to
ventricular tachycardia

Strip 9-74
Rhythm: Basic rhythm regular; irregular with PVC
Rate: Basic rhythm rate 100
P waves: Sinus P waves with basic rhythm
PR interval: 0.14 to 0.16 seconds
QRS: 0.08 seconds (basic rhythm); 0.12 seconds
(PVC)
Rhythm interpretation: Normal sinus rhythm with
one PVC (5th complex)

Strip 9-75
Rhythm: Regular
Rate: 50
P waves: Sinus
PR interval: 0.16–0.18 seconds
QRS: 0.12–0.14 seconds
Rhythm interpretation: Sinus bradycardia with
bundle branch block

Strip 9-76
Rhythm: 0
Rate: 0 (no QRS complexes)
P waves: Sinus P waves present
PR interval: Not measurable
QRS: Absent
Rhythm interpretation: Ventricular standstill

Strip 9-77
Rhythm: Regular
Rate: 41
P waves: Absent
PR interval: Not measurable
QRS: 0.12 seconds
Rhythm interpretation: Idioventricular rhythm

Strip 9-78
Rhythm: 0 (only 1 QRS complex)
Rate: 0 (only 1 QRS complex)
P waves: None identified
PR interval: Not measurable
QRS: 0.14 seconds
Rhythm interpretation: One ventricular complex
followed by ventricular standstill

Strip 9-79
Rhythm: 0
Rate: 0
P waves: Absent; wave deflections are chaotic and
vary in height, size, and shape
PR interval: Not measurable
QRS: Absent
Rhythm interpretation: Ventricular fibrillation
changing to ventricular standstill

Strip 9-80
Rhythm: First rhythm regular; second rhythm
regular
Rate: 94 (first rhythm); 75 (second rhythm)
P waves: Sinus P waves present with first rhythm
PR interval: 0.16 seconds
QRS: 0.12 seconds (first rhythm); 0.12 seconds
(second rhythm)
Rhythm interpretation: Normal sinus rhythm with
bundle branch block changing to accelerated
idioventricular rhythm and back to NSR; T wave
inversion is present

Strip 9-81
Rhythm: Regular atrial rhythm; ventricular rhythm
cannot be determined for sure (only one cardiac
cycle)
Rate: Atrial: 94; Ventricular: 40
P waves: Sinus P waves present; bear no
relationship to QRS
PR interval: Varies greatly
QRS: 0.14 seconds
Rhythm interpretation: Third-degree AV block
changing to ventricular standstill

Strip 9-82
Rhythm: Regular
Rate: 72
P waves: Sinus P waves are present
PR interval: 0.16 seconds
QRS: 0.12 seconds
Rhythm interpretation: Normal sinus rhythm with
bundle branch block

Strip 9-83
Rhythm: First rhythm regular; second rhythm
irregular, chaotic
Rate: 214 (first rhythm)
P waves: None identified
PR interval: Not measurable
QRS: 0.16 to 0.18 seconds (first rhythm)
Rhythm interpretation: Ventricular tachycardia
changing to ventricular fibrillation

Strip 9-84
Rhythm: Regular
Rate: 32
P waves: Absent
PR interval: Not measurable
QRS: 0.20 seconds
Rhythm interpretation: Idioventricular rhythm

Strip 9-85
Rhythm: Regular with basic rhythm; irregular with
PVCs
Rate: Basic rhythm rate 125
P waves: Sinus with basic rhythm
PR interval: 0.12 seconds
QRS: 0.06–0.08 seconds (basic rhythm); 0.12
seconds (PVCs)
Rhythm interpretation: Sinus tachycardia with
multifocal paired PVCs (8th, 9th complexes)

Strip 9-86
Rhythm: P waves are regular; (no QRS complexes)
Rate: Atrial: 52; Ventricular: 0
P waves: Sinus P waves present
PR interval: Not measurable
QRS: Absent
Rhythm interpretation: Ventricular standstill

Strip 9-87
Rhythm: First rhythm regular; second rhythm irregular
Rate: 68 (first rhythm); about 80 (second rhythm)
P waves: Sinus P waves with first rhythm
PR interval: 0.12 to 0.14 seconds
QRS: 0.08 seconds (first rhythm); 0.12 seconds
(second rhythm)
Rhythm interpretation: Normal sinus rhythm
changing to accelerated idioventricular rhythm

Strip 9-88
Rhythm: Regular
Rate: 167
P waves: Not identified
PR interval: Not measurable
QRS: 0.16 to 0.20 seconds
Rhythm interpretation: Ventricular tachycardia
(torsades de pointes)

Strip 9-89
Rhythm: Basic rhythm regular; irregular with PVCs
Rate: Basic rhythm rate 125
P waves: Sinus with basic rhythm
PR interval: 0.12 seconds
QRS: 0.06–0.08 seconds (basic rhythm); 0.12
seconds (PVCs)
Rhythm interpretation: Sinus tachycardia with
paired PVCs (7th and 8th complexes)

Strip 9-90
Rhythm: Regular atrial rhythm
Rate: Atrial: 72; ventricular: 0 (no QRS complexes)
P waves: Sinus P waves present
PR interval: Not measurable
QRS: Absent
Rhythm interpretation: Ventricular standstill

Strip 9-91
Rhythm: Regular
Rate: 188
P waves: Sinus P waves seen between QRS
complexes but not associated with QRS
PR interval: Not measurable
QRS: 0.18–0.20 seconds or wider
Rhythm interpretation: Ventricular tachycardia

Strip 9-92
Rhythm: Chaotic
Rate: 0
P waves: Wave deflections chaotic—vary in size,
shape, direction
PR interval: Not measurable
QRS: Absent
Rhythm interpretation: Ventricular fibrillation; 60-
cycle (electrical) interference is noted on baseline

Strip 9-93
Rhythm: Regular
Rate: 28
P waves: None
PR interval: Not measurable
QRS: 0.20 seconds or wider
Rhythm interpretation: Idioventricular rhythm

Strip 9-94
Rhythm: Regular
Rate: 79
P waves: Sinus P waves present
PR interval: 0.18 to 0.20 seconds
QRS: 0.12 seconds
Rhythm interpretation: Normal sinus rhythm with
bundle branch block

Strip 9-95
Rhythm: Basic rhythm regular
Rate: Basic rhythm rate 68
P waves: Sinus P waves with basic rhythm
PR interval: 0.16 to 0.18 seconds
QRS: 0.06 to 0.08 seconds
Rhythm interpretation: Normal sinus rhythm with
one interpolated PVC (7th complex). Interpolated
PVCs are sandwiched between two sinus beats and
have no compensatory pause. ST segment
depression and T wave inversion are present

Strip 9-96
Rhythm: Basic rhythm regular; irregular with PVCs
Rate: Basic rhythm rate 72
P waves: Sinus P waves are present with basic
rhythm
PR interval: 0.12 to 0.14 seconds
QRS: 0.08 seconds (basic rhythm); 0.12–0.14
seconds (PVCs)
Rhythm interpretation: Normal sinus rhythm with
PVCs in a trigeminal pattern

Strip 10-1
Automatic interval rate: 72
Analysis: The first four beats are paced beats
followed by one patient beat and three paced beats
Interpretation: Normal pacemaker function

Strip 10-2
Automatic interval rate: 84
Analysis: The first three beats are paced beats,
followed by two patient beats, a pacer spike
occuring too early, a patient beat, a fusion beat, and
two paced beats
Interpretation: Undersensing malfunction

Strip 10-3
Automatic interval rate: 72
Analysis: All beats are pacemaker-induced
Interpretation: Pacemaker rhythm

Strip 10-4

Automatic interval rate: 68

Analysis: First two beats are paced followed by a failure to capture spike, paced beat, failure to capture spike, pt beat, paced beat, failure to capture spike, and patient beat

Interpretation: Frequent failure to capture

Strip 10-5

Automatic interval rate: 72

Analysis: No patient or paced beats are seen

Interpretation: Failure to capture in the presence of ventricular standstill (asystole)

Strip 10-6

Automatic interval rate: 72

Analysis: First five beats are patient beats followed by two paced beats, two patient beats and one paced beat

Interpretation: Normal pacemaker function: Underlying rhythm is NSR with frequent PVCs (multifocal)

Strip 10-7

Automatic interval rate: 50

Analysis: The first two beats are pacemaker induced, followed by a pseudofusion beat, two patient beats, and one paced beat

Interpretation: Normal pacemaker function

Strip 10-8

Automatic interval rate: 72

Analysis: All beats are pacemaker-induced

Interpretation: Pacemaker rhythm

Strip 10-9

Automatic interval rate: 63

Analysis: The first two beats are paced beats followed by a pacing spike which occurs on time but doesn't capture, a native beat, three paced beats, and a native beat

Interpretation: Failure to capture

Strip 10-10

Automatic interval rate: 72

Analysis: All beats are pacemaker induced

Interpretation: Pacemaker rhythm

Strip 10-11

Automatic interval rate: 72

Analysis: First three beats are paced beats followed by one patient beat, a pacing spike that occurs too early, one patient beat, a paced beat that occurs too early and 3 paced beats

Interpretation: Undersensing malfunction

Strip 10-12

Automatic interval rate: 72

Analysis: First six beats are patient beats followed by two paced beats and two patient beats

Interpretation: Normal pacemaker function; underlying rhythm is atrial fibrillation

Strip 10-13

Automatic interval rate: 60

Analysis: All beats are pacemaker induced

Interpretation: Pacemaker rhythm

Strip 10-14

Automatic interval rate: 72

Analysis: The first three beats are paced beats followed by two patient beats, and two paced beats, one patient beat, and one paced beat

Interpretation: Normal pacemaker function

Strip 10-15

Automatic interval rate: 84

Analysis: The first three beats are paced beats; when the pacemaker is turned off the underlying rhythm is ventricular standstill. Two paced beats are seen when the pacemaker is turned back on

Interpretation: This strip shows an indication for permanent pacemaker implantation if the underlying rhythm does not resolve

Strip 10-16

Automatic interval rate: 72

Analysis: First two beats are paced beats followed by one patient beat, a pacing spike that occurs on time but doesn't capture, two paced beats, two patient beats and one paced beat

Interpretation: Failure to capture

Strip 10-17

Automatic interval rate: 72

Analysis: The first two beats are paced followed by a fusion beat (note spike in native QRS with decrease in height); two native beats; a spike that occurs too early; a native beat; a spike that occurs too early; a native beat; a paced beat that occurs too early; and a paced beat

Interpretation: Undersensing malfunction (spikes too early following 5th and 6th complex and a paced beat too early following 7th complex)

Strip 10-18

Automatic interval rate: 72

Analysis: The first two beats are patient beats followed by a spike that occurs on time but doesn't capture, a patient beat, and five paced beats

Interpretation: Failure to capture

Strip 10-19
Automatic interval rate: 60
Analysis: First four beats are paced beats followed by one patient beat (PVC) and three paced beats
Interpretation: Normal pacemaker function

Strip 10-20
Automatic interval rate: 72
Analysis: All beats are pacemaker induced
Interpretation: Pacemaker rhythm

Strip 10-21
Automatic interval rate: 72
Analysis: All beats are pacemaker induced
Interpretation: Pacemaker Rhythm

Strip 10-22
Automatic interval rate: Cannot be determined (only one paced beat)
Analysis: One paced beat with rhythm changing to ventricular tachycardia
Interpretation: One paced beat changing to ventricular tachycardia (torsades de pointes)

Strip 10-23
Automatic interval rate: 63
Analysis: The first four beats are paced beats followed by a patient beat (PVC), a pacing spike that occurs too early, a fusion beat, and a paced beat
Interpretation: Undersensing malfunction (pacing spike occurs too early following 5th complex)

Strip 10-24
Automatic interval rate: 72
Analysis: The first beat is paced followed by one failure to capture spike, one patient beat, one failure to capture spike, one patient beat, one paced beat, one failure to capture spike, one patient beat, one failure to capture spike, and one patient beat
Interpretation: Frequent failure to capture

Strip 10-25
Automatic interval rate: 63
Analysis: All beats are pacemaker induced
Interpretation: Pacemaker rhythm

Strip 10-26
Automatic interval rate: 72
Analysis: The first two beats are paced beats followed by one PVC, two paced beats, one pseudofusion beat, one patient beat, and two paced beats
Interpretation: Normal pacemaker function

Strip 10-27
Automatic interval rate: 84
Analysis: The first two beats are paced beats followed by two failure to capture spikes, one paced beat, two failure to capture spikes, two paced beats, and one failure to capture spike
Interpretation: Frequent failure to capture

Strip 10-28
Automatic interval rate: 72
Analysis: The first three beats are paced beats followed by one patient beat, two paced beats, one pseudofusion beat (spike superimposed on R wave), and two paced beats
Interpretation: Normal pacemaker function

Strip 10-29
Automatic interval rate: 72
Analysis: The first two beats are paced beats followed by three patient beats (second a PVC), and three paced beats
Interpretation: Normal pacemaker function; underlying rhythm is atrial fibrillation

Strip 10-30
Automatic interval rate: 65
Analysis: The first two beats are patient beats followed by three pseudofusion beats, and four patient beats
Interpretation: Normal pacemaker function

Strip 10-31
Automatic interval rate: Cannot be determined for sure since there aren't two consecutively paced beats present
Analysis: Strip shows six patient beats and 5 failure to capture spikes. No paced beats are seen
Interpretation: Complete failure to capture

Strip 10-32
Automatic interval rate: 72
Analysis: The first beat is paced followed by one patient beat, one fusion beat, two patient beats (second a PVC), one paced beat that occurs too early, two paced beats, one patient beat (PVC), one paced beat occuring too early, one patient beat (PVC), and a spike occuring too early
Interpretation: Frequent undersensing malfunction; this strip shows a sensing malfunction with capture (sixth and tenth QRS) and without capture (spike after 11th QRS)

Strip 10-33
Automatic interval rate: 65
Analysis: First two beats are paced beats followed by two patient beats, one fusion beat and two paced beats
Interpretation: Normal pacemaker function

Strip 10-34
Automatic interval rate: 72
Analysis: All beats are pacemaker induced
Interpretation: Pacemaker rhythm

Strip 10-35
Automatic interval rate: 56
Analysis: The first two beats are paced beats followed by one patient beat, one paced beat, one patient beat, one paced beat that occurs too early, two paced beats, and one patient beat
Interpretation: Undersensing malfunction

Strip 11-1
Rhythm: Regular
Rate: 107
P waves: Sinus P waves are present
PR interval: 0.12 seconds
QRS: 0.06 to 0.08 seconds
Rhythm interpretation: Sinus tachycardia

Strip 11-2
Rhythm: Regular
Rate: 58
P waves: Sinus P waves are present
PR interval: 0.12 to 0.14 seconds
QRS: 0.12 seconds
Rhythm interpretation: Sinus bradycardia with bundle branch block; ST segment depression is present

Strip 11-3
Rhythm: Regular atrial and ventricular rhythm
Rate: Atrial: 42; Ventricular: 21
P waves: Two sinus P waves to each QRS
PR interval: 0.32 to 0.36 seconds (remain constant)
QRS: 0.12 seconds
Rhythm interpretation: Second-degree AV block, Mobitz II; clinical correlation is suggested to diagnose Mobitz II when 2 : 1 conduction is present; ST segment elevation is present

Strip 11-4
Rhythm: Irregular
Rate: 100
P waves: Fibrillatory waves are present—some flutter waves are seen mixed with the fibrillatory waves
PR interval: Not measurable
QRS: 0.04 seconds
Rhythm interpretation: Atrial fibrillation; ST segment depression is present

Strip 11-5
Rhythm: Regular
Rate: 48
P waves: Hidden in QRS
PR interval: Not measurable
QRS: 0.08 seconds
Rhythm interpretation: Junctional rhythm; ST segment depression is present

Strip 11-6
Rhythm: Regular
Rate: 188
P waves: Hidden in preceding T waves
PR interval: Not measurable
QRS: 0.10 seconds
Rhythm interpretation: Paroxysmal atrial tachycardia

Strip 11-7
Automtic interval rate: 72
Analysis: First four beats are paced followed by two patient beats, one paced beat, and two patient beats
Rhythm interpretation: Normal pacemaker function

Strip 11-8
Rhythm: Regular atrial and ventricular rhythm
Rate: Atrial: 75; Ventricular: 26
P waves: Sinus P waves present—bear no constant relationship to QRS complexes
PR interval: Varies
QRS: 0.14–0.16 seconds
Rhythm interpretation: Third-degree AV block; ST segment elevation is present

Strip 11-9
Rhythm: Regular
Rate: 188
P waves: Not discernible
PR interval: Not discernible
QRS: 0.16 to 0.20 seconds
Rhythm interpretation: Ventricular tachycardia

Strip 11-10
Rhythm: Regular
Rate: 42
P waves: Absent
PR interval: Not measurable
QRS: 0.16 seconds
Rhythm interpretation: Idioventricular rhythm

Strip 11-11
Rhythm: Basic rhythm regular
Rate: Basic rhythm rate 56
P waves: Sinus P waves present (appear notched which may indicate left atrial hypertrophy)
PR interval: 0.16 seconds
QRS: 0.06 seconds (basic rhythm); 0.16 seconds (PVC)
Rhythm interpretation: Sinus bradycardia with one interpolated PVC; ST segment depression is present

Strip 11-12
Rhythm: Regular
Rate: 84
P waves: Inverted before each QRS
PR interval: 0.10 seconds
QRS: 0.06–0.08 seconds
Rhythm interpretation: Accelerated junctional rhythm

Strip 11-13
Rhythm: Regular
Rate: Atrial: 232; Ventricular: 58
P waves: Four flutter waves before each QRS
PR interval: Not measurable
QRS: 0.06–0.08 seconds
Rhythm interpretation: Atrial flutter with 4 : 1 AV conduction

Strip 11-14
Rhythm: Regular
Rate: 88
P waves: Sinus
PR interval: 0.20 seconds
QRS: 0.08–0.10 seconds
Rhythm interpretation: Normal sinus rhythm

Strip 11-15
Rhythm: Regular
Rate: 88
P waves: Absent
PR interval: Not measurable
QRS: 0.14–0.16 seconds
Rhythm interpretation: Accelerated idioventricular rhythm

Strip 11-16
Rhythm: Basic rhythm regular; irregular with pause
Rate: Basic rhythm 75
P waves: Sinus P waves present with basic rhythm; one premature, abnormal P wave with QRS (after 5th QRS)
PR interval: 0.24 to 0.28 seconds
QRS: 0.06 to 0.08 seconds
Rhythm interpretation: Normal sinus rhythm with first-degree AV block and one nonconducted PAC (follows 5th QRS)

Strip 11-17
Rhythm: Regular
Rate: 115
P waves: Sinus P waves are present
PR interval: 0.14 to 0.16 seconds
QRS: 0.06 seconds
Rhythm interpretation: Sinus tachycardia

Strip 11-18
Rhythm: Regular
Rate: 48
P waves: Sinus
PR interval: 0.12 seconds
QRS: 0.08–0.10 seconds
Rhythm interpretation: Sinus bradycardia; ST segment elevation is present

Strip 11-19
Rhythm: Basic rhythm regular; irregular with premature beats
Rate: Basic rhythm rate 72
P waves: Sinus with basic rhythm; inverted with premature beats
PR interval: 0.12–0.14 seconds (basic rhythm); 0.08 seconds (premature beats)
QRS: 0.08 seconds
Rhythm interpretation: Normal sinus rhythm with two premature junctional contractions (4th and 6th complexes)

Strip 11-20
Rhythm: Regular
Rate: 63
P waves: Vary in size, shape, and position
PR interval: 0.12 to 0.14 seconds
QRS: 0.06 to 0.08 seconds
Rhythm interpretation: Wandering atrial pacemaker; ST segment depression is present

Strip 11-21
Rhythm: Chaotic
Rate: 0 (no QRS complexes)
P waves: No P waves; wave deflections are chaotic, irregular and vary in height, size, and shape
PR interval: Not measurable
QRS: Absent
Rhythm interpretation: Ventricular fibrillation

Strip 11-22
Rhythm: Regular
Rate: 107
P waves: Inverted before each QRS
PR interval: 0.08 seconds
QRS: 0.04 to 0.06 seconds
Rhythm interpretation: Junctional tachycardia

Strip 11-23
Rhythm: Irregular atrial rhythm
Rate: Atrial, 40; ventricular, 0
P waves: Sinus P waves are present
PR interval: Not measurable
QRS: Absent
Rhythm interpretation: Ventricular standstill

Strip 11-24
Rhythm: Irregular
Rate: 70
P waves: Sinus
PR interval: 0.44–0.48 seconds
QRS: 0.08–0.10 seconds
Rhythm interpretation: Sinus arrhythmia with first degree AV block; ST segment elevation is present

Strip 11-25
Rhythm: Regular
Rate: 188
P waves: Not discernible
PR interval: Unmeasurable
QRS: 0.16 to 0.20 seconds
Rhythm interpretation: Ventricular tachycardia; ST segment elevation is present

Strip 11-26
Rhythm: Atrial: regular; Ventricular: irregular
Rate: Atrial (72); Ventricular (40)
P waves: Sinus
PR interval: Lengthens from 0.20–0.28 seconds
QRS: 0.04–0.06 seconds
Rhythm interpretation: Second degree AV block, Mobitz I; ST segment depression is present

Strip 11-27
Rhythm: Regular
Rate: 72
P waves: Sinus
PR interval: 0.20 seconds
QRS: 0.08–0.10 seconds
Rhythm interpretation: Normal sinus rhythm; ST segment depression and T wave inversion is present

Strip 11-28
Rhythm: Basic rhythm regular; irregular with pause
Rate: Basic rhythm 72 (rate slows to 63 during first cycle following pause; rate suppression can occur for several cycles following an interruption in the basic rhythm)
P waves: Sinus P waves are present
PR interval: 0.16 to 0.18 seconds
QRS: 0.04 to 0.06 seconds
Rhythm interpretation: Normal sinus rhythm with sinus arrest

Strip 11-29
Rhythm: Basic rhythm regular; irregular with premature beats
Rate: Basic rhythm rate 63
P waves: Sinus with basic rhythm; premature, pointed P wave with premature beat
PR interval: 0.14–0.16 (basic rhythm); 0.12 seconds (Premature beat)
QRS: 0.08 seconds
Rhythm interpretation: Normal sinus rhythm with one PAC (5th complex)

Strip 11-30
Rhythm: Basic rhythm regular; irregular with PVCs
Rate: Basic rhythm rate 72
P waves: Sinus P waves are present
PR interval: 0.12 to 0.14 seconds
QRS: 0.12 seconds (basic rhythm and PVCs)
Rhythm interpretation: Normal sinus rhythm with bundle branch block and paired PVCs; a U wave is present

Strip 11-31
Rhythm: Atrial: regular; Ventricular: regular
Rate: Atrial: 240; Ventricular: 60
P waves: 4 Flutter waves to each QRS
PR interval: Not measurable
QRS: 0.04–0.06 seconds
Rhythm interpretation: Atrial flutter with 4 : 1 AV conduction

Strip 11-32

Rhythm: Basic rhythm regular; irregular with pause
Rate: Basic rhythm rate 54
P waves: Sinus with basic rhythm; no P waves with 4th and 5th complexes
PR interval: 0.18–0.20 seconds (basic rhythm)
QRS: 0.06–0.08 seconds
Rhythm interpretation: Sinus bradycardia with sinus arrest and 2 junctional escape beats during pause

Strip 11-33

Rhythm: Regular
Rate: 25
P waves: None identified
PR interval: Not measurable
QRS: 0.24 seconds or greater
Rhythm interpretation: Idioventricular rhythm

Strip 11-34

Automatic interval rate: 63
Analysis: The first three beats are paced beats followed by a pacing spike that doesn't capture, one patient beat, and 2 paced beats
Rhythm interpretation: Failure to capture

Strip 11-35

Rhythm: Regular
Rate: 84
P waves: Not identified
PR interval: Not measurable
QRS: 0.12–0.14 seconds
Rhythm interpretation: Accelerated idioventricular rhythm

Strip 11-36

Rhythm: Chaotic
Rate: 0
P waves: Absent; wave deflections are chaotic, irregular and vary in size, shape, and height
PR interval: Not measurable
QRS: Absent
Rhythm interpretation: Ventricular fibrillation followed by electrical shock and return to ventricular fibrillation

Strip 11-37

Rhythm: Regular
Rate: 52
P waves: Sinus P waves are present
PR interval: 0.18 to 0.20 seconds
QRS: 0.06 to 0.08 seconds
Rhythm interpretation: Sinus bradycardia; a U wave is present

Strip 11-38

Rhythm: Regular
Rate: 94
P waves: Inverted before each QRS
PR interval: 0.08–0.10 seconds
QRS: 0.08 seconds
rhythm interpretation: Accelerated junctional rhythm; baseline artifact is present

Strip 11-39

Rhythm: Irregular
Rate: 60
P waves: Fibrillatory waves are present
PR interval: Not measurable
QRS: 0.12 seconds
Rhythm interpretation: Atrial fibrillation with bundle branch block; ST segment depression and T wave inversion are present

Strip 11-40

Automatic interval rate: 72
Analysis: All beats are pacemaker induced
Rhythm interpretation: Pacemaker rhythm

Strip 11-41

Rhythm: P waves occur regularly
Rate: Atrial: 88; Ventricular: 0
P waves: P waves present
PR interval: Not measurable
QRS: Absent
Rhythm interpretation: Ventricular standstill

Strip 11-42

Rhythm: Basic rhythm regular; irregular with premature beats
Rate: Basic rhythm rate 63
P waves: Sinus with basic rhythm
PR interval: 0.12–0.14 seconds
QRS: 0.08 seconds (basic rhythm); 0.12–0.16 seconds (PVCs)
Rhythm interpretation: Normal sinus rhythm with paired multifocal PVCs (4th, 5th complexes)

Strip 11-43

Rhythm: Basic rhythm regular; irregular with PAC
Rate: Basic rhythm rate 136
P waves: Sinus with basic rhythm; premature pointed P waves with premature beats
PR interval: 0.16–0.20 seconds
QRS: 0.06–0.08 seconds
Rhythm interpretation: Sinus tachycardia with 2 PACs (4th and 8th complexes)

Strip 11-44
Rhythm: Basic rhythm regular; irregular with pause
Rate: Basic rhythm rate 84—rate slows after pause but returns to basic rate after 4 cycles
P waves: Sinus
PR interval: 0.20 seconds
QRS: 0.08 seconds
Rhythm interpretation: Normal sinus rhythm with sinus arrest; ST segment depression and T wave inversion are present

Strip 11-45
Rhythm: 0
Rate: 0
P waves: No P waves present; pacing spikes seen
PR interval: Not measurable
QRS: No QRS complexes are present
Rhythm interpretation: Failure to capture in presence of ventricular standstill (asystole)

Strip 11-46
Automatic interval rate: 72
Analysis: First four beats are paced beats, followed by one patient beat, a pacing spike that occurs too early, a patient beat, a fusion beat, and two paced beats
Rhythm interpretation: Sensing malfunction

Strip 11-47
Rhythm: Regular
Rate: 42
P waves: Hidden in QRS
PR interval: Not measurable
QRS: 0.08 to 0.10 seconds
Rhythm interpretation: Junctional rhythm

Strip 11-48
Rhythm: Atrial: regular; Ventricular: irregular
Rate: Atrial: 79; Ventricular: 50
P waves: Sinus P waves present
PR interval: Lengthens from 0.20–0.32 seconds
QRS: 0.08–0.10 seconds
Rhythm interpretation: Second degree AV block Mobitz I

Strip 11-49
Rhythm: Basic rhythm regular; irregular with premature beat
Rate: 107
P waves: Inverted before each QRS (except 9th QRS which has a premature, pointed P wave)
PR interval: 0.08–0.10 seconds (basic rhythm); 0.10 seconds (premature beat)
QRS: 0.08–0.10 seconds
Rhythm interpretation: Junctional tachycardia with one PAC (9th complex)

Strip 11-50
Rhythm: Regular atrial and ventricular rhythm
Rate: Atrial: 84; Ventricular: 28
P waves: Sinus P waves are present; bear no relationship to QRS complexes
PR interval: Varies greatly
QRS: 0.12 seconds
Rhythm interpretation: Third degree AV block; ST segment depression is present

Strip 11-51
Rhythm: Irregular
Rate: 50
P waves: Sinus P waves are present
PR interval: 0.12 to 0.14 seconds
QRS: 0.08 seconds
Rhythm interpretation: Sinus arrhythmia; sinus bradycardia; a U wave is present

Strip 11-52
Rhythm: Basic rhythm regular; irregular with premature beats
Rate: Basic rhythm rate 72
P waves: Sinus with basic rhythm
PR interval: 0.16 seconds
QRS: 0.10 seconds
Rhythm interpretation: Normal sinus rhythm with unifocal PVCs in a trigeminal pattern. ST segment depression and T wave inversion are present

Strip 11-53
Rhythm: Regular
Rate: Atrial 93; ventricular 31
P waves: 3 sinus P waves to each QRS (one hidden in T wave)
PR interval: 0.36 seconds (remains constant)
QRS: 0.08 seconds
Rhythm interpretation: Second-degree AV block, Mobitz II

Strip 11-54
Rhythm: Basic rhythm regular; irregular with PVCs
Rate: Basic rhythm rate 72
P waves: Sinus P waves present with basic rhythm
PR interval: 0.12 to 0.14 seconds
QRS: 0.08 seconds (basic rhythm); 0.14–0.16 seconds (PVCs)
Rhythm interpretation: Normal sinus rhythm with multifocal PVCs

Strip 11-55
Rhythm: Regular atrial and ventricular rhythm
Rate: Atrial: 62; Ventricular: 31
P waves: Two sinus P waves before each QRS
PR interval: 0.44 seconds (remains constant)
QRS: 0.14–0.16 seconds
Rhythm interpretation: Second degree AV block
Mobitz II

Strip 11-56
Rhythm: Regular
Rate: 65
P waves: Inverted before each QRS
PR interval: 0.10 seconds
QRS: 0.04 seconds
Rhythm interpretation: Accelerated junctional
rhythm; ST segment elevation is present

Strip 11-57
Rhythm: Basic rhythm regular; irregular with pause
Rate: Basic rhythm rate 68
P waves: Sinus P waves
PR interval: 0.22–0.24 seconds
QRS: 0.08–0.10 seconds
Rhythm interpretation: Normal sinus rhythm with
first degree AV block and sinus arrest; ST segment
elevation is present

Strip 11-58
Automatic Interval Rate: Cannot be determined for sure
since there are no two consecutive paced beats or two
consecutive pacing spikes (estimated to be 75 when
measured from beat immediately preceding each spike)
Analysis: All beats are patient beats—four pacing
spikes appear at appropriate intervals for capture to
occur but capture doesn't occur
Rhythm interpretation: Complete failure to capture

Strip 11-59
Rhythm: Regular
Rate: 188
P waves: Not identified
PR interval: Not measurable
QRS: 0.06 to 0.08 seconds
Rhythm interpretation: Paroxysmal atrial tachycardia

Strip 11-60
Rhythm: Irregular
Rate: 30
P waves: None present
PR interval: Not measurable
QRS: 0.16 seconds
Rhythm interpretation: Idioventricular rhythm;
ST segment depression is present

Strip 11-61
Rhythm: Atrial: regular; Ventricular: irregular
Rate: Atrial: 125; Ventricular: 80
P waves: Sinus
PR interval: Lengthens from 0.12–0.24 seconds
QRS: 0.06–0.08 seconds
Rhythm interpretation: Second degree AV block
Mobitz I; T wave inversion is present

Strip 11-62
Rhythm: Basic rhythm regular; irregular with
nonconducted PAC
Rate: Basic rhythm rate 100
P waves: Sinus P waves present; two premature
abnormal P waves without QRS (following 4th and
8th complexes)
PR interval: 0.12 seconds
QRS: 0.06 to 0.08 seconds
Rhythm interpretation: Normal sinus rhythm with two
nonconducted PACs; T wave inversion is present

Strip 11-63
Rhythm: Regular
Rate: 75
P waves: Sinus
PR interval: 0.16–0.18 seconds
QRS: 0.12–0.14 seconds
Rhythm interpretation: Normal sinus rhythm with
bundle branch block; ST segment elevation is present

Strip 11-64
Rhythm: Regular
Rate: 50
P waves: Sinus
PR interval: 0.16 seconds
QRS: 0.06–0.08 seconds
Rhythm interpretation: Sinus bradycardia; a
U wave is present

Strip 11-65
Automatic Interval rate: 72
Analysis: All beats are pacemaker induced
Rhythm interpretation: Pacemaker rhythm

Strip 11-66
Rhythm: Regular
Rate: Atrial, 78; ventricular, 39
P waves: Two sinus P waves to each QRS complex
PR interval: 0.24 with a constant relationship to the
QRS complexes
QRS: 0.12 to 0.14 seconds
Rhythm interpretation: Second-degree AV block,
Mobitz II. Clinical correlation is suggested to
diagnose Mobitz II when 2 : 1 conduction is present

Strip 11-67

Rhythm: Basic rhythm regular
Rate: Basic rhythm rate: 54
P waves: Sinus P waves with basic rhythm; no P waves seen with 3rd, 4th complexes
PR interval: 0.20 seconds
QRS: 0.06–0.08 seconds
Rhythm interpretation: Sinus bradycardia with two junctional escape beats (3rd, 4th beat)

Strip 11-68

Rhythm: Irregular and chaotic
Rate: 0
P waves: Absent
PR interval: Unmeasurable
QRS: Absent
Rhythm interpretation: Loss of pacemaker capture in the presence of ventricular fibrillation

Strip 11-69

Rhythm: Regular
Rate: 115
P waves: Inverted before each QRS
PR interval: 0.08 to 0.10 seconds
QRS: 0.06 to 0.08 seconds
Rhythm interpretation: Junctional tachycardia

Strip 11-70

Rhythm: Basic rhythm regular; irregular with PJC
Rate: Basic rhythm rate 58
P waves: Sinus P waves present (basic rhythm); inverted P waves with PJC
PR interval: 0.14 to 0.16 seconds (basic rhythm); 0.10 seconds (PJC)
QRS: 0.08 seconds
Rhythm interpretation: Sinus bradycardia with one PJC

Strip 11-71

Rhythm: Basic rhythm regular; irregular with nonconducted PAC
Rate: Basic rhythm rate 63
P waves: Sinus P waves (basic rhythm); one premature, abnormal P wave without QRS complex (follows 4th complex)
PR interval: 0.28 to 0.32 seconds
QRS: 0.12 seconds
Rhythm interpretation: Normal sinus rhythm with first-degree AV block and bundle branch block with one nonconducted PAC following 4th QRS; ST segment elevation and T wave inversion are present

Strip 11-72

Rhythm: Basic rhythm regular; irregular with PVC
Rate: Basic rate: 50
P waves: Sinus with basic rhythm
PR interval: 0.12–0.14 seconds
QRS: 0.08 seconds (basic rhythm); 0.18 seconds (PVC)
Rhythm interpretation: Sinus bradycardia with one PVC (follows 3rd QRS); ST segment elevation is present

Strip 11-73

Automatic interval rate: 79
Analysis: First two beats are paced beats followed by one fusion beat, one pseudofusion beat (note spike at beginning of R wave), three patient beats, pacing spike that occurs too early, a patient beat followed by a pacing spike that occurs too early, and another patient beat followed by an early pacing spike
Rhythm interpretation: Sensing malfunction

Strip 11-74

Rhythm: Regular
Rate: 50
P waves: None identified
PR interval: Not measurable
QRS: 0.04–0.06 seconds
Rhythm interpretation: Junctional rhythm; ST segment depression and T wave inversion is present

Strip 11-75

Rhythm: Irregular atrial rhythm
Rate: Atrial: 40 ventricular 0
P waves: Sinus P waves are present
PR interval: Not measurable
QRS: Absent
Rhythm interpretation: Ventricular standstill

Strip 11-76

Rhythm: Irregular
Rate: 60
P waves: Sinus
PR interval: 0.12–0.14 seconds
QRS: 0.08–0.10 seconds
Rhythm interpretation: Sinus arrhythmia; ST segment elevation is present

Strip 11-77

Rhythm: Regular
Rate: 68
P waves: P waves vary in size, shape, position
PR interval: 0.14 to 0.16 seconds
QRS: 0.06 to 0.08 seconds
Rhythm interpretation: Wandering atrial pacemaker; T wave inversion is present

Strip 11-78
Rhythm: Regular
Rate: 214
P waves: Hidden
PR interval: Not measurable
QRS: 0.06–0.08 seconds
Rhythm interpretation: Paroxysmal atrial
tachycardia

Strip 11-79
Rhythm: First rhythm regular; second rhythm
regular
Rate: 94 (first rhythm); 136 (second rhythm)
P waves: Sinus P waves (first rhythm)
PR interval: 0.18 to 0.20 seconds (first rhythm)
QRS: 0.06 to 0.08 seconds (first rhythm); 0.12
seconds (second rhythm)
Rhythm interpretation: Normal sinus rhythm
changing to ventricular tachycardia

Strip 11-80
Rhythm: Basic rhythm regular
Rate: Basic rhythm rate 107
P waves: Sinus with basic rhythm
PR interval: 0.14–0.16 seconds
QRS: 0.06–0.08 seconds (basic rhythm); 0.12
seconds (ventricular beats)
Rhythm interpretation: Sinus tachycardia with a
four-beat burst of ventricular tachycardia and
paired, unifocal PVCs

Strip 11-81
Rhythm: Irregular
Rate: Atrial, 260; ventricular, 70
P waves: Flutter waves present
PR interval: Not measurable
QRS: 0.06 to 0.08 seconds
Rhythm interpretation: Atrial flutter with variable
block

Strip 11-82
Rhythm: Regular
Rate: 88
P waves: Sinus
PR interval: 0.12 seconds
QRS: 0.04–0.06 seconds
Rhythm interpretation: Normal sinus rhythm

Strip 11-83
Automatic interval rate: 63
Analysis: First two beats are paced beats followed
by one patient beat, two paced beats, one patient
beat, and two paced beats
Rhythm interpretation: Normal pacemaker function

Strip 11-84
Rhythm: Regular
Rate: 136
P waves: Sinus
PR interval: 0.12–0.14 seconds
QRS: 0.06–0.08 seconds
Rhythm interpretation: Sinus tachycardia

Strip 11-85
Rhythm: Regular
Rate: 54
P waves: Sinus
PR interval: 0.24–0.26 seconds
QRS: 0.04–0.06 seconds
Rhythm interpretation: Sinus bradycardia with first
degree AV block

Strip 11-86
Rhythm: Regular atrial and ventricular rhythm
Rate: Atrial: 94; Ventricular: 37
P waves: Sinus P waves present—bear no
relationship to QRS complexes
PR interval: Varies
QRS: 0.12–0.14 seconds
Rhythm interpretation: Third degree AV block

Strip 11-87
Rhythm: Regular
Rate: 150
P waves: None identified
PR interval: Not measurable
QRS: 0.12–0.14 seconds
Rhythm interpretation: Ventricular tachycardia

Strip 11-88
Rhythm: Basic rhythm regular; irregular with pause
Rate: Basic rhythm rate: 56
P waves: Sinus with basic rhythm; absent during
pause
PR interval: 0.16–0.18 seconds
QRS: 0.08–0.10 seconds
Rhythm interpretation: Sinus bradycardia with
sinus arrest; ST segment depression and T wave
inversion are present

Strip 11-89
Rhythm: 0
Rate: 0
P waves: Absent
PR interval: Not measurable
QRS: Absent
Rhythm interpretation: Ventricular standstill

Strip 11-90
Rhythm: Regular
Rate: 88
P waves: Sinus
PR interval: 0.16 seconds
QRS: 0.06–0.08 seconds
Rhythm interpretation: Normal sinus rhythm;
ST segment depression and T wave inversion are
present

Strip 11-91
Rhythm: Basic rhythm regular; irregular with PVC
Rate: 115 (basic rhythm)
P waves: Inverted before each QRS
PR interval: 0.08 to 0.10 seconds
QRS: 0.04 to 0.06 seconds; 0.12 (premature beat)
Rhythm interpretation: Junctional tachycardia with
one premature ventricular contraction

Strip 11-92
Rhythm: Regular
Rate: 188
P waves: Hidden in T waves
PR interval: Not measurable
QRS: 0.06 to 0.08 seconds
Rhythm interpretation: Paroxysmal atrial
tachycardia; ST segment depression is present

Strip 11-93
Rhythm: Chaotic
Rate: 0
P waves: Absent—fibrillatory waves present
PR interval: Not measurable
QRS: Absent
Rhythm interpretation: Ventricular fibrillation

Strip 11-94
Rhythm: Irregular
Rate: 80
P waves: Vary in size, shape, and position
PR interval: 0.14 to 0.16 seconds
QRS: 0.06 to 0.08 seconds
Rhythm interpretation: Wandering atrial
pacemaker; T wave inversion is present

Strip 11-95
Rhythm: Regular
Rate: 100
P waves: Inverted before each QRS
PR interval: 0.08 seconds
QRS: 0.06 to 0.08 seconds
Rhythm interpretation: Accelerated junctional
rhythm

Strip 11-96
Rhythm: Regular atrial rhythm; irregular ventricular
rhythm
Rate: Atrial: 84; Ventricular: 70
P waves: Sinus
PR interval: Lengthens from 0.20–0.36 seconds
QRS: 0.08–0.10 seconds
Rhythm interpretation: Second degree AV block
Mobitz I; ST segment depression is present

Strip 11-97
Rhythm: Irregular
Rate: 100
P waves: Fibrillatory waves present
PR interval: Not measurable
QRS: 0.06–0.08 seconds (basic rhythm); 0.12
seconds (PVC)
Rhythm interpretation: Atrial fibrillation with one PVC

Strip 11-98
Automatic interval rate: 63
Analysis: First two beats are paced beats followed
by one patient beat, two paced beats, loss of capture
spike, one patient beat, and 1 paced beat
Rhythm interpretation: Loss of capture

Strip 11-99
Rhythm: Basic rhythm regular; irregular with
premature beat
Rate: Basic rhythm rate 125
P waves: Sinus
PR interval: 0.12 seconds
QRS: 0.04–0.06 seconds
Rhythm interpretation: Sinus tachycardia with one
PAC (12th complex)

Strip 11-100
Rhythm: Regular
Rate: Atrial: 272; Ventricular: 136
P waves: Two flutter waves to each QRS
PR interval: Not measurable
QRS: 0.04 seconds
Rhythm interpretation: Atrial flutter with 2 : 1 AV
conduction

Strip 11-101
Rhythm: Irregular
Rate: 60
P waves: Sinus
PR interval: 0.14–0.16 seconds
QRS: 0.08 seconds
Rhythm interpretation: Sinus arrhythmia

Strip 11-102
Rhythm: Regular
Rate: 48
P waves: Sinus
PR interval: 0.14–0.16 seconds
QRS: 0.08 seconds
Rhythm interpretation: Sinus bradycardia; a
U wave is present

Strip 11-103
Rhythm: Regular
Rate: 214
P waves: None identified
PR interval: Not measurable
QRS: 0.16 seconds or greater
Rhythm interpretation: Ventricular tachycardia

Strip 11-104
Rhythm: Irregular
Rate: 60
P waves: Fibrillatory waves present
PR interval: Not measurable
QRS: 0.06–0.08 seconds
Rhythm interpretation: Atrial fibrillation

Strip 11-105
Rhythm: Basic rhythm regular
Rate: Basic rhythm rate 72
P waves: Sinus P waves present
PR interval: 0.16 to 0.18 seconds
QRS: 0.06 to 0.08 seconds (basic rhythm); 0.12
seconds (PVC)
Rhythm interpretation: Normal sinus rhythm with one
interpolated PVC; ST segment depression is present

Strip 11-106
Rhythm: Basic rhythm regular; irregular with PJC
Rate: Basic rhythm rate 65
P waves: Sinus P waves with basic rhythm; inverted
P wave with PJC
PR interval: 0.12 to 0.16 seconds (basic rhythm);
0.10 seconds (PJC)
QRS: 0.06 to 0.08 seconds
Rhythm interpretation: Normal sinus rhythm with
one PJC; a U wave is present

Strip 11-107
Rhythm: Basic rhythm regular; irregular with PVC
Rate: Basic rhythm rate 88
P waves: Sinus
PR interval: 0.12–0.14 seconds
QRS: 0.04–0.06 seconds
Rhythm interpretation: Normal sinus rhythm with
three PVCs